The Role of Nutrition in Cardiometabolic Health: Experimental, Clinical, and Community-Based Evidence

The Role of Nutrition in Cardiometabolic Health: Experimental, Clinical, and Community-Based Evidence

Editors

Abeer M. Mahmoud
Shane A. Phillips

MDPI • Basel • Beijing • Wuhan • Barcelona • Belgrade • Manchester • Tokyo • Cluj • Tianjin

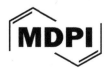

Editors
Abeer M. Mahmoud
University of Illinois at Chicago
USA

Shane A. Phillips
University of Illinois at Chicago
USA

Editorial Office
MDPI
St. Alban-Anlage 66
4052 Basel, Switzerland

This is a reprint of articles from the Special Issue published online in the open access journal *Nutrients* (ISSN 2072-6643) (available at: https://www.mdpi.com/journal/nutrients/special_issues/ nutrition_in_cardiometabolic_health).

For citation purposes, cite each article independently as indicated on the article page online and as indicated below:

LastName, A.A.; LastName, B.B.; LastName, C.C. Article Title. *Journal Name* **Year**, *Volume Number*, Page Range.

ISBN 978-3-0365-4837-1 (Hbk)
ISBN 978-3-0365-4838-8 (PDF)

Contents

About the Editors

Abeer M. Mahmoud

Abeer M. Mahmoud, MD, PhD, is an Assistant Professor in the Department of Medicine, UIC. She received her MD degree and training as a Pathologist from Assiut University, Egypt. She served as a surgical pathologist at South Egypt Cancer Institute (2002–2008), before realizing her true passion was in biomedical research. She earned her Ph.D. in Pathology (College of Medicine, UIC, 2013), in which she studied chemoprevention in prostate cancer. For her postdoctoral research (College of Applied Health Sciences, UIC, 2013–2017), she studied the physiological and molecular outcomes of lifestyle interventions. She is funded by the National Institute of Health to study epigenetic modifications in morbidly obese patients and their impact on cardiometabolic functions. She also studies the role of adipose tissue secretions and exosomes in diabetes-associated vascular dysfunction and has conducted several exercise and nutrition trials to mitigate obesity- and diabetes-associated co-morbidities.

Shane A. Phillips

Shane A. Phillips, PT, PhD, FAHA, is Professor and Associate Head in the Department of Physical Therapy at the University of Illinois in Chicago. Phillips has clinical expertise in physical therapy and cardiovascular rehabilitation. His PhD degree in physiology was completed at the Medical College of Wisconsin, and he completed his post-doctoral training in Cardiovascular Medicine. He is the Director of the Vascular Biology Laboratory in the College of Applied Health Sciences, where he studies obesity, hypertension, and the control of blood flow and responses of the microcirculation to surgery, diet, and exercise interventions. His other research interests include the impact of cardiovascular risk factors such as high blood pressure, alcohol, and high cholesterol on macro- and microcirculatory function. His laboratory is funded by the National Institute of Health.

Preface to "The Role of Nutrition in Cardiometabolic Health: Experimental, Clinical, and Community-Based Evidence"

Cardiometabolic disease is a major health and economic burden worldwide, and its prevalence is expected to rise. Excess body fat, dyslipidemia, poor glucose metabolism, and elevated blood pressure are just a few of the many cardiometabolic risk factors that can be influenced by diet. As the rates of these factors continue to rise, a healthy lifestyle that includes proper nutrition should be a public health goal. In this book, renowned researchers provide cutting-edge scientific evaluations of the impacts of diet and lifestyle on cardiometabolic health.

This book contains 11 chapters which cover a wide range of topics, such as biological mechanisms governing food intake, lifestyle and surgical approaches to weight loss, nutritional aspects for optimal cardiometabolic health, the association between macronutrients, micronutrients, whole foods, and dietary patterns with obesity, diabetes, and cardiovascular risk factors. The effects of vitamin D and low-carbohydrate diets on microvascular function in morbidly obese people are addressed in Chapters 1 and 2, respectively, whereas the influence of fat-based versus sugar-based Western diets on cardiac remodeling is discussed in Chapter 3. The ANCHORS A-WHEY and African-PREDICT clinical trials, which provide data on the cardiovascular effects of supplements (whey protein) and medicinal drugs (marinobufagenin), are discussed in Chapters 4 and 5, respectively. Chapters 6 and 7 provide a comprehensive summary of the dietary characteristics that contribute to an increased cardiovascular risk and micronutrient deficiencies following various modalities of bariatric surgery. Chapters 8 and 9 cover homocysteine, a byproduct of one-carbon metabolism, and its epigenetic and vascular consequences in obese people. Finally, Chapters 10 and 11 present new findings and a review of the literature on the mechanisms by which the bile acid receptor, TGR5, maintains glucose homeostasis.

We are grateful to all of the scientists and researchers who contributed to this book's diverse, impactful, and insightful themes. We hope that this book will provide nutrition and healthcare professionals with an authoritative summary of the present state of knowledge about the impact of diet on cardiometabolic health.

Abeer M. Mahmoud and Shane A. Phillips
Editors

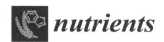

Article

Vitamin D Improves Nitric Oxide-Dependent Vasodilation in Adipose Tissue Arterioles from Bariatric Surgery Patients

Abeer M. Mahmoud [1,2,3,*], Mary Szczurek [2], Chandra Hassan [4], Mario Masrur [4], Antonio Gangemi [4] and Shane A. Phillips [1,2,3]

[1] Division of Endocrinology, Diabetes and Metabolism, Department of Medicine, University of Illinois at Chicago, Chicago, IL 60612, USA; shanep@uic.edu

[2] Department of Physical Therapy, University of Illinois at Chicago, Chicago, IL 60612, USA; mszczurek@uic.edu

[3] Integrative Physiology Laboratory, College of Applied Health Sciences, University of Illinois at Chicago, Chicago, IL 60612, USA

[4] Department of Surgery, University of Illinois at Chicago, Chicago, IL 60612, USA; chandrar@uic.edu (C.H.); mmasrur@uic.edu (M.M.); gangemi@uic.edu (A.G.)

[*] Correspondence: amahmo4@uic.edu; Tel.: +1-(312)-355-8099

Received: 6 September 2019; Accepted: 15 October 2019; Published: 18 October 2019

Abstract: There is a high prevalence of vitamin-D deficiency in obese individuals that could be attributed to vitamin-D sequestration in the adipose tissue. Associations between vitamin-D deficiency and unfavorable cardiometabolic outcomes were reported. However, the pathophysiological mechanisms behind these associations are yet to be established. In our previous studies, we demonstrated microvascular dysfunction in obese adults that was associated with reduced nitric oxide (NO) production. Herein, we examined the role of vitamin D in mitigating microvascular function in morbidly obese adults before and after weight loss surgery. We obtained subcutaneous (SAT) and visceral adipose tissue (VAT) biopsies from bariatric patients at the time of surgery (n = 15) and gluteal SAT samples three months post-surgery (n = 8). Flow-induced dilation (FID) and acetylcholine-induced dilation (AChID) and NO production were measured in the AT-isolated arterioles ± NO synthase inhibitor N(ω)-nitro-L-arginine methyl ester (L-NAME), hydrogen peroxide (H_2O_2) inhibitor, polyethylene glycol-modified catalase (PEG-CAT), or 1,25-dihydroxyvitamin D. Vitamin D improved FID, AChID, and NO production in AT-isolated arterioles at time of surgery; these effects were abolished by L-NAME but not by PEG-CAT. Vitamin-D-mediated improvements were of a higher magnitude in VAT compared to SAT arterioles. After surgery, significant improvements in FID, AChID, NO production, and NO sensitivity were observed. Vitamin-D-induced changes were of a lower magnitude compared to those from the time of surgery. In conclusion, vitamin D improved NO-dependent arteriolar vasodilation in obese adults; this effect was more significant before surgery-induced weight loss.

Keywords: vitamin D; obesity; microvascular; bariatric surgery; weight loss; nitric oxide

---

1. Introduction

Obesity and vitamin-D deficiency are two major global public health concerns that affect over one-third of the population. A body mass index of more than 30 kg/m^2 is associated with lower serum vitamin-D levels compared with non-obese individuals [1]. Several mechanisms that contribute to the high incidence of vitamin-D deficiency in obese people were suggested. Ultraviolet radiation from sunlight exposure is required for cutaneous production of vitamin D [2]. It was proposed that obese individuals, overall, have suboptimal levels of vitamin D because they tend to participate in fewer outdoor activities and, accordingly, have less exposure to sunlight. Vitamin D is a lipid-soluble vitamin, and it is thought that the lower bioavailability of vitamin D in obese individuals, compared to lean individuals, is due to vitamin-D sequestration within the adipose tissues [3]. Lastly, vitamin-D deficiency may also be due to inadequate dietary intake or malabsorption of vitamin D [4,5]. Obesity is a well-established risk factor for the development of cardiovascular disease (CVD), and several mechanisms may contribute to this link. However, a role of vitamin-D deficiency in obesity-associated cardiovascular (CV) risk is yet to be established.

Epidemiological data reported associations between vitamin D deficiency and left ventricular hypertrophy, hypertension, increased arterial stiffness, and endothelial dysfunction [4,6–12]. The pathophysiological underpinnings of these associations remain mostly unexplained. The most reliable and convincing evidence for the involvement of vitamin D in the pathogenesis of CVD comes from studies demonstrating an association between vitamin-D deficiency and hypertension [13]. Vitamin-D deficiency is associated with a higher risk for preeclampsia, a condition that is characterized by hypertension [14]. Also, a significant inverse association was reported between vitamin-D serum levels and arterial blood pressure in the elderly [15]. An interventional study demonstrated that one month of vitamin-D intake (1,5000 IU/day) reduced tissue sensitivity to the stimulation of the renin–angiotensin system manifested by improved renal blood flow and reduced mean arterial pressure during an infusion of angiotensin II [16]. Moreover, vitamin-D intake (2000 IU/day) for 14 days in healthy adults reduced augmentation index, a measure of arterial stiffness that contributes to the development of hypertension [17].

The discovery of vitamin-D receptor (VDR) widened the scope of biological effects that vitamin D plays in human health [18]. VDR is a transcription factor that enters the nucleus upon binding to vitamin D, where it attaches to specific DNA regions and activates the transcription of a myriad of genes that coordinate several biological responses [18]. VDR is widely expressed throughout the human body in almost all cells and tissues, including vascular smooth muscle cells, cardiomyocytes, and endothelial cells [19]. Animal studies found that loss of VDR signaling increased arterial stiffness and elevated systolic and diastolic blood pressure, independent of the renin–angiotensin–aldosterone system [20]. Another study found that VDR knockout mice have increased arterial stiffness through decreased bioavailability of nitric oxide (NO) [21]. These and other studies proposed that the leading mechanism for the association between vitamin-D deficiency and CVD is related to endothelial dysfunction and impaired endothelial-dependent NO production [22–24].

Despite this accumulating evidence of the role of vitamin D in vascular function, direct mechanistic evidence of this role in the microvasculature of morbidly obese population and how it might be modified following massive weight loss are largely unexplored. The purpose of the current study is to investigate the effects of vitamin D on the microvasculature isolated from both subcutaneous (SAT) and visceral adipose tissue (VAT) in morbidly obese adults before and after bariatric surgery-induced weight loss. The central hypothesis is that vitamin D would improve microvascular function in obese adults via improving flow-mediated NO production, and this effect would be of a greater magnitude before compared to after weight loss. In our previous work, we found that flow-induced dilation (FID) is impaired in morbidly obese individuals due to an imbalance of NO and H_2O_2 [25,26]. H_2O_2 may serve as a compensatory mechanism for vasodilation during pathological conditions such as obesity [27]. Using the proposed ex vivo system in this study, we are able to explore the contributing vasoactive mediators of vitamin-D effects on microvascular function, mainly NO and H_2O_2.

2. Methods

2.1. Human Participants

Subjects were 15 men ($n = 2$) and women ($n = 13$), who underwent laparoscopic bariatric surgery at the University of Illinois Medical Center. The age of subjects ranged from 21 to 49 years old, and all the women were premenopausal. The eligibility criteria included a body mass index (BMI) of at least 40 kg/m^2 and the absence of significant chronic morbidities or inflammatory conditions that may have confounding effects on the study outcomes. Excluded subjects included pregnant women and individuals with current diabetes mellitus (type I or II), heart disease, liver disease, kidney disease, gallbladder disease, cancer, or acute or chronic inflammatory diseases such as rheumatoid arthritis. Four subjects were taking vitamin D supplementation (10,000–50,000 IU vitamin D/week). Determination of the subject's eligibility criteria was completed before the pre-surgery evaluation clinical visit. At the clinical visit, eligible subjects were informed about the study details, and those who were interested in participating provided written informed consent. The study protocol and procedures were approved by the University of Illinois at Chicago Institutional Review Board and followed the standards set by the latest revision of the Declaration of Helsinki. A post-surgery visit at the University of Illinois Clinical Interface Core (UIC CIC) was established with each subject during the time of written consent. The study flowchart detailing subject numbers, the timeline for biopsy, and clinical data collection is displayed in Figure 1.

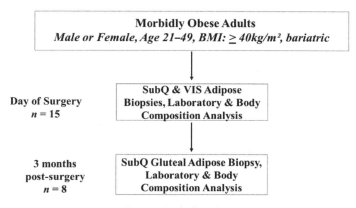

Figure 1. Study flow chart.

2.2. Physical and Cardiometabolic Measurements

Physical characteristics, including age, gender, body weight, height, BMI, waist circumference, and cardiometabolic risk factors, were assessed. Fasting blood samples were obtained before biopsy acquisition for measuring biochemical parameters (lipid profile and glucose metabolism).

2.3. Sample Acquisition

On the day of bariatric surgery, blood samples were collected before the administration of anesthesia. After the administration of anesthesia, adipose tissue samples (SAT and VAT) were collected by the surgeon. All samples were immediately placed in cold 2-(4-(2-hydroxyethyl) piperazin-1-yl) ethanesulfonic acid (HEPES) buffer solution to maintain the viability of the tissue. In the post-surgery visit, all subjects fasted for 12 hours before the study visit. At the visit, subjects' anthropometric measurements, blood pressure, and heart rate were measured. A fasting blood draw was obtained for total cholesterol, triglycerides, glucose, and insulin measurements. During the post-surgery visit, a SAT biopsy was obtained by a certified nurse practitioner from the gluteal region under local anesthesia. The biopsy was immediately placed in cold HEPES buffer solution.

2.4. Microvascular Preparation

Adipose tissues were dissected, and resistance arterioles were isolated and cleaned of excess fat and connective tissues. Arterioles were then washed and prepared for measuring changes in the internal diameter in response to flow and acetylcholine (Ach) as previously described [26,28,29]. In summary, isolated arterioles were cannulated using glass micropipettes in an organ perfusion chamber, and both ends were secured using a 10-0 nylon Ethilon monofilament suture. Cannulated arterioles within the organ chamber were then placed on the stage of an inverted microscope attached to a video camera, a video monitor, and a video measuring device (model VIA-100; Boeckeler, Madison, WI, USA). The organ chamber was perfused with heated physiological salt solution (Krebs buffer) that contained the following components (mM): 4.4 KCL, 123 NaCl, 2.5 $CaCl_2$, 20 $NaHCO_3$, 1.2 $MgSO_4$, 1.2 KH_2PO_4, and 11 glucose. The pH of the solution was kept at 7.4 ± 0.05, and the temperature was maintained at 37 °C. The buffer was also supplied with air mixture of 21% O_2, 5% CO_2, and 74% N_2. Each end of the cannulated arteriole was connected via silicon tubes to a physiological buffer-containing reservoir, and the intraluminal pressure gradient (10–100 cm H_2O) was established by modifying the distance between both reservoirs in equal and opposite directions [30].

2.5. Measurements of Flow-Induced Dilation

Arterioles were constricted with endothelin-1 (Peninsula, San Carlos, CA, USA), and those constricted less than 30% were excluded from the study. The internal diameter of the cannulated arterioles was measured at baseline and during gradual increases of the intraluminal pressure gradient (10–100 cm H_2O) or acetylcholine concentration (ACh; 10^{-9} to 10^{-4} M) [26]. Measurements were repeated after incubations with 1,25-dihydroxyvitamin D (1-25(OH)$_2$D; vitamin D, 1 nM), the eNOS (endothelial nitric oxide synthase) inhibitor L-NAME (10^{-4} M), the H_2O_2 scavenger PEG-CAT (500U/mL), L-NAME plus vitamin D, or PEG-CAT plus vitamin D. Treatments were added to the physiological bathing solution in 30 minutes before FID and acetylcholine-induced dilation (AchID) measurements were obtained. Papaverine (10^{-4} M) was used at the end of each experiment to measure maximal vasodilation. We reported percentage vasodilation as the percentage increase in the arteriolar diameter after each treatment condition relative to the endothelin-1 (ET-1)-constricted state.

2.6. Measurements of Arteriolar NO

Nitric oxide produced by freshly isolated microvessels was measured as previously described [31] using Enzo Life Sciences NO Detection Kit (ThermoFisher Scientific, MA, USA). NO measurements were performed in cannulated vessels in the organ chambers. In order to stimulate NO production, vessels were exposed to a pressure gradient of Δ60 cm H_2O during which they were incubated with the NO detection reagents. This step was followed by vessel excision, washing, and mounting on microscopic coverslips. Images were taken immediately using fluorescence microscopy (Eclipse TE 2000, Nikon, Japan) at 650/670 nm. All incubations and staining and detection protocols were fixed in all experiments. The acquired images were then analyzed for the intensity of the fluorescent signal in arbitrary units using National Institute of Health (NIH) Image J software (NIH, Bethesda, MD, USA).

2.7. Statistical Analyses

All results are reported as means ± standard error, and $p < 0.05$ was considered statistically significant. Fluorescent images were analyzed for fluorescence intensity after correcting for background autofluorescence using NIH Image J software (NIH, Bethesda, MD, USA). Paired measurements for FID, AChID, NO fluorescence, physical characteristics, and cardiometabolic parameters were assessed using Student's paired *t*-test for within-group comparisons. One-way ANOVA followed by an appropriate post hoc test was used when there were more than two comparisons among different vessel treatments. Dilation in dose–response data was presented as a percentage increase in the arteriolar diameter after each treatment condition relative to the ET-1-constricted state. Analyses were performed using SPSS statistical package (version 18.0; SPSS Inc, Chicago, IL, USA).

3. Results

3.1. Physical and Cardiometabolic Parameters

Table 1 summarizes age, gender, and anthropometric characteristics of all participants. Fifteen subjects (13 females and two males; age: 37 ± 8 years) were enrolled in the study. Eight subjects (seven female and one male; age: 35 ± 6 years) participated in the post-surgery visit. Study participants lost 13.3 kg of their body weight on average, and their BMI and waist circumference decreased by 13.6% and 12%, respectively. Table 2 summarizes the cardiometabolic parameters we measured in the study, including blood pressure, heart rate, lipid profile, and glucose metabolism. After surgery, both systolic and diastolic blood pressures decreased significantly. On average, total cholesterol and glucose decreased by ~10% and 4%, respectively, three months after surgery compared to the day of surgery. Serum levels of vitamin D increased significantly (31.8%, $p = 0.0003$) after bariatric surgery.

Table 1. Physical characteristics of study participants at the time of surgery ($n = 15$) and three months post-surgery ($n = 8$).

	Surgery ($n = 15$)	Post-Surgery ($n = 8$)	p-Value
Age (years)	37 ± 6	35 ± 6	0.455
Sex	2 ♂, 13 ♀	1 ♂, 7 ♀	
Height (cm)	164.9 ± 6.0	166.8 ± 7.7	0.518
Body weight (kg)	132.5 ± 10.4	119.2 ± 3.5 *	0.002
BMI (kg/m^2)	47.1 ± 6.3	40.7 ± 5.6 *	0.025
Waist circumference (cm)	131.1 ± 12.6	115.4 ± 13.8 *	0.012

* p-value < 0.05; BMI, body mass index.

Table 2. Cardiometabolic risk factors of participants at the time of surgery ($n = 15$) and three months post-surgery ($n = 8$). 1-25(OH)$_2$D—1,25-dihydroxyvitamin D.

	Surgery ($n = 15$)	Post-Surgery ($n = 8$)	p-Value
Systolic BP (mm Hg)	130.3 ± 13.5	119.6 ± 9.8 *	0.042
Diastolic BP (mm Hg)	78.1 ± 9.1	66.7 ± 3.7 *	0.003
Heart rate (beats/min)	85.2 ± 12.9	84.5 ± 10.8	0.897
Total cholesterol (mg/dL)	185.9 ± 20.8	168.7 ± 19.3 *	0.044
Triglycerides (mg/dL)	78.8 ± 10.2	77.3 ± 16.5	0.789
Glucose (mg/dL)	87.4 ± 15.4	83.8 ± 13.3 *	0.047
Insulin (μIU/mL)	10.1 ± 2.0	9.7 ± 1.3	0.616
1-25(OH)$_2$D (ng/mL)	13.8 ± 1.8	18.1 ± 2.2 *	0.0003

* p-value < 0.05; BP, blood pressure.

3.2. Effect of Vitamin D on Arteriolar FID, AchID, and NO Production before Weight Loss (at Time of Surgery)

Vitamin D enhanced the FID and AChID measurements in arterioles ($n = 15$) isolated from both VAT (Figure 2A,B) and SAT (Figure 2C,D) compared to baseline. These improvements were of a higher magnitude in the VAT compared to SAT arterioles. At $\Delta 60$ cm H$_2$O, the average FID increased by 60% in VAT arterioles and 14% in SAT arterioles. Similar results were obtained in response to Ach. Also, vasodilation improvements in VAT arterioles were obtained at lower pressure gradient ($\Delta 40$) compared to SAT arterioles where significant improvements were only achieved at $\Delta 60$ and higher. These findings could be explained by the lower baseline FID and AchID measurements in VAT compared to SAT arterioles. These impaired measurements provide a chance for a more perceptible magnitude of improvement in the VAT arterioles in response to vitamin D. Previous data from our lab [32] recapitulated the same phenomenon of impaired dilation responses of VAT arterioles in response to flow and acetylcholine compared to SAT arterioles. Moreover, unlike the significant reduction in FID and AChID observed in SAT arterioles in response to endothelial nitric oxide synthase (eNOS) inhibition by L-NAME (Figure 3C,D), no significant response was observed in VAT arterioles (Figure 3A,B). The observed low sensitivity of VAT arterioles to NO inhibition might indicate a disruption in the NO-dependent vasodilation mechanism in these arterioles.

Our data show an enhanced NO sensitivity in VAT arterioles in response to vitamin D as evident by significant reductions in FID and AchID in vitamin-D-treated VAT arterioles in response to L-NAME (Figure 3A,B). Vitamin-D-induced FID and AChID improvements were also abolished in SAT arterioles in response to L-NAME. Unlike VAT arterioles, the magnitude of L-NAME-induced inhibition in vitamin-D-treated SAT arterioles is comparable to that of the untreated SAT arterioles, indicating a lesser effect of vitamin D on improving NO pathway in SAT arterioles (Figure 3A–D).

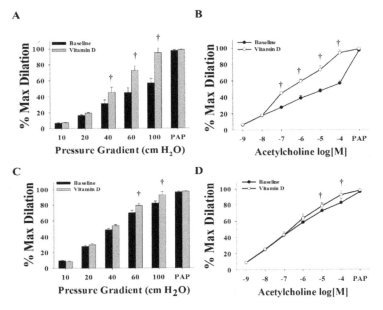

Figure 2. Effect of vitamin D on flow-induced dilation (FID) and acetylcholine-induced dilation (AChID) in adipose tissue resistance arterioles collected on the day of surgery ($n = 15$ subjects). FID measurements in visceral adipose tissue (VAT) arterioles (**A**) and subcutaneous adipose tissue (SAT) arterioles (**C**) corresponding to increasing intraluminal pressure gradients of 10–100 cm H_2O. AchID measurements in VAT arterioles (**B**) and SAT arterioles (**D**) corresponding to increasing concentrations of acetylcholine (Ach) (10^{-9} to 10^{-4} M). All measurements are presented as means ± standard error (SE); † $p < 0.05$ comparing vitamin D with baseline.

It was established that H_2O_2 is a vasoactive mediator that is released from the endothelium as a compensatory mechanism for impaired NO-mediated vasodilation [27,33,34]. This compensatory mechanism mediates vasodilation, at least partly, in conditions characterized by inflammation and increased production of reactive oxygen species (ROS) such as obesity, hypertension, and coronary artery disease [26,31]. Our data show that scavenging H_2O_2 via PEG-CAT decreased FID significantly in both VAT (Figure 4A) and SAT (Figure 4B) arterioles, indicating a possible contribution of H_2O_2 in the arteriolar FID in the obese subjects of this study. On the other hand, vitamin-D-treated vessels lost the response to the H_2O_2 scavenger, PEG-CAT (Figure 4A,B), which might refer to an effect of vitamin D in reducing ROS production or arteriolar dependence on H_2O_2 as a vasodilator. In the four subjects who were administered prescribed vitamin-D supplementation before surgery (10000 IU, $n = 1$; 5,0000 IU, $n = 3$), we observed no differences in arteriolar FID compared to those who were not taking vitamin-D supplementation (Figure 5A,B). Also, the effect of L-NAME on inhibiting vasodilation in participants taking vitamin-D supplementation (Figure 5C,D) followed the same patterns observed in all participants (Figure 3).

Consistent with the FID and AchID data, NO production was attenuated in response to L-NAME incubation, albeit to a greater extent in SAT (−64%) compared to VAT (−20%) arterioles. In the presence of vitamin D, the production of NO increased in both VAT and SAT arterioles (Figure 6A,B, respectively). This increase was of a higher magnitude in VAT (75%) than SAT (50%) arterioles, which follows the pattern of FID changes we presented above. These increases in NO production were abolished by L-NAME, albeit to a greater extent in SAT (−57%) compared to VAT (−29%) arterioles. PEG-CAT did not induce any significant effects on NO production in either SAT or VAT arterioles. In summary, vasodilation in SAT arterioles is more dependent on NO and more sensitive to NO inhibition than VAT arterioles, and the average baseline NO production in VAT arterioles was lower than SAT arterioles. Therefore, by improving NO production, vitamin D enhanced vasodilation of VAT arterioles to a greater extent than SAT arterioles and increased their sensitivity to NO inhibition.

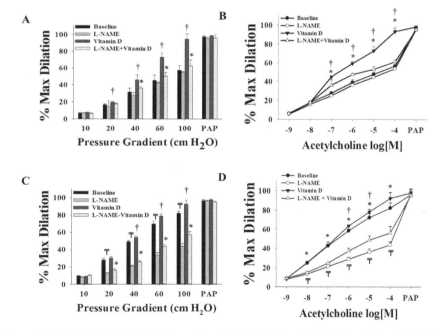

Figure 3. Effect of endothelial nitric oxide synthase (eNOS) inhibition via L-NAME on FID and AchID in adipose tissue resistance arterioles collected on the day of surgery (n = 15 subjects). FID measurements corresponding to intraluminal pressure gradients of 10–100 cm H_2O in VAT arterioles (**A**) and SAT arterioles (**C**) with and without vitamin D incubation. AchID measurements corresponding to increasing Ach concentrations (10^{-9} to 10^{-4} M) in VAT arterioles (**B**) and SAT arterioles (**D**) with and without vitamin-D incubation. All measurements are presented as means ± standard error (SE); $\overline{T}$ $p < 0.05$ comparing L-NAME with baseline, † $p < 0.05$ comparing vitamin D with baseline, and * $p < 0.05$ comparing L-NAME + vitamin D with vitamin D alone.

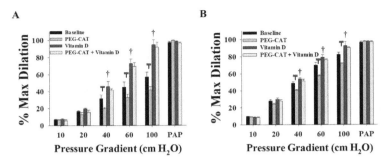

Figure 4. Effect of scavenging H_2O_2 via PEG-CAT on FID in adipose tissue resistance arterioles collected on the day of surgery ($n = 15$). FID measurements corresponding to intraluminal pressure gradients of 10–100 cm H_2O in VAT arterioles (**A**) and SAT arterioles (**B**) with and without vitamin-D incubation. All measurements are presented as means ± standard error (SE); $\overline{T}\ p < 0.05$ comparing L-NAME with baseline, and $†\ p < 0.05$ comparing vitamin D with baseline.

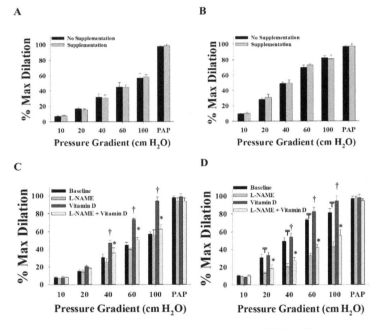

Figure 5. Effect of vitamin-D supplementation prior to surgery on FID in adipose tissue resistance arterioles collected on the day of surgery. FID measurements corresponding to intraluminal pressure gradients of 10–100 cm H_2O in VAT arterioles (**A**) and SAT arterioles (**B**) from subjects who administered vitamin-D supplements before surgery ($n = 4$) and subjects who did not ($n = 11$). Effect of L-NAME and vitamin-D incubation on FID in VAT arterioles (**C**) and SAT arterioles (**D**) from subjects who administered vitamin-D supplements before surgery ($n = 4$). All measurements are presented as means ± standard error (SE); $\overline{T}\ p < 0.05$ comparing L-NAME with baseline, $†\ p < 0.05$ comparing vitamin D with baseline, and $*\ p < 0.05$ comparing L-NAME + vitamin D with vitamin D alone.

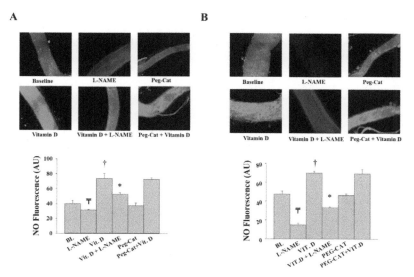

Figure 6. Nitric oxide (NO) production in isolated adipose tissue arterioles collected on the day of surgery. Representative images by fluorescence microscopy of NO generation conditions at baseline and after incubation with L-NAME, PEG-CAT, vitamin D, vitamin D plus L-NAME, and vitamin D plus PEG-CAT in VAT arterioles (**A**) and SAT arterioles (**B**). Charts represent NO fluorescent signals that were measured and expressed in arbitrary units using NIH Image J software. All measures are represented as means ± SE; $\overline{T}$ $p < 0.05$ comparing L-NAME with baseline, † $p < 0.05$ comparing vitamin D with baseline, * $p < 0.05$ comparing L-NAME + vitamin D with vitamin D alone.

3.3. Effect of Vitamin D on Arteriolar FID, AchID, and NO Production after Weight Loss (Three Months after Surgery)

Post-surgery SAT arterioles showed minimal to no improvements in FID (Figure 7A) or AChID (Figure 7B) in response to vitamin D. Baseline arteriolar dilation was attenuated in response to NO inhibition via L-NAME, to a higher degree (−67% in Δ60) than that in arterioles obtained during surgery (−52% in Δ60). These findings might indicate a role of surgical weight loss in improving NO generation in SAT arterioles. The H_2O_2 scavenger, PEG-CAT, reduced the FID in post-surgery SAT arterioles to a lesser extent (−9% at Δ60, Figure 7C) than those obtained at the time of surgery (−20% at Δ60, Figure 4B), indicating less dependence on H_2O_2 as a vasodilator after surgical weight loss. This effect was further enhanced by vitamin-D incubation as evident by a complete loss of response to PEG-CAT in these arterioles (Figure 7C).

When compared to those collected on the day of surgery, post-surgery SAT arterioles demonstrated improved FID (Figure 8A) at baseline and an enhanced response to the eNOS inhibitor, L-NAME (Figure 8B). This effect can also be observed when comparing the percentage of FID reduction after L-NAME in the post-surgery arterioles (Δ60, −68%, Figure 7A) to that in the surgery arterioles (Δ60, −57%, Figure 3C). After incubation with vitamin D, FID in surgery and post-surgery SAT arterioles was comparable even though FID in post-surgery SAT arterioles did not improve in response to vitamin D (Figure 8C). These results may indicate that the effect of vitamin D on improving FID before weight loss is comparable to the effect of weight loss three months after bariatric surgery. Furthermore, additional augmentation by vitamin D could not be achieved following weight loss surgery. Enhanced sensitivity of SAT arterioles to L-NAME was observed in response to a combined effect of weight loss and vitamin D compared to the sole effect of vitamin D (Figure 8D). In post-surgery arterioles, the response to Ach mirrored that of FID (Figure 9).

Nitric oxide fluorescence was higher in SAT arterioles obtained post-surgery compared to arterioles obtained during surgery, and a more significant reduction in NO production in response to L-NAME was observed in post-surgery SAT arterioles (Figure 10A). Similar to FID data, NO production was comparable in SAT arterioles obtained during and after surgery and incubated with vitamin D (Figures 6A and 10B). In the presence of a combined weight loss and vitamin D, a greater reduction in NO production in response to L-NAME was observed in SAT arterioles from post-surgery (−69%) vs. surgery (−54%) (Figures 6B and 10B). When arterioles from surgery samples were incubated with vitamin D, there was an enhancement in NO production (40%); however, after weight loss surgery, vitamin-D-induced improvements in NO production were significantly lower (15%). In summary, both NO and H_2O_2 play a role in vasodilation in SAT arterioles at the time of surgery in obese bariatric patients. After surgical weight loss, the NO vasodilatory component is enhanced, and the H_2O_2 compensatory component is reduced. Vitamin D has a more prominent effect in improving vasodilation and NO production and sensitivity in SAT arterioles obtained before weight loss compared to those collected after weight loss.

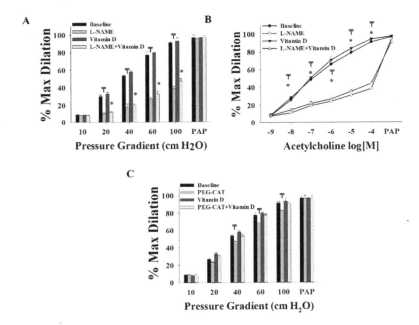

Figure 7. Effect of vitamin D, L-NAME, and PEG-CAT on vasodilation of SAT arterioles collected three months after bariatric surgery ($n = 8$). FID measurements corresponding to intraluminal pressure gradients of 10–100 cm H_2O in SAT arterioles at baseline and after incubation with L-NAME, PEG-CAT, vitamin D, vitamin D plus L-NAME, and vitamin D plus PEG-CAT (**A,C**). AchID measurements corresponding to increasing Ach concentrations (10^{-9} to 10^{-4} M) in SAT arterioles at baseline and after incubation with L-NAME, vitamin D, and vitamin D plus L-NAME (**B**). All measures are represented as means ± SE; $\overline{T}$ $p < 0.05$ comparing L-NAME or PEG-CAT with baseline, and * $p < 0.05$ comparing L-NAME + vitamin D with vitamin D alone.

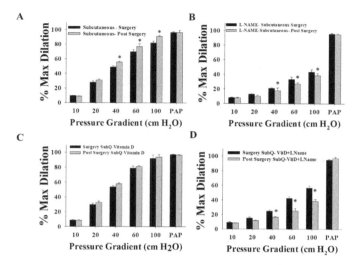

Figure 8. Comparison of the FID between SAT arterioles collected on the day of bariatric surgery and those collected three months after surgery. FID measurements corresponding to intraluminal pressure gradients of 10–100 cm H_2O in SAT arterioles at baseline (**A**) and after incubation with L-NAME (**B**), vitamin D (**C**), and vitamin D plus L-NAME (**D**). All measures are represented as means ± SE; * $p < 0.05$ comparing post-surgery with surgery-obtained arterioles.

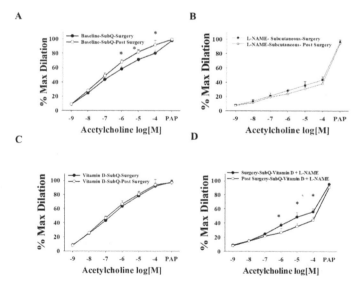

Figure 9. Comparison of the AchID between SAT arterioles collected on the day of bariatric surgery and those collected three months after surgery. AchID measurements corresponding to increasing Ach concentrations (10^{-9} to 10^{-4} M) in SAT arterioles at baseline (**A**) and after incubation with L-NAME (**B**), vitamin D (**C**), and vitamin D plus L-NAME (**D**). All measures are represented as means ± SE; * $p < 0.05$ comparing post-surgery with surgery-obtained arterioles.

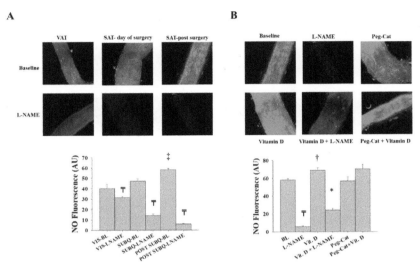

Figure 10. NO production in isolated adipose tissue arterioles. (**A**) Representative images by fluorescence microscopy of NO generation conditions at baseline and after incubation with L-NAME in adipose tissue arterioles collected on the day of surgery (VAT and SAT day of surgery) and three months after surgery (SAT post-surgery). (**B**) Representative fluorescence microscopy images of NO generation conditions at baseline and after incubation with L-NAME, PEG-CAT, vitamin D, vitamin D plus L-NAME, and vitamin D plus PEG-CAT in SAT arterioles collected three months after surgery. Charts represent NO fluorescent signals that were measured and expressed in arbitrary units using NIH Image J software. All measures are represented as means ± SE; $\overline{T}$ $p < 0.05$ comparing L-NAME with corresponding baseline in VAT, SAT day of surgery, and SAT post-surgery, ‡ $p < 0.05$ comparing SAT day of surgery and SAT post-surgery, † $p < 0.05$ comparing vitamin D with baseline, and * $p < 0.05$ comparing L-NAME + vitamin D with vitamin D alone.

4. Discussion

The main findings of the current study are that vitamin D improved FID and AChID and increased NO production in resistance arterioles from SAT and VAT. These effects were abolished by eNOS inhibition via L-NAME but not by H_2O_2 scavenging via PEG-CAT. In comparing the measures from pre- and post-surgery, the primary findings of the study are that (1) subjects lost a significant percentage of their body weight three months after bariatric surgery, (2) SAT arterioles from post-surgery biopsies demonstrated improved FID and AChID at baseline, increased NO production, enhanced sensitivity to L-NAME, and reduced effect of PEG-CAT compared to SAT arterioles from the day of surgery sample, (3) in post-surgery SAT arterioles, vitamin D did not induce any further enhancements in vasodilation or NO production, and (4) a synergistic interaction between weight loss and vitamin-D incubation was observed in relation to arteriolar sensitivity to eNOS inhibition via L-NAME.

The findings that vitamin D improves FID, AChID, and NO fluorescence in SAT and VAT support the notion that vitamin D is a regulator of endothelial function [35,36]. Our findings are consistent with previous studies suggesting that vitamin D is a transcriptional regulator of eNOS, effectively increasing the production of NO, the most potent vasodilator within the vasculature [37,38]. Previous studies showed that vitamin-D receptors play a critical role in maintaining vascular health, and this assumption was supported by data showing reduced NO production, endothelial dysfunction, increased arterial stiffness, increased aortic impedance, and structural remodeling of the aorta in mice with mutant vitamin-D receptors [21]. Also, earlier studies demonstrated hypertension and myocardial hypertrophy in vitamin-D receptor knockout mice [39]. In vitro experiments conducted by

Martínez-Miguel et al. [40] also supported the role of vitamin-D supplementation in inducing eNOS transcription and activity in endothelial cells. In addition to the effect of vitamin D on inducing eNOS expression, it was suggested that vitamin D improves vascular function via reducing the production of NO-scavenging oxygen radicals and subsequently improving NO bioavailability [41–43].

In addition to its role in inducing eNOS expression and activity, vitamin D was shown to reduce nuclear factor kappa B (NF-κB) activity and inhibit the production of several pro-inflammatory cytokines such as tumor necrosis factor-α (TNF-α), interferon gamma (IFN-γ), interleukin 1 beta (IL-1β), and IL-8, while upregulating the anti-inflammatory cytokine, IL-10 [44]. Previous studies showed that vitamin D inhibits cytokine-mediated endothelial cell activation and the production of surface adhesion molecules [45]. Furthermore, vitamin D's protective effect against atherosclerosis and hypertension was explained by its ability to decrease the proliferation of vascular smooth muscle, decrease calcium influx into endothelial cells, decrease vascular resistance, and regulate the renin–angiotensin system [46,47].

In addition to the experimental evidence, several epidemiological studies linked low vitamin-D levels with high blood pressure, coronary artery disease, myocardial infarction, and heart failure [48–50]. Despite this experimental and epidemiological evidence, results from clinical trials investigating the effect of vitamin-D supplementation on improving vascular function and reducing cardiovascular risk were less encouraging. In a metanalysis by Beveridge et al. [51], effects of vitamin-D supplementation on flow-mediated dilatation of the brachial artery, pulse wave velocity, augmentation index, central blood pressure, microvascular function, and reactive hyperemia index were assessed using data from 31 trials (2751 participants). This metanalysis showed no significant improvements in macrovascular function and modest improvements in microvascular function in response to vitamin-D administration in a daily dose that ranged from 900 to 5000 IU for a duration of four weeks to 12 months. Other metanalyses showed a similar lack of significant effects of vitamin-D supplementation on vascular function [52–54]. It is important to note that most of the trials included in these studies did not account for variations in biologic availability of the administered vitamin D that might be caused by different body compositions. It is possible that the lack of response to vitamin-D supplementation is due to low blood serum levels of vitamin D secondary to its sequestration within the adipose tissue. In support of this notion, previous studies reported lower serum bioavailability of vitamin-D supplementation in obese individuals [55,56]. Accordingly, it would be challenging to measure the systemic effects of vitamin D if it is sequestered in the body fat. In the current study, we sought to test the effect of direct exposure to vitamin D in endothelial function and the contributing vasoactive mediators in isolated human arterioles. Furthermore, we sought to test the effect of fat mass reduction after bariatric surgery on microvascular function and response to vitamin-D exposure.

The demonstrated vascular improvements in response to exogenous (ex vivo) application of vitamin D on isolated blood vessels in the current study suggests that the lack of in vivo effects in previous clinical trials could be related to vitamin-D inaccessibility to vascular tissues. This supposition might also explain the observed lack of any significant differences in microvascular function between subjects who administered vitamin D before surgery and those who did not in the current study. Our findings also highlighted the mechanism via which vitamin D enhanced the microvascular function, which was found to be mainly mediated by a restoration of the production and sensitivity of the most potent endothelial-dependent vasodilator, NO. The effect of vitamin D on abolishing any dependence of microvascular dilation on H_2O_2, a compensatory mechanism for compromised NO pathways, indicates the role of vitamin D in reestablishing healthier vascular milieu and vasodilation mechanisms. The phenomenon of shifting the primary vasoactive mediator from NO to H_2O_2 under conditions characterized by inflammation and oxidative stress was reported by our research group and by others [26,27,31,57,58]. Despite being a vasodilator, H_2O_2 possesses proinflammatory, prothrombotic, and proatherogenic properties that eventually exacerbate vascular dysfunction [59]. Accordingly, the reduced sensitivity of arteriolar vasodilation to H_2O_2 scavenging might indicate a reduction in inflammation or ROS production or improved anti-oxidative mechanisms. However, future studies are required to confirm this assumption and explore the exact mechanism via which vitamin D reduces the dependence on H_2O_2 as a vasodilator.

The findings that baseline FID, AChID, and NO fluorescence improved in SAT arterioles three months post-surgery and that no further improvements could be achieved in response to exogenous vitamin-D incubation suggest increased accessibility of vitamin D to vascular tissues after weight loss. This assumption is supported by the significant elevation of serum vitamin-D levels after surgery. However, this does not rule out other non-vitamin-D-related, weight loss-induced biological changes that might have contributed to the observed vascular improvements. Some of the previously suggested mechanisms could include an improved lipid profile and glucose metabolism and reduced systemic inflammation [60,61]. It is conceivable that the effect of weight loss in improving microvascular function is multifactorial; however, the results from the current study indicate a potential role of vitamin D in restoring vascular health after weight loss. We recently demonstrated the effect of dietary-induced weight loss in promoting microvascular health and endothelial-mediated NO production [29]. In the current study, we present evidence that vitamin D contributes, at least partially, to weight loss-associated vascular improvements.

Findings from previous studies suggest that loss of visceral adipose tissue after weight loss interventions is easier and greater than subcutaneous adipose tissue [62,63] and that the latter is the primary storage site for cutaneously produced vitamin D [64]. In our study, weight loss three months post-surgery may not have affected the amount of subcutaneous adipose tissue significantly. Therefore, a significant amount of vitamin D sequestered in those tissues may not have been released into the serum. Accordingly, future studies with long-term follow-up are required to detect robust improvements in circulating vitamin D and vascular function. The response of FID to PEG-CAT decreased in the arterioles isolated after surgery compared to arterioles from the day of surgery. These findings are consistent with previous evidence indicating that in chronic diseases and morbid obesity, other endothelium-derived vasodilators, such as H_2O_2, may compensate for the lack of NO [26,27,34,65]. Yet, the current study is the first to demonstrate the effectiveness of surgical weight loss in shifting the major vasodilator back to NO and minimizing the dependence on H_2O_2 in human adipose tissue resistance arterioles.

Although, consecutive to bariatric surgery, vitamin-D levels improved (Table 2), these levels are still considered less than adequate (>20 ng/mL) [66]. A growing body of evidence demonstrates a state of malabsorption and vitamin deficiencies following certain types of bariatric surgeries as reviewed by Lespessailles et al. [67]. For instance, bypassing the jejunum in the Roux-en-Y gastric bypass (RYGB) surgery and bile salt deficiency associated with bariatric surgery procedures affect vitamin-D absorption and bioavailability in post-bariatric patients [68,69]. Based on these facts, the 2008 interdisciplinary European guidelines on metabolic and bariatric surgery recommended the inclusion of vitamin D as a routine laboratory test that should be evaluated annually after bariatric surgery [70]. Also, the latest recommendations of the American Association of Clinical Endocrinologists, the Obesity Society, and American Society for Metabolic and Bariatric Surgery are to measure vitamin-D blood levels before and after bariatric surgery and to treat patients with 3000 IU of vitamin D daily after bariatric surgery to obtain a level greater than 30 ng/mL [71]. Obesity on one hand and post-bariatric malabsorption on the other hand might cause vitamin-D deficiency; therefore, future studies that investigate long-term vascular outcomes after bariatric surgery with and without vitamin-D supplementation are required.

There were several limitations to this study. Firstly, this study was limited to a young morbidly obese male and premenopausal female population, thereby limiting the generalizability of the findings to the population at large. Secondly, we had a relatively small sample size (pre-surgery: $n = 15$, post-surgery: $n = 8$), which carries with it the risk of a type II error due to low statistical power. Thirdly, the study design made it not possible to control for the menstrual cycle in the female subjects during sample acquisition. Hormonal changes during the menstrual cycle were shown to affect the macrovasculature, but its influence on the microcirculation is unknown. The surgery date could not be scheduled to control for this as a confounder a priori. Moreover, only eight of the 15 recruited subjects returned after their surgery for their second visit. No post-surgery VAT sample was obtained, as this biopsy was unattainable in the absence of general anesthesia. Another limitation of the current study is that pre- and post-surgery SAT samples were obtained from different adipose depots (abdominal vs. gluteal SAT). However, previous studies showed that mechanisms of dilations in SAT depots are not dependent on the region of biopsy [26]. In addition, the follow-up after surgery was for a short term (three months), which imposes difficulty in identifying long-term consequences of surgical weight loss. Thus, future investigations to evaluate the long-term vascular effects of weight loss after bariatric surgery are warranted. Finally, one of the main limitations of our study is the unbalanced female-to-male ratio. Although this study was not designed to determine gender- or racial/ethnic-specific differences in response to bariatric surgery, future studies are required to determine the influence of such variables on microvascular function.

In summary, this is the first study to explore the effects of surgical weight loss and vitamin D on microvascular function and the leading mechanisms of vasodilation in human isolated SAT and VAT resistance arterioles. The results of this study suggest a role of vitamin D in maintaining vascular health. It also suggests that weight loss is an integral component of enhancing vitamin-D bioavailability and its effects on enhancing microvascular function and, subsequently, the reduction of cardiovascular risk in morbidly obese individuals.

Author Contributions: A.M.M., conceptualization, data acquisition, editing, and reviewing final draft; M.S., data acquisition, editing, and reviewing final draft; C.H., data acquisition, editing, and reviewing final draft; M.M., data acquisition, editing, and reviewing final draft; A.G., data acquisition, editing, and reviewing final draft; S.A.P., conceptualization, editing, and reviewing final draft.

Funding: The authors were supported by research funding from the National Heart, Lung, and Blood Institute (NHLBI), grants HL095701 (S.A.P.) and K99HL140049 and 4 R00 HL140049-03 (A.M.M.). The project described was supported by the National Center for Advancing Translational Sciences, National Institutes of Health, through Grant UL1TR002003. The content is solely the responsibility of the authors and does not necessarily represent the official views of the National Institutes of Health.

Acknowledgments: We would like to thank Maryann Holtcamp M.S., A.P.N. and the rest of the staff at the Center for Clinical and Translational Science (CCTS) for their support with the study. We would like to thank Jing-Tan Bian for his technical assistance in the study. The content is solely the responsibility of the authors and does not necessarily represent the official views of the National Institutes of Health.

Conflicts of Interest: The authors declare no conflict of interest.

References

1. Daniel, D.; Hardigan, P.; Bray, N.; Penzell, D.; Savu, C. The incidence of vitamin D deficiency in the obese: A retrospective chart review. *J. Community Hosp. Intern. Med. Perspect.* **2015**, *5*, 26069. [CrossRef] [PubMed]
2. Compston, J.; Vedi, S.; Ledger, J.; Webb, A.; Gazet, J.C.; Pilkington, T.R. Vitamin D status and bone histomorphometry in gross obesity. *Am. J. Clin. Nutr.* **1981**, *34*, 2359–2363. [CrossRef] [PubMed]
3. Hengist, A.; Perkin, O.; Gonzalez, J.T.; Betts, J.A.; Hewison, M.; Manolopoulos, K.N.; Jones, K.S.; Koulman, A.; Thompson, D. Mobilising vitamin D from adipose tissue: The potential impact of exercise. *Nutr. Bull.* **2019**, *44*, 25–35. [CrossRef]
4. Pittas, A.G.; Chung, M.; Trikalinos, T.; Mitri, J.; Brendel, M.; Patel, K.; Lichtenstein, A.H.; Lau, J.; Balk, E.M. Systematic review: Vitamin D and cardiometabolic outcomes. *Ann. Intern. Med.* **2010**, *152*, 307–314. [CrossRef] [PubMed]
5. Al Mheid, I.; Patel, R.; Murrow, J.; Morris, A.; Aznaouridis, K.; Rahman, A.; Fike, L.; Kavtaradze, N.; Ahmed, Y.; Uphoff, I.; et al. Vitamin D Status is Associated with Arterial Stiffness and Vascular Dysfunction in Healthy Humans. *J. Am. Coll. Cardiol.* **2011**, *57*, E2049. [CrossRef]
6. Al Mheid, I.; Patel, R.S.; Tangpricha, V.; Quyyumi, A.A. Vitamin D and cardiovascular disease: Is the evidence solid? *Eur. Hear. J.* **2013**, *34*, 3691–3698. [CrossRef]
7. Chitalia, N.; Recio-Mayoral, A.; Kaski, J.C.; Banerjee, D. Vitamin D deficiency and endothelial dysfunction in non-dialysis chronic kidney disease patients. *Atheroscler* **2012**, *220*, 265–268. [CrossRef]

8. Judd, S.; Nanes, M.S.; Ziegler, T.R.; Wilson, P.W.F.; Tangpricha, V. Optimal vitamin D status attenuates the age-associated increase in systolic blood pressure in white Americans: Results from the third National Health and Nutrition Examination Survey. *Am. J. Clin. Nutr.* **2008**, *87*, 136–141. [CrossRef]

9. London, G.M.; Guérin, A.P.; Verbeke, F.H.; Pannier, B.; Boutouyrie, P.; Marchais, S.J.; Metivier, F. Mineral Metabolism and Arterial Functions in End-Stage Renal Disease: Potential Role of 25-Hydroxyvitamin D Deficiency. *J. Am. Soc. Nephrol.* **2007**, *18*, 613–620. [CrossRef]

10. Motiwala, S.R.; Wang, T.J. Vitamin D and cardiovascular disease. *Curr. Opin. Nephrol. Hypertens.* **2011**, *20*, 345–353. [CrossRef]

11. Scragg, R.; Sowers, M.; Bell, C. Serum 25-hydroxyvitamin D, Ethnicity, and Blood Pressure in the Third National Health and Nutrition Examination Survey. *Am. J. Hypertens.* **2007**, *20*, 713–719. [CrossRef] [PubMed]

12. Yiu, Y.-F.; Chan, Y.-H.; Yiu, K.-H.; Siu, C.-W.; Li, S.-W.; Wong, L.-Y.; Lee, S.W.L.; Tam, S.; Wong, E.W.K.; Cheung, B.M.Y.; et al. Vitamin D Deficiency Is Associated with Depletion of Circulating Endothelial Progenitor Cells and Endothelial Dysfunction in Patients with Type 2 Diabetes. *J. Clin. Endocrinol. Metab.* **2011**, *96*, 830–835. [CrossRef] [PubMed]

13. Pilz, S.; Tomaschitz, A.; Ritz, E.; Pieber, T.R. Vitamin D status and arterial hypertension: A systematic review. *Nat. Rev. Cardiol.* **2009**, *6*, 621–630. [CrossRef] [PubMed]

14. Bodnar, L.M.; Simhan, H.N.; Catov, J.M.; Roberts, J.M.; Platt, R.W.; Diesel, J.C.; Klebanoff, M.A. Maternal vitamin D status and the risk of mild and severe preeclampsia. *Epidemiology* **2014**, *25*, 207–214. [CrossRef] [PubMed]

15. Almirall, J.; Vaqueiro, M.; Baré, M.L.; Anton, E. Association of low serum 25-hydroxyvitamin D levels and high arterial blood pressure in the elderly. *Nephrol. Dial. Transplant.* **2010**, *25*, 503–509. [CrossRef] [PubMed]

16. Vaidya, A.; Sun, B.; Larson, C.; Forman, J.P.; Williams, J.S. Vitamin D_3 therapy corrects the tissue sensitivity to angiotensin ii akin to the action of a converting enzyme inhibitor in obese hypertensives: An interventional study. *J. Clin. Endocrinol. Metab.* **2012**, *97*, 2456–2465. [CrossRef] [PubMed]

17. Al-Dujaili, E.A.S.; Munir, N.; Iniesta, R.R. Effect of vitamin D supplementation on cardiovascular disease risk factors and exercise performance in healthy participants: A randomized placebo-controlled preliminary study. *Ther. Adv. Endocrinol. Metab.* **2016**, *7*, 153–165. [CrossRef] [PubMed]

18. Bouillon, R.; Carmeliet, G.; Verlinden, L.; Van Etten, E.; Verstuyf, A.; Luderer, H.F.; Lieben, L.; Mathieu, C.; DeMay, M. Vitamin D and human health: Lessons from vitamin D receptor null mice. *Endocr. Rev.* **2008**, *29*, 726–776. [CrossRef]

19. Haussler, M.R.; Haussler, C.A.; Bartik, L.; Whitfield, G.K.; Hsieh, J.-C.; Slater, S.; Jurutka, P.W. Vitamin D receptor: Molecular signaling and actions of nutritional ligands in disease prevention. *Nutr. Rev.* **2008**, *66*, 98–112. [CrossRef]

20. Elliott, P.; McKenna, W. Hypertrophic cardiomyopathy: A 50th anniversary. *Heart* **2008**, *94*, 1247–1248. [CrossRef]

21. Andrukhova, O.; Slavic, S.; Zeitz, U.; Riesen, S.C.; Heppelmann, M.S.; Ambrisko, T.D.; Markovic, M.; Kuebler, W.M.; Erben, R.G. Vitamin D is a regulator of endothelial nitric oxide synthase and arterial stiffness in mice. *Mol. Endocrinol.* **2014**, *28*, 53–64. [CrossRef] [PubMed]

22. Al-Daghri, N.M.; Bukhari, I.; Yakout, S.M.; Sabico, S.; Khattak, M.N.K.; Aziz, I.; Alokail, M.S. Associations of Serum Nitric Oxide with Vitamin D and Other Metabolic Factors in Apparently Healthy Adolescents. *Biomed. Res. Int.* **2018**, *2018*, 1489132. [CrossRef] [PubMed]

23. Arfian, N.; Kusuma, M.H.; Anggorowati, N.; Nugroho, D.B.; Jeffilano, A.; Suzuki, Y.; Ikeda, K.; Emoto, N. Vitamin D upregulates endothelin-1, ETBR, eNOS mRNA expression and attenuates vascular remodelling and ischemia in kidney fibrosis model in mice. *Physiol. Res.* **2018**, *67*, 137–147. [CrossRef] [PubMed]

24. Molinari, C.; Uberti, F.; Grossini, E.; Vacca, G.; Carda, S.; Invernizzi, M.; Cisari, C. 1alpha,25-dihydroxycholecalciferol induces nitric oxide production in cultured endothelial cells. *Cell Physiol. Biochem.* **2011**, *27*, 661–668. [CrossRef]

25. Robinson, A.T.; Szczurek, M.; Bian, J.T.; Cavka, A.; Grizelj, I.; Phillips, S. Mitochondrial reactive oxygen species contribute to impaired flow-induced dilation in visceral but not subcutaneous adipose tissue resistance arteries in human obesity. *FASEB J.* **2013**, *27*, 687.

26. Phillips, S.A.; Hatoum, O.A.; Gutterman, D.D. The mechanism of flow-induced dilation in human adipose arterioles involves hydrogen peroxide during CAD. *Am. J. Physiol. Circ. Physiol.* **2007**, *292*, 93–100. [CrossRef]

27. Matoba, T.; Shimokawa, H. Hydrogen peroxide is an endothelium-derived hyperpolarizing factor in animals and humans. *J. Pharmacol. Sci.* **2003**, *92*, 1–6. [CrossRef]

28. Mahmoud, A.M.; Szczurek, M.R.; Blackburn, B.K.; Mey, J.T.; Chen, Z.; Robinson, A.T.; Bian, J.-T.; Unterman, T.G.; Minshall, R.D.; Brown, M.D.; et al. Hyperinsulinemia augments endothelin-1 protein expression and impairs vasodilation of human skeletal muscle arterioles. *Physiol. Rep.* **2016**, *4*, e12895. [CrossRef]

29. Mahmoud, A.M.; Hwang, C.-L.; Szczurek, M.R.; Bian, J.-T.; Ranieri, C.; Gutterman, D.D.; Phillips, S.A. Low-Fat Diet Designed for Weight Loss but not Weight Maintenance Improves Nitric Oxide-Dependent Arteriolar Vasodilation in Obese Adults. *Nutrition* **2019**, *11*, 1339. [CrossRef]

30. Miura, H.; Wachtel, R.E.; Liu, Y.; Loberiza, F.R.; Saito, T.; Miura, M.; Gutterman, D.D. Flow-induced dilation of human coronary arterioles: Important role of Ca (2+)-activated K (+) channels. *Circulation* **2001**, *103*, 1992–1998. [CrossRef]

31. Robinson, A.T.; Franklin, N.C.; Norkeviciute, E.; Bian, J.T.; Babana, J.C.; Szczurek, M.R.; Phillips, S.A. Improved arterial flow-mediated dilation after exertion involves hydrogen peroxide in overweight and obese adults following aerobic exercise training. *J. Hypertens.* **2016**, *34*, 1309–1316. [CrossRef] [PubMed]

32. Grizelj, I.; Cavka, A.; Bian, J.-T.; Szczurek, M.; Robinson, A.; Shinde, S.; Nguyen, V.; Braunschweig, C.; Wang, E.; Drenjancevic, I.; et al. Reduced flow- and acetylcholine-induced dilations in visceral compared to subcutaneous adipose arterioles in human morbid obesity. *Microcirculation* **2015**, *22*, 44–53. [CrossRef] [PubMed]

33. Thengchaisri, N.; Kuo, L. Hydrogen peroxide induces endothelium-dependent and -independent coronary arteriolar dilation: Role of cyclooxygenase and potassium channels. *Am. J. Physiol. Circ. Physiol.* **2003**, *285*, 2255–2263. [CrossRef] [PubMed]

34. Matoba, T.; Shimokawa, H.; Kubota, H.; Morikawa, K.; Fujiki, T.; Kunihiro, I.; Mukai, Y.; Hirakawa, Y.; Takeshita, A. Hydrogen Peroxide is an Endothelium-Derived Hyperpolarizing Factor in Human Mesenteric Arteries. *Biochem. Biophys. Res. Commun.* **2002**, *290*, 909–913. [CrossRef] [PubMed]

35. Wong, M.S.K.; Delansorne, R.; Man, R.Y.K.; Vanhoutte, P.M. Vitamin D derivatives acutely reduce endothelium—Dependent contractions in the aorta of the spontaneously hypertensive rat. *Am. J. Physiol. Circ. Physiol.* **2008**, *295*, 289–296. [CrossRef] [PubMed]

36. Capitanio, S.; Sambuceti, G.; Giusti, M.; Morbelli, S.; Murialdo, G.; Garibotto, G.; Lara, V.; Pietro, A.; Barbara, R.; Mehrdad, N.; et al. 1,25-Dihydroxy vitamin D and coronary microvascular function. *Eur. J. Nucl. Med. Mol. Imaging* **2013**, *40*, 280–289. [CrossRef] [PubMed]

37. Merke, J.; Milde, P.; Lewicka, S.; Hügel, U.; Klaus, G.; Mangelsdorf, D.J.; Haussler, M.R.; Rauterberg, E.W.; Ritz, E. Identification and regulation of 1,25-dihydroxyvitamin D_3 receptor activity and biosynthesis of 1,25-dihydroxyvitamin D_3. Studies in cultured bovine aortic endothelial cells and human dermal capillaries. *J. Clin. Investig.* **1989**, *83*, 1903–1915. [CrossRef]

38. Zehnder, D.; Bland, R.; Williams, M.C.; McNinch, R.W.; Howie, A.J.; Stewart, P.M.; Hewison, M. Extrarenal expression of 25-hydroxyvitamin D_3-1 α-hydroxylase. *J. Clin. Endocrinol. Metab.* **2001**, *86*, 888–894. [CrossRef]

39. Li, Y.C.; Kong, J.; Wei, M.; Chen, Z.-F.; Liu, S.Q.; Cao, L.-P. 1,25-Dihydroxyvitamin D_3 is a negative endocrine regulator of the renin-angiotensin system. *J. Clin. Investig.* **2002**, *110*, 229–238. [CrossRef]

40. Martínez-Miguel, P.; Valdivielso, J.M.; Medrano-Andrés, D.; Román-García, P.; Cano-Peñalver, J.L.; Rodríguez-Puyol, M.; Rodríguez-Puyol, D.; López-Ongil, S. The active form of vitamin D, calcitriol, induces a complex dual upregulation of endothelin and nitric oxide in cultured endothelial cells. *Am. J. Physiol. Metab.* **2014**, *307*, 1085–1096. [CrossRef]

41. Khan, A.; Dawoud, H.; Malinski, T. Nanomedical studies of the restoration of nitric oxide/peroxynitrite balance in dysfunctional endothelium by 1,25-dihydroxy vitamin D_3—Clinical implications for cardiovascular diseases. *Int. J. Nanomed.* **2018**, *13*, 455–466. [CrossRef]

42. Jia, X.; Xu, J.; Gu, Y.; Gu, X.; Li, W.; Wang, Y. Vitamin D suppresses oxidative stress-induced microparticle release by human umbilical vein endothelial cells. *Boil. Reprod.* **2017**, *96*, 199–210. [CrossRef]

43. Xu, J.; Jia, X.; Gu, Y.; Lewis, D.F.; Gu, X.; Wang, Y. Vitamin D Reduces Oxidative Stress—Induced Procaspase-3/ROCK1 Activation and MP Release by Placental Trophoblasts. *J. Clin. Endocrinol. Metab.* **2017**, *102*, 2100–2110. [CrossRef] [PubMed]

44. Hoe, E.; Nathanielsz, J.; Toh, Z.Q.; Spry, L.; Marimla, R.; Balloch, A.; Mulholland, K.; Licciardi, P.V. Anti-Inflammatory Effects of Vitamin D on Human Immune Cells in the Context of Bacterial Infection. *Nutrition* **2016**, *8*, 806. [CrossRef]

45. Naeini, A.E.; Moeinzadeh, F.; Vahdat, S.; Ahmadi, A.; Hedayati, Z.P.; Shahzeidi, S. The Effect of Vitamin D Administration on Intracellular Adhesion Molecule-1 and Vascular Cell Adhesion Molecule-1 Levels in Hemodialysis Patients: A Placebo-controlled, Double-blinded Clinical Trial. *J. Res. Pharm. Pract.* **2017**, *6*, 16–20.

46. Min, B. Effects of Vitamin D on Blood Pressure and Endothelial Function. *Korean J. Physiol. Pharmacol.* **2013**, *17*, 385–392. [CrossRef]

47. Carbone, F.; Mach, F.; Vuilleumier, N.; Montecucco, F. Potential pathophysiological role for the vitamin D deficiency in essential hypertension. *World J. Cardiol.* **2014**, *6*, 260–276. [CrossRef] [PubMed]

48. Autier, P.; Boniol, M.; Pizot, C.; Mullie, P. Vitamin D status and ill health: A systematic review. *Lancet Diabetes Endocrinol.* **2014**, *2*, 76–89. [CrossRef]

49. Theodoratou, E.; Tzoulaki, I.; Zgaga, L.; Ioannidis, J.P. Vitamin D and multiple health outcomes: Umbrella review of systematic reviews and meta-analyses of observational studies and randomised trials. *BMJ* **2014**, *348*, 2035. [CrossRef]

50. Beveridge, L.A.; Witham, M.D. Vitamin D and the cardiovascular system. *Osteoporos. Int.* **2013**, *24*, 2167–2180. [CrossRef]

51. Beveridge, L.A.; Khan, F.; Struthers, A.D.; Armitage, J.; Barchetta, I.; Bressendorff, I.; Cavallo, M.G.; Clarke, R.; Dalan, R.; Dreyer, G.; et al. Effect of Vitamin D Supplementation on Markers of Vascular Function: A Systematic Review and Individual Participant Meta-Analysis. *J. Am. Hear. Assoc.* **2018**, *7*, e008273. [CrossRef] [PubMed]

52. Beveridge, L.A.; Struthers, A.D.; Khan, F.; Jorde, R.; Scragg, R.; Macdonald, H.M.; Alvarez, J.A.; Boxer, R.S.; Dalbeni, A.; Gepner, A.D.; et al. Effect of Vitamin D Supplementation on Blood Pressure: A Systematic Review and Meta-Analysis Incorporating Individual Patient Data. *JAMA Intern Med.* **2015**, *175*, 45–54. [CrossRef] [PubMed]

53. Hussin, A.M.; Ashor, A.W.; Schoenmakers, I.; Hill, T.; Mathers, J.C.; Siervo, M. Effects of vitamin D supplementation on endothelial function: A systematic review and meta-analysis of randomised clinical trials. *Eur. J. Nutr.* **2017**, *56*, 1095–1104. [CrossRef] [PubMed]

54. Upala, S.; Sanguankeo, A.; Congrete, S.; Jaruvongvanich, V. Effect of cholecalciferol supplementation on arterial stiffness: A systematic review and meta-analysis. *Scand. Cardiovasc. J.* **2016**, *50*, 230–235. [CrossRef]

55. Wortsman, J.; Matsuoka, L.Y.; Chen, T.C.; Lu, Z.; Holick, M.F. Decreased bioavailability of vitamin D in obesity. *Am. J. Clin. Nutr.* **2000**, *72*, 690–693. [CrossRef]

56. Zhou, J.C.; Zhu, Y.M.; Chen, Z.; Mo, J.L.; Xie, F.Z.; Wen, Y.H.; Guo, P.; Peng, J.; Xu, J.; Wang, J.; et al. Oral vitamin D supplementation has a lower bioavailability and reduces hypersecretion of parathyroid hormone and insulin resistance in obese Chinese males. *Public Health Nutr.* **2015**, *18*, 2211–2219. [CrossRef]

57. Durand, M.J.; Dharmashankar, K.; Bian, J.T.; Das, E.; Vidovich, M.; Gutterman, D.D.; Phillips, S.A. Acute exertion elicits a H_2O_2-dependent vasodilator mechanism in the microvasculature of exercise-trained but not sedentary adults. *Hypertension* **2015**, *65*, 140–145. [CrossRef]

58. Beyer, A.M.; Durand, M.J.; Hockenberry, J.; Gamblin, T.C.; Phillips, S.A.; Gutterman, D.D. An acute rise in intraluminal pressure shifts the mediator of flow-mediated dilation from nitric oxide to hydrogen peroxide in human arterioles. *Am. J. Physiol. Circ. Physiol.* **2014**, *307*, 1587–1593. [CrossRef]

59. Cai, H. Hydrogen peroxide regulation of endothelial function: Origins, mechanisms, and consequences. *Cardiovasc. Res.* **2005**, *68*, 26–36. [CrossRef]

60. Bigornia, S.J.; Mott, M.M.; Hess, D.T.; Apovian, C.M.; McDonnell, M.E.; Duess, M.-A.; Kluge, M.A.; Fiscale, A.J.; Vita, J.A.; Gokce, N. Long-term successful weight loss improves vascular endothelial function in severely obese individuals. *Obesity* **2010**, *18*, 754–759. [CrossRef]

61. Brook, R.D. Obesity, Weight Loss, and Vascular Function. *Endocrine* **2006**, *29*, 21–26. [CrossRef]

62. Chaston, T.B.; Dixon, J.B. Factors associated with percent change in visceral versus subcutaneous abdominal fat during weight loss: Findings from a systematic review. *Int. J. Obes.* **2008**, *32*, 619–628. [CrossRef] [PubMed]

63. Pinho, C.P.S.; da Silva Diniz, A.; de Arruda, I.K.G.; Leite, A.P.D.L.; Rodrigues, I.G. Effects of weight loss on adipose visceral and subcutaneous tissue in overweight adults. *Clin. Nutr.* **2018**, *37*, 1252–1258. [CrossRef] [PubMed]

64. Didriksen, A.; Burild, A.; Jakobsen, J.; Fuskevåg, O.M.; Jorde, R. Vitamin D_3 increases in abdominal subcutaneous fat tissue after supplementation with vitamin D_3. *Eur. J. Endocrinol.* **2015**, *172*, 235–241. [CrossRef] [PubMed]

65. Miura, H.; Bosnjak, J.J.; Ning, G.; Saito, T.; Miura, M.; Gutterman, D.D. Role for hydrogen peroxide in flow-induced dilation of human coronary arterioles. *Circ. Res.* **2003**, *92*, 31–40. [CrossRef] [PubMed]

66. Kennel, K.A.; Drake, M.T.; Hurley, D.L. Vitamin D Deficiency in Adults: When to Test and How to Treat. *Mayo Clin. Proc.* **2010**, *85*, 752–758. [CrossRef] [PubMed]

67. Lespessailles, E.; Toumi, H. Vitamin D alteration associated with obesity and bariatric surgery. *Exp. Boil. Med.* **2017**, *242*, 1086–1094. [CrossRef]

68. Riedt, C.S.; Brolin, R.E.; Sherrell, R.M.; Field, M.P.; Shapses, S.A. True fractional calcium absorption is decreased after Roux-en-Y gastric bypass surgery. *Obesity* **2006**, *14*, 1940–1948. [CrossRef]

69. Shaker, J.L.; Norton, A.J.; Woods, M.F.; Fallon, M.D.; Findling, J.W. Secondary hyperparathyroidism and osteopenia in women following gastric exclusion surgery for obesity. *Osteoporos. Int.* **1991**, *1*, 177–181. [CrossRef]

70. Fried, M.; Yumuk, V.; Oppert, J.M.; Scopinaro, N.; Torres, A.; Weiner, R.; Yashkov, Y.; Frühbeck, G. Interdisciplinary European Guidelines on metabolic and bariatric surgery. *Obes. Surg.* **2013**, *24*, 42–55. [CrossRef]

71. Mechanick, J.I.; Youdim, A.; Jones, D.B.; Garvey, W.T.; Hurley, D.L.; McMahon, M.; Heinberg, L.J.; Kushner, R.; Adams, T.D.; Shikora, S.; et al. Clinical Practice Guidelines for the Perioperative Nutritional, Metabolic, and Nonsurgical Support of the Bariatric Surgery Patient—2013 Update: Cosponsored by American Association of Clinical Endocrinologists, The Obesity Society, and American Society for Metabolic & Bariatric Surgery. *Obesity* **2013**, *21*, 1–27.

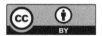

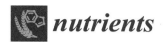

Article

Temporal Measures in Cardiac Structure and Function During the Development of Obesity Induced by Different Types of Western Diet in a Rat Model

Danielle Fernandes Vileigas [1,†], Cecília Lume de Carvalho Marciano [1,†],
Gustavo Augusto Ferreira Mota [1], Sérgio Luiz Borges de Souza [1], Paula Grippa Sant'Ana [1],
Katashi Okoshi [1], Carlos Roberto Padovani [2] and Antonio Carlos Cicogna [1,*]

[1]   Department of Internal Medicine, Botucatu Medical School, São Paulo State University, UNESP,
     Botucatu 18618687, Brazil; dani.vileigas@gmail.com (D.F.V.); cecilialcm3@gmail.com (C.L.d.C.M.);
     gamota@alunos.fmb.unesp.br (G.A.F.M.); enfeborges@gmail.com (S.L.B.d.S.);
     paulagrippa@yahoo.com.br (P.G.S.); katashi.okoshi@unesp.br (K.O.)
[2]   Department of Biostatistics, Institute of Biosciences, São Paulo State University, Botucatu 18618970, Brazil;
     cr.padovani@unesp.br
*   Correspondence: ac.cicogna@unesp.br; Tel.: +55-14-3880-1618
†   These authors contributed equally to this work.

Received: 18 November 2019; Accepted: 23 December 2019; Published: 26 December 2019

Abstract: Obesity is recognized worldwide as a complex metabolic disorder that has reached epidemic proportions and is often associated with a high incidence of cardiovascular diseases. To study this pathology and evaluate cardiac function, several models of diet-induced obesity (DIO) have been developed. The Western diet (WD) is one of the most widely used models; however, variations in diet composition and time period of the experimental protocol make comparisons challenging. Thus, this study aimed to evaluate the effects of two different types of Western diet on cardiac remodeling in obese rats with sequential analyses during a long-term follow-up. Male Wistar rats were distributed into three groups fed with control diet (CD), Western diet fat (WDF), and Western diet sugar (WDS) for 41 weeks. The animal nutritional profile and cardiac histology were assessed at the 41st week. Cardiac structure and function were evaluated by echocardiogram at four different moments: 17, 25, 33, and 41 weeks. A noninvasive method was performed to assess systolic blood pressure at the 33rd and 41st week. The animals fed with WD (WDF and WDS) developed pronounced obesity with an average increase of 86.5% in adiposity index at the end of the experiment. WDF and WDS groups also presented hypertension. The echocardiographic data showed no structural differences among the three groups, but WDF animals presented decreased endocardial fractional shortening and ejection fraction at the 33rd and 41st week, suggesting altered systolic function. Moreover, WDF and WFS animals did not present hypertrophy and interstitial collagen accumulation in the left ventricle. In conclusion, both WD were effective in triggering severe obesity in rats; however, only the WDF induced mild cardiac dysfunction after long-term diet exposure. Further studies are needed to search for an appropriate DIO model with relevant cardiac remodeling.

Keywords: cardiac remodeling; cardiac dysfunction; echocardiogram; obese rats; high-fat high-sugar diet

---

1. Introduction

Obesity is a complex metabolic disorder recognized worldwide as a significant health concern, and its prevalence has reached epidemic proportions [1]. In 2016, more than 1.9 billion adults were overweight; of these, over 650 million were obese [2]. The etiology of obesity is complex and multifactorial, especially involving environmental and genetic factors. However, the modern obesity epidemic is undoubtedly the result of environmental determinants and is often associated with a reduction in physical activity and increased intake of diets high in saturated fat and sugars, commonly termed Western diet [3,4]. Excessive body fat is the leading risk factor for numerous comorbidities, most notably gastrointestinal diseases, type 2 diabetes mellitus, certain types of cancer, and cardiovascular disease (CVD) [5].

A number of clinical and animal studies have generated convincing evidence that hemodynamic, neurohormonal, and metabolic alterations, which are commonly found in obesity, contribute to changes in cardiac morphology that may predispose to impaired ventricular function and heart failure [6,7]. For a better understanding of the mechanisms underlying cardiac dysfunction in obesity and to assess potential treatments for this pathology, several experimental animal models have been developed, and one of the most commonly used is the diet-induced obesity (DIO) model [8]. Among the various types of experimental diets, such as high-fat, cafeteria, and high-fructose, many studies have preferably used the Western diet (WD) due to its relative similarity to the human consumption responsible for the obesity epidemic [9,10].

In WD, various sources of fat and sugar are used in different proportions, sometimes higher in fat or higher in sugar, and there is no consensus on which one is the most effective to cause cardiac dysfunction; moreover, the duration of experimental studies ranges widely [11–16]. Thus, a considerable divergence of results concerning heart function is observed among different studies making comparisons challenging. Despite the existence of these several investigations regarding Western diet-induced cardiac dysfunction in animal models, a direct comparison between different patterns of WD on cardiac structure and function over time has not been adequately evaluated so far. Therefore, this study aimed to assess the effects of two types of the Western diet, one with high fat (50% fat, 35% carbohydrate) and one with high carbohydrate (34% fat, 49% carbohydrate) content, on cardiac remodeling in obese rats with sequential analyses during a long-term follow-up. This proposal may be useful to determine an adequate obesity model with functional impairment of the heart so that pathophysiological mechanisms or preventive and therapeutic strategies can be investigated in future studies.

2. Material and Methods

2.1. Animals

Male *Wistar* rats (60 days old) were obtained from our breeding colony and housed in individual cages under a controlled environment with 12 h light/dark cycle at room temperature (24 °C ± 2 °C) and 55 ± 5% humidity with water and food ad libitum. All animal experiments and procedures were performed according to the Guide for the Care and Use of Laboratory Animals published by U.S. National Institutes of Health [17] and were approved by the Ethics Committee on Animal Experiments of the Botucatu Medical School, São Paulo State University, UNESP (protocol 1119/2015-CEUA).

2.2. Experimental Design

The experimental timeline for this study was conducted as shown in Figure 1. Randomized rats were fed with a control diet (CD), Western diet fat (WDF), or Western diet sugar (WDS) for 41 weeks ($n = 10$ for each group). The echocardiographic analysis was performed 17 weeks after the beginning of the study and repeated every 2 months until completion at 41 weeks.

After 41 weeks of experimental protocol, following the echocardiogram and systolic blood pressure evaluation, the animals were fasted overnight (12 h), anesthetized (50 mg/kg ketamine; 10 mg/kg xylazine; intraperitoneal injection), and sacrificed by decapitation. The heart was rapidly isolated; perfused with phosphate-buffered saline (PBS) to remove blood; and then the left and right ventricles, atria, and papillary muscle were dissected for further analysis. White adipose tissues (WATs) were also isolated, dissected, and weighed for nutritional profile assessment.

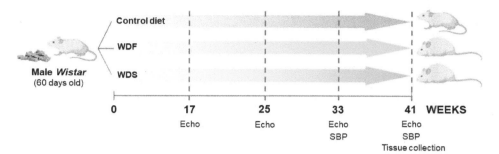

Figure 1. Schematic representation of the experimental design for the study of the effects of dietary interventions using a rat model. WDF and WDS: Western diet fat and sugar, respectively. Echo: echocardiographic analysis. SBP: systolic blood pressure.

2.3. Diet Composition

Diets were developed at the Experimental Research Unit (UNIPEX-UNESP) using the following ingredients: soybean meal, soybean hull, corn bran, dextrin, sucrose, fructose, soybean oil, palm oil, palm kernel oil, lard, salt, and vitamin and mineral premix. The CD was custom-formulated with the same ingredients as the WDF and WDS except for fructose, sucrose, palm oil, and lard added only in the WDF and WDS, and soybean oil added only in the CD to produce three different diets in fat, protein, and carbohydrate contents (Table 1 and Figure 2). The CD and WDF have been used in our previous study [18].

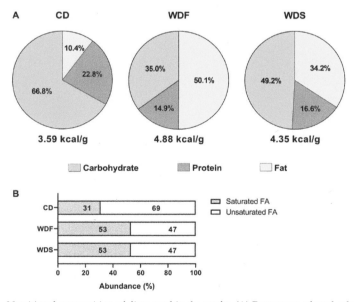

Figure 2. Nutritional composition of diets used in the study. (**A**) Percentage of total calories from carbohydrate (orange), protein (blue), and fat (yellow) in the Control diet (CD), Western diet fat (WDF), and Western diet sugar (WDS). (**B**) Relative abundance of saturated and unsaturated fatty acids (FA) in all diets.

Table 1. Ingredients of Control diet (CD), Western diet fat (WDF), and Western diet sugar (WDS).

Ingredients (g/kg)	CD	WDF	WDS
Soybean bran	335	344	340
Soybean hull	189	117	117
Corn bran	278	80	80
Dextrin	147	20	20
Fructose	–	100	180
Sucrose	–	50	80
Soybean oil	14	–	–
Palm oil	–	40	30
Palm kernel oil	9	80	49
Lard	–	140	75
Salt	4	8	8
Vitamin and mineral premix	25	25	25

2.4. Nutritional Profile of the Animals

The nutritional profile was assessed according to the following parameters: energy intake, feed efficiency, body weight, white adipose tissues (WATs) weight, and adiposity index (AI).

Calorie consumption was determined by multiplying the energy value of each diet by the food intake (g × kcal). The feed efficiency was calculated to analyze the animal's capacity to convert consumed food energy in body weight, dividing the total body weight gain (g) by total energy intake (kcal). The animals were weighed once a week. The WATs were determined by the sum of epididymal, retroperitoneal, and visceral fat pad weights. To calculate the AI, the WATs was divided by the final body weight as follows: (WATs/final body weight) × 100. This index is an easy and consistent method to evaluate the amount of body fat in rodents and several authors have used it [9,19,20].

2.5. Systolic Blood Pressure Evaluation

Systolic blood pressure (SBP) was measured in conscious rats at the 33rd and 41st week using the noninvasive tail-cuff method with an electro-sphygmomanometer, Narco Bio-System (International Biomedical, Austin, TX, USA), as previously described [21]. The rats were warmed in a wooden box between 38 and 40 °C with heat generated by two incandescent lamps for 4 min to cause vasodilation of tail artery. Then, they were transferred to a cylindrical iron support that was specially designed to allow total exposure of the animal's tail. A sensor coupled to the electro-sphygmomanometer was placed in the proximal region of the tail. The arterial pulsations were recorded in a computerized data acquisition system (AcqKnowledge ® MP100, Biopac Systems Inc., Santa Barbara, CA, USA). The average of two readings was recorded for each measurement.

2.6. Echocardiographic Study

The first echocardiographic analysis was performed at the 17th week of dietary treatment and evaluated every 2 months until the 41st week, totaling four moments of study (17, 25, 33, and 41 weeks). The analysis was performed using commercially available echocardiography (General Electric Medical Systems, Vivid S6, Tirat Carmel, Israel) equipped with a 5–11.5 MHz multi-frequency transducer, as previously described [22]. Rats were anesthetized by intraperitoneal injection of a mixture of ketamine (50 mg/kg) and xylazine (1 mg/kg). Two-dimensionally guided M-mode images were obtained from short-axis views of the LV at or just below the tip of the mitral valve leaflets and at the level of the aortic valve and left atrium. Flow evaluation (E and A waves) and tissue Doppler were performed in the apical four-chamber view. The parameters used to calculate the Tei index were obtained in the apical five-chamber view. M-mode images of the LV were printed on a black and white thermal printer (Sony UP-890MD) at a sweep speed of 100 mm/sec. The same observer manually measured all LV structures according to the method of the American Society of Echocardiography [23]. The measurements obtained were the mean of at least five cardiac cycles on the M-mode tracings.

The following LV structural parameters were analyzed: LV diastolic diameter (LVDD), LV diastolic posterior wall thickness (DPWT), LV relative wall thickness (RWT), and diameters of the left atrium (LA) and aorta (AO). LV function was assessed by the following parameters: endocardial fractional shortening (EFS), ejection fraction (EF) calculated by the Cube method, and early and late diastolic mitral inflow velocities (E and A waves) ratio. A combined diastolic and systolic LV function was measured, calculating the myocardial performance index (Tei index). The study was complemented using tissue Doppler imaging (TDI) to evaluate early diastolic (E′) velocity of the mitral annulus (arithmetic average of the lateral and septal walls) and the ratio E/E′.

2.7. Cardiac Morphological Profile

The following parameters determined macroscopic cardiac remodeling: heart, atria, and left and right ventricle weights, as well as their ratio with tibia length. Additionally, frozen LV samples were used for histological analysis, as previously described [22]. LV transverse sections were cut at 5 μm thickness in a cryostat cooled to −20 °C and then stained with hematoxylin and eosin to determine transverse myocyte diameter, which was measured in at least 50–70 myocytes from each LV as the shortest distance between borders drawn across the nucleus. Collagen interstitial fraction was also determined using picrosirius red staining of LV sections and, on average, 20 microscopic fields were used to quantify interstitial collagen fractional area. Perivascular collagen was excluded from this analysis. All measurements were performed using a Leica microscope (magnification 40×) attached to a video camera and connected to a computer equipped with image analysis software (Image-Pro Plus 3.0, Media Cybernetics, Silver Spring, MD, USA).

2.8. Statistical Analysis

All data were tested for normality before statistical analysis using the Shapiro-Wilk test. The results were analyzed using One-way ANOVA followed by Tukey post hoc test (parametric distribution of data) or Kruskal-Wallis test followed by Dunn's (non-parametric distribution). Two-way ANOVA with repeated measures followed by Bonferroni post hoc test was used to determine statistical differences in body weight evolution, SBP, and echocardiogram. Data are expressed as mean ± s.e.m. (standard error of the mean) or median (maximum [Max] and minimum [Min] values). All statistical analyses were performed using SigmaPlot 12.0 (Systat Software, Inc., San Jose, CA, USA), and graphics were generated using GraphPad Prism 8 (GraphPad Software Inc., San Diego, CA, USA). The differences were considered statistically significant when $p < 0.05$.

3. Results

3.1. Nutritional Profile of the Animals

Over the 41 weeks, both WD induced a progressive increase in body weight gain. The rats fed with WDS became heavier than those fed with CD diet from the 12th week of dietary treatment until the end of the study, while rats fed with WDF showed higher body weight than CD rats only after the 15th week (Figure 3).

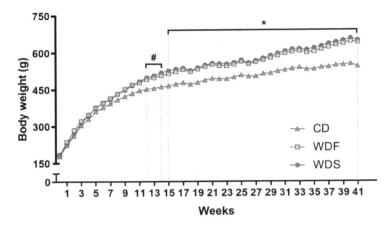

Figure 3. Body weight evolution during dietary intervention with Control diet (CD), Western diet fat (WDF), and Western diet sugar (WDS) for 41 weeks. Data are presented as mean ± s.e.m. Two-way repeated-measures ANOVA and Bonferroni's multiple comparisons test. # $p < 0.05$ Control vs. WDS; * $p < 0.05$ Control vs. WDF and WDS ($n = 10$ rats per group).

As observed in Table 2, the energy intake (kcal per rat) was similar in all groups. After 41 weeks, the rats receiving WDF and WDS showed an average increase of 18% in body weight, 126% in WATs, and 86% in adiposity index, indicating that both diets were equally significant in triggering severe obesity in comparison to CD. Moreover, the feed efficiency was higher in rats fed with WDF and WDS, even though these rats did not consume more calories than rats fed CD, suggesting that weight gain occurred regardless of energy intake.

Table 2. Nutritional profile of the animals.

Variables	CD ($n = 10$)	WDF ($n = 10$)	WDS ($n = 10$)
Energy intake, kcal/day	92.1 ± 2.7	85.2 ± 2.2	86.8 ± 2.6
Feed efficiency, %	1.39 ± 0.03	1.88 ± 0.05 ***	1.85 ± 0.07 ***
Initial body weight, g	179 ± 8	183 ± 7	186 ± 8
Final body weight, g	544 ± 10	643 ± 20 **	649 ± 24 **
Total body weight gain, g	366 ± 6	460 ± 17 **	463 ± 26 **
Epididymal fat, g	11.1 ± 0.9	19.3 ± 1.9 *	21.5 ± 2.8 **
Retroperitoneal fat, g	12.1 (8.8–16.3)	33.2 (18.9–78.9) **	34.7 (6.5–63.1) **
Visceral fat, g	8.5 ± 0.6	17.1 ± 1.8 **	15.0 ± 1.9 *
WATs, g	32.2 ± 2.2	73.6 ± 9.0 **	72.0 ± 9.3 **
Adiposity index, %	5.9 ± 0.4	11.2 ± 1.0 ***	10.8 ± 1.1 **

Data are presented as mean ± s.e.m. (One-way ANOVA with Tukey *post-hoc* test) or median (Min–Max) (Kruskal-Wallis followed by Dunn's *post-hoc* test). * $p < 0.05$, ** $p < 0.01$, and *** $p < 0.001$ vs. Control. Abbreviations: CD: control diet; WDF: Western diet fat; WDS: Western diet sugar; WATs: white adipose tissues.

3.2. Systolic Blood Pressure Evaluation

The SBP was higher in WDF-fed animals than their respective controls at 33 and 41 weeks. In the WDS group, there was a trend toward increased SBP ($p = 0.052$) at 33 weeks and significant elevation of the SBP at 41 weeks compared to the CD. These findings indicate that both WD were able to trigger hypertension in the animals (Figure 4).

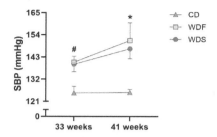

Figure 4. Systolic blood pressure (SBP) at 33rd and 41st week of dietary intervention with Control diet (CD), Western diet fat (WDF), and Western diet sugar (WDS). Data are presented as mean ± s.e.m. Two-way repeated-measures ANOVA and Bonferroni's multiple comparisons test. * $p < 0.05$ Control vs. WDF and WDS; # $p < 0.05$ Control vs. WDF ($n = 7$–10 rats per group).

3.3. Cardiac Structural and Functional Assessment

Illustrative LV M-mode echocardiograms are shown in Figure 5. Structural analysis of the heart performed by echocardiogram revealed no significant changes among the CD, WDF, and WDS groups for all variables (Figure 6). Regarding the evaluated moments, LVDD was increased in the WDF group at the 25th and 33rd weeks when compared to the 17th week (Figure 6A). DPWT was increased at 41 weeks compared to 17 weeks in CD and WDF groups; moreover, this variable increased from the 25th week to 41st week in the WDF and WDS groups (Figure 6B). RWT showed a decrease from week 17 to week 25 and augmented from weeks 25 and 33 to week 41 in the WDF group (Figure 6C). AO enlarged at weeks 25 and 33 compared to week 17 in WDF-fed rats; furthermore, this variable increased from the 17th week to the 41st week in all groups (Figure 6D). LA expanded from week 17 to weeks 33 and 41 only in the WDF group (Figure 5E). No changes were observed over time for all groups when LA was normalized by AO (Figure 6F). Overall, most of the observed changed reflect the growth of animals over time, with no significant effect of obesogenic diets on the cardiac structure.

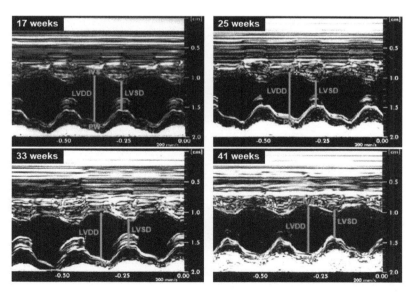

Figure 5. Illustrative left ventricle M-mode echocardiograms from rats at 17th, 25th, 33rd, and 41st week. LVDD and LVSD: left ventricular diastolic and systolic diameters, respectively; PW: left ventricle posterior wall; IVS: interventricular septum.

Regarding cardiac function, no statistical differences were detected among the three groups for the Tei index and E/A and E/E' ratios (Figure 7B,E,F). HR was higher at the 33rd and 41st weeks in the WDS group compared to CD (Figure 7A). EFS was lower at weeks 33 and 41 in the WDF group in comparison to CD and WDS (Figure 7C). EF also decreased at the 33rd week in the WDF group compared to CD and WDS; however, this variable was reduced more at week 41 in the WDF group than in CD, showing a trend toward declined values concerning WDS ($p = 0.059$) (Figure 7D). In the comparisons among the moments, the HR was lower in the 41st week compared to the 17th and 33rd week in the WDF group; this variable decreased over time in the CD group, being different between the weeks 17 and 41 (Figure 7A). The E/A ratio was reduced at weeks 25, 33, and 41 concerning week 17 in the WDF group (Figure 7E). The E/E ratio decreased significantly from the 17th week to 25th in the CD group (Figure 7F). There was no difference among the moments for the Tei index, EFS, and EF in the three groups (Figure 7B–D).

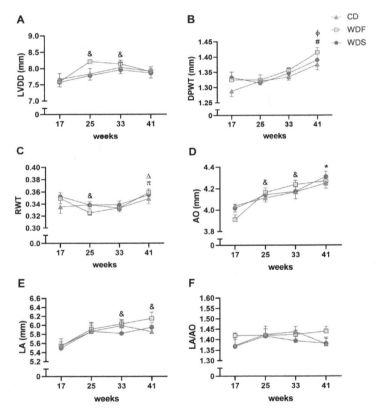

Figure 6. Serial echocardiographic structural assessment. The analysis was performed at the 17th, 25th, 33rd, and 41st week of dietary intervention with Control diet (CD), Western diet fat (WDF), and Western diet sugar (WDS). (**A**) Left ventricle (LV) diastolic diameter (LVDD). (**B**) LV diastolic posterior wall thickness (DPWT). (**C**) Relative wall thickness (RWT). (**D**) Aortic diameter (AO). (**E**) Left atrial diameter (LA). (**F**) LA/AO ratio. Data are presented as mean ± s.e.m. Two-way repeated-measures ANOVA and Bonferroni post hoc test. Symbols indicate differences between the moments fixed the group. & $p < 0.05$ vs. 17 weeks for WDF; Δ vs. 33 weeks for WDF; Φ $p < 0.01$ vs. 25 weeks for WDF and WDS; * vs. 17 weeks for C, WDF, and WDS; # $p < 0.001$ vs. 17 weeks for C and WDF; π vs. 25 weeks for WDF ($n = 10$ per group).

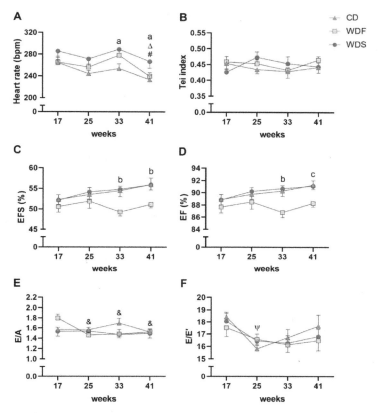

Figure 7. Serial echocardiographic functional assessment. The analysis was performed at 17th, 25th, 33rd, and 41st week of dietary intervention with Control diet (CD), Western diet fat (WDF), and Western diet sugar (WDS). (**A**) Heart rate. (**B**) Tei index. (**C**) Endocardial fractional shortening (EFS). (**D**) Ejection fraction (EF). (**E**) early (E) and late (A) diastolic mitral inflow velocities ratio. (**F**) E and tissue Doppler imaging (TDI) of early mitral annulus diastolic velocity (E') ratio. Data are presented as mean ± s.e.m. Two-way repeated-measures ANOVA and Bonferroni post hoc test. Symbols indicate differences between the moments fixed the group. Letters indicate differences between the groups fixed the moment. [#] $p < 0.001$ vs. 17 weeks for C and WDF; [Δ] $p < 0.05$ vs. 33 weeks for WDF; [&] vs. 17 weeks for WDF; [Ψ] vs. 17 weeks for C; [a] C vs. WDS, [b] C and WDS vs. WDF; and [c] C vs. WDF ($n = 10$ per group).

3.4. Cardiac Morphological Evaluation

Post-mortem cardiac macroscopic structure data for the three groups are presented in Table 3. The WDF group showed increased RVW/T and a trend toward increased HW/T ($p = 0.067$) in relation to the CD.

Table 3. Macroscopic cardiac remodeling.

Variables	CD (*n* = 10)	WDF (*n* = 10)	WDS (*n* = 10)
Tibia, cm	4.49 ± 0.02	4.54 ± 0.04	4.53 ± 0.06
HW/T, mg/cm	263 ± 5	285 ± 8	271 ± 6
ATW/T, mg/cm	24.7 ± 1.1	25.2 ± 1.1	24.0 ± 0.8
LVW/T, mg/cm	193 ± 5	202 ± 5	195 ± 4
RVW/T, mg/cm	48.7 ± 1.1	57.8 ± 3.3 *	52.4 ± 2.0

Data are presented as mean ± s.e.m. (one-way ANOVA with Tukey *post-hoc* test). * $p < 0.05$ vs. CD. Abbreviations: CD: control diet; WDF: Western diet fat; WDS: Western diet sugar; HW, ATW, LVW, and RVW: heart, atria, left, and right ventricles weights, respectively.

Regarding the LV histological analysis (Figure 8), our results showed that the rats receiving WDF and WDS had no change in the transverse myocyte diameter and interstitial collagen fraction. These results indicate that the obese rats did not develop cardiac hypertrophy and interstitial collagen accumulation. Of note, there was a tendency to higher values of interstitial collagen fraction in the WDS group compared to the CD ($p = 0.059$).

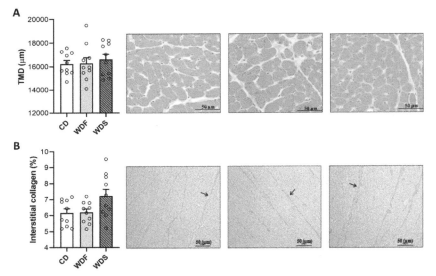

Figure 8. Left ventricle histologic analysis at the 41st week of dietary intervention with Control diet (CD), Western diet fat (WDF), and Western diet sugar (WDS). (**A**) Transverse myocyte diameter (TMD). (**B**) Collagen interstitial fraction (evidenced with arrows). Data are presented as mean ± s.e.m. One-way ANOVA with Tukey post-hoc test (*n* = 10 rats per group).

4. Discussion

Obesity is a metabolic disease associated with several comorbidities, including CVD, and its epidemic has reached alarming levels worldwide. Thus, pre-clinically, experimental models of DIO have been widely studied. One of the most commonly used diets is the WD, which may change in the proportion of fat and sugar, as well as in the time-course of obesity and CVD induction, making it challenging to find the most appropriate model. Therefore, in the present study we have directly assessed the effects of two types of WD, one with a higher quantity of fat (WDF) and another higher in sugar (WDS), on cardiac remodeling in obese rats during a long-term follow-up. The main findings of our study were that although both WD (WDF and WDS) caused pronounced obesity and hypertension, only the WDF was able to induce mild cardiac systolic dysfunction after 33 and 41 weeks of dietary treatment without any sign of cardiac hypertrophy.

As expected, both WD substantially triggered obesity in animals after 41 weeks of the dietary treatment since these animals showed increased body weight and WATs compared to control animals. Although measures related to body fat were only obtained at the end of the study, differences in body weight were early observed from the 12th week for WDS group and from the 15th week for WDF. It has been previously showed that body weight changes reflect body fat in rodents [24]. Despite similar energy intake among the three groups studied, the animals fed with WDS and WDF became obese, suggesting that the nutritional quality of the diet is more related to obesity induction than the calories per se. Similarly, Bortolin et al. [9] showed that WD-fed rats gained more weight and adipose tissue than rats fed a control diet, even though the WD group consumed calories resembling a control group, which proposes that weight gain occurred regardless of calorie consumption. This fact could be explained by the fact that saturated fatty acids are usually less oxidized than unsaturated ones, and the nutrients present different thermogenesis, thus favoring fat deposition [25–27]. Taken together, our findings evidence that both Western diets, i.e., regardless of the proportion of fat and carbohydrate, were effective in promoting excessive adipose tissue accumulation, which characterizes obesity, in consensus with other studies [9,12,16,28].

Excess adipose tissue is a major contributor to hypertension [29]. In agreement, the results showed that our DIO models increased systolic blood pressure regardless of the higher predominance of fat or sugar in the diet. Several mechanisms are involved in the pathogenesis of obesity-induced hypertension, including adipokine release, insulin resistance, and stimulation of sympathetic nervous system and renin-angiotensin system [30,31]. However, the renin-angiotensin system overactivity has been described as a crucial factor since excessive and dysfunctional adipose tissue leads to increased release of angiotensin II in circulation [32].

Our main goal was to evaluate the effects of two types of WD on cardiac function in rats during a follow-up of 41 weeks to establish an appropriate model for future studies. Surprisingly, our data revealed that only the WDF was able to induce a mild systolic cardiac dysfunction at the 33rd and 41st week, presenting lower values of EFS and EF, and without any change in structural parameters or presence of hypertrophy or fibrosis. Our present findings did not support the expectation that WD would result in pronounced impairment of diastolic and systolic functions over the 41-week experimental period. The cardiac performance in vivo, evaluated by echocardiogram, may be influenced by many factors, such as heart rate, contractility, preload, and afterload [33]. Thus, a possible explanation for the decreased systolic function observed in WDF-fed rats could be related to elevated afterload since these rats presented hypertension. However, the WDS-fed animals also showed increased SBP and yet no functional change in the heart was observed. Therefore, we believe that the alterations observed in the WDF group str related to contractile muscle properties due to excessive fatty acid supply in this diet. Indeed, lipid overload in the heart is associated with cardiac dysfunction by several mechanisms due to lipotoxicity, including alterations in energy metabolism, especially fatty acid β-oxidation, de novo ceramide synthesis, oxidative stress, inflammation, endoplasmic reticulum stress, among others [34].

The idea that a WD is harmful to cardiac function is based on a growing body of evidence. However, studies have also presented controversial dysfunction pattern, because of different variables, such as animal models, dietary composition, cardiac function analysis methodology, and experimental duration. These points should be taken into consideration for the divergent findings when comparing them. The majority of studies that used WD with higher fat predominance, regardless of the experiment duration, demonstrated an important functional impairment of the heart, assessed by isolated heart preparation, hemodynamic evaluation, isolated cardiomyocyte measurements, and cardiac magnetic resonance imaging [11,12,16,35,36]. However, there was no functional alteration when the analysis was performed by echocardiogram [37,38]. These findings reveal the importance of choosing the method in the cardiac functional outcome. Among the studies that employed WD with high carbohydrate content, authors did not show cardiac dysfunction by echocardiographic or hemodynamic evaluation, independently of experimental protocol duration [39–41]. Conversely, authors evidenced the presence of relevant systolic and diastolic dysfunction, evaluated by echocardiogram, when the WD high in carbohydrate was associated with 25% fructose or sucrose in drinking water, suggesting a crucial role of sugars [14,42–45]. Indeed, elevated sugar intake has been associated with greater risks of developing cardiovascular disease [46]. However, experimental studies with high sugar added in the diet [38,47,48] or in the drinking water [49–51] have also shown conflicting results regarding the cardiac dysfunction due to the heterogeneity of the experimental protocol. Future investigations should be of reasonable duration, use defined animal models, and improve comparisons concerning results of relevant doses of nutrients on specific outcomes to better understand the effect of sugar consumption in the absence of potential confounding factors. We believe that the synergy between sugar added in drinking water and the Western diet has a more relevant effect on cardiac remodeling in obesity.

Of note, investigations also showed that WD with a balance between fat and carbohydrate and without sugar in drinking water impairs both systolic and diastolic function [13] or causes slight cardiac systolic dysfunction when assessed by echocardiogram. These discrepant outcomes with other authors cited above may be due to protocol duration, animal model or amount and source of fat and sugar.

Regarding the above remarks, it is noteworthy that the lack of cardiac dysfunction at the whole heart level does not necessarily imply a lack of subtle alterations in cardiomyocyte function. Perhaps a functional analysis at the level of isolated heart, myocyte preparations, or papillary muscle could detect cardiac dysfunction that was not observed in our study. The ex vivo functional evaluations could minimize neurohumoral influences that can compensate for changes in heart performance. Dietary modifications, such as introducing sugar into drinking water, could also modify the outcomes found. Therefore, further studies are needed to search for an appropriate DIO model with cardiac dysfunction, widely exploring different techniques of functional analysis of the heart, animal models, diets, and exposure time.

In conclusion, both WD used in the current study (WDF and WDS) were effective in triggering obesity in animals characterized by the high body weight and adiposity; however, only the WDF induced mild cardiac systolic dysfunction after long-term exposure to diet.

Author Contributions: D.F.V., C.L.d.C.M. and A.C.C. designed the study; D.F.V., C.L.d.C.M., G.A.F.M., P.G.S. and K.O. performed the experiments; D.F.V., C.L.d.C.M., S.L.B.d.S. and C.R.P. analyzed the data; D.F.V., C.L.d.C.M. and A.C.C. wrote the manuscript. All authors have read and agreed to the published version of the manuscript.

Funding: This work was supported by the São Paulo Research Foundation-FAPESP (grants: 2014/22152-0, 2015/10782-1, and 2015/16934-8).

Acknowledgments: The authors are grateful to Dijon Henrique Salomé de Campos (São Paulo State University-UNESP) for his support in the systolic blood pressure analysis and the Biotron Zootecnica® company (Rio Claro, SP, Brazil) for kindly supplying some of the ingredients of the diets.

Conflicts of Interest: The authors declare no conflict of interest.

References

1. NCD Risk Factor Collaboration. Trends in adult body-mass index in 200 countries from 1975 to 2014: A pooled analysis of 1698 population-based measurement studies with 19·2 million participants. *Lancet* **2016**, *387*, 1377–1396. [CrossRef]
2. World Health Organization. Fact Sheets: Obesity and Overweight. Available online: http://www.who.int/ news-room/fact-sheets/detail/obesity-and-overweight (accessed on 29 October 2019).
3. Swinburn, B.A.; Sacks, G.; Hall, K.D.; McPherson, K.; Finegood, D.T.; Moodie, M.L.; Gortmaker, S.L. The global obesity pandemic: Shaped by global drivers and local environments. *Lancet* **2011**, *378*, 804–814. [CrossRef]
4. Varlamov, O. Western-style diet, sex steroids and metabolism. *Biochim. Biophys. Acta Mol. Basis Dis.* **2017**, *1863*, 1147–1155. [CrossRef] [PubMed]
5. Upadhyay, J.; Farr, O.; Perakakis, N.; Ghaly, W.; Mantzoros, C. Obesity as a Disease. *Med. Clin. N. Am.* **2018**, *102*, 13–33. [CrossRef] [PubMed]

6.   Alpert, M.A.; Karthikeyan, K.; Abdullah, O.; Ghadban, R. Obesity and Cardiac Remodeling in Adults: Mechanisms and Clinical Implications. *Prog. Cardiovasc. Dis.* **2018**, *61*, 114–123. [CrossRef]

7.   Abel, E.D.; Litwin, S.E.; Sweeney, G. Cardiac remodeling in obesity. *Physiol. Rev.* **2008**, *88*, 389–419. [CrossRef]

8.   Nilsson, C.; Raun, K.; Yan, F.; Larsen, M.O.; Tang-Christensen, M. Laboratory animals as surrogate models of human obesity. *Acta Pharmacol. Sin.* **2012**, *33*, 173–181. [CrossRef]

9.   Bortolin, R.C.; Vargas, A.R.; Gasparotto, J.; Chaves, P.R.; Schnorr, C.E.; Martinello, K.B.; Silveira, A.K.; Rabelo, T.K.; Gelain, D.P.; Moreira, J.C.F. A new animal diet based on human Western diet is a robust diet-induced obesity model: Comparison to high-fat and cafeteria diets in term of metabolic and gut microbiota disruption. *Int. J. Obes.* **2018**, *42*, 525–534. [CrossRef]

10.   Reuter, T.Y. Diet-induced models for obesity and type 2 diabetes. *Drug Discov. Today Dis. Model.* **2007**, *4*, 3–8. [CrossRef]

11.   Gonçalves, N.; Silva, A.F.; Rodrigues, P.G.; Correia, E.; Moura, C.; Eloy, C.; Roncon-Albuquerque, R., Jr.; Falcão-Pires, I.; Leite-Moreira, A.F. Early cardiac changes induced by a hypercaloric Western-type diet in "subclinical" obesity. *Am. J. Physiol. Heart Circ. Physiol.* **2016**, *310*, H655–H666. [CrossRef]

12.   Wilson, C.R.; Tran, M.K.; Salazar, K.L.; Young, M.E.; Taegtmeyer, H. Western diet, but not high fat diet, causes derangements of fatty acid metabolism and contractile dysfunction in the heart of Wistar rats. *Biochem. J.* **2007**, *406*, 457–467. [CrossRef] [PubMed]

13.   Carbone, S.; Mauro, A.G.; Mezzaroma, E.; Kraskauskas, D.; Marchetti, C.; Buzzetti, R.; Van Tassell, B.W.; Abbate, A.; Toldo, S. A high-sugar and high-fat diet impairs cardiac systolic and diastolic function in mice. *Int. J. Cardiol.* **2015**, *198*, 66–69. [CrossRef] [PubMed]

14.   Panchal, S.K.; Poudyal, H.; Waanders, J.; Brown, L. Coffee extract attenuates changes in cardiovascular and hepatic structure and function without decreasing obesity in high-carbohydrate, high-fat diet-fed male rats. *J. Nutr.* **2012**, *142*, 690–697. [CrossRef] [PubMed]

15.   Verboven, M.; Deluyker, D.; Ferferieva, V.; Lambrichts, I.; Hansen, D.; Eijnde, B.O.; Bito, V. Western diet given to healthy rats mimics the human phenotype of diabetic cardiomyopathy. *J. Nutr. Biochem.* **2018**, *61*, 140–146. [CrossRef] [PubMed]

16.   Akki, A.; Seymour, A.-M.L. Western diet impairs metabolic remodelling and contractile efficiency in cardiac hypertrophy. *Cardiovasc. Res.* **2009**, *81*, 610–617. [CrossRef]

17.   National Research Council. *Guide for the Care and Use of Laboratory Animals*, 8th ed.; National Academies Press: Washington, DC, USA, 2011.

18.   Vileigas, D.F.; Harman, V.M.; Freire, P.P.; Marciano, C.L.C.; Sant'Ana, P.G.; de Souza, S.L.B.; Mota, G.A.F.; da Silva, V.L.; Campos, D.H.S.; Padovani, C.R.; et al. Landscape of heart proteome changes in a diet-induced obesity model. *Sci. Rep.* **2019**, *9*, 18050. [CrossRef]

19.   Vileigas, D.F.; de Deus, A.F.; da Silva, D.C.T.; de Tomasi, L.C.; de Campos, D.H.S.; Adorni, C.S.; de Oliveira, S.M.; Sant'Ana, P.G.; Okoshi, K.; Padovani, C.R.; et al. Saturated high-fat diet-induced obesity increases adenylate cyclase of myocardial β-adrenergic system and does not compromise cardiac function. *Physiol. Rep.* **2016**, *4*, e12914. [CrossRef]

20.   Song, J.-X.; Ren, H.; Gao, Y.-F.; Lee, C.-Y.; Li, S.-F.; Zhang, F. Dietary Capsaicin Improves Glucose Homeostasis and Alters the Gut Microbiota in Obese Diabetic ob/ob Mice. *Front. Physiol.* **2017**, *8*, 602. [CrossRef]

21.   Deus, A.F.; Vileigas, D.F.; Silva, D.C.T.; Tomasi, L.C.; Campos, D.H.S.; Okoshi, K.; Padovani, C.R.; Cicogna, A.C. Cardiac function and intracellular Ca^{2+} handling proteins are not impaired by high-saturated-fat diet-induced obesity. *Braz. J. Med. Biol. Res.* **2019**, *52*, e8085. [CrossRef]

22.   Rosa, C.M.; Gimenes, R.; Campos, D.H.S.; Guirado, G.N.; Gimenes, C.; Fernandes, A.A.H. Apocynin influence on oxidative stress and cardiac remodeling of spontaneously hypertensive rats with diabetes mellitus. *Cardiovasc. Diabetol.* **2016**, *15*, 126. [CrossRef]

23.   Lang, R.M.; Bierig, M.; Devereux, R.B.; Flachskampf, F.A.; Foster, E.; Pellikka, P.A.; Picard, M.H.; Roman, M.J.; Seward, J.; Shanewise, J.S.; et al. Recommendations for chamber quantification: A report from the American Society of Echocardiography's Guidelines and Standards Committee and the Chamber Quantification Writing Group, developed in conjunction with the European Association of Echocardiograph. *J. Am. Soc. Echocardiogr.* **2005**, *18*, 1440–1463. [CrossRef] [PubMed]

24.   Rogers, P.; Webb, G.P. Estimation of body fat in normal and obese mice. *Br. J. Nutr.* **1980**, *43*, 83–86. [CrossRef] [PubMed]

25. Casas-Agustench, P.; López-Uriarte, P.; Bulló, M.; Ros, E.; Gómez-Flores, A.; Salas-Salvadó, J. Acute effects of three high-fat meals with different fat saturations on energy expenditure, substrate oxidation and satiety. *Clin. Nutr.* **2009**, *28*, 39–45. [CrossRef] [PubMed]

26. Krishnan, S.; Cooper, J.A. Effect of dietary fatty acid composition on substrate utilization and body weight maintenance in humans. *Eur. J. Nutr.* **2014**, *53*, 691–710. [CrossRef] [PubMed]

27. Jéquier, E. Pathways to obesity. *Int. J. Obes. Relat. Metab. Disord.* **2002**, *26* (Suppl. S2), S12. [CrossRef]

28. Neves, F.A.; Cortez, E.; Bernardo, A.F.; Mattos, A.B.M.; Vieira, A.K.; Malafaia, T.O. Heart energy metabolism impairment in Western-diet induced obese mice. *J. Nutr. Biochem.* **2014**, *25*, 50–57. [CrossRef] [PubMed]

29. Kurukulasuriya, L.R.; Stas, S.; Lastra, G.; Manrique, C.; Sowers, J.R. Hypertension in obesity. *Endocrinol. Metab. Clin. N. Am.* **2008**, *37*, 647–662. [CrossRef]

30. Seravalle, G.; Grassi, G. Obesity and hypertension. *Pharmacol. Res.* **2017**, *122*, 1–7. [CrossRef]

31. Dorresteijn, J.A.N.; Visseren, F.L.J.; Spiering, W. Mechanisms linking obesity to hypertension. *Obes. Rev.* **2012**, *13*, 17–26. [CrossRef]

32. Schütten, M.T.J.; Houben, A.J.H.M.; de Leeuw, P.W.; Stehouwer, C.D.A. The Link between Adipose Tissue Renin-Angiotensin-Aldosterone System Signaling and Obesity-Associated Hypertension. *Physiology* **2017**, *32*, 197–209. [CrossRef]

33. Bers, D.M.; Borlaug, B.A. Mechanisms of Cardiac Contraction and Relaxation. In *Braunwald's Heart Disease: A Textbook of Cardiovascular Medicine*, 11th ed.; Elsevier: Philadelphia, PA, USA, 2019; pp. 418–441.

34. Sletten, A.C.; Peterson, L.R.; Schaffer, J.E. Manifestations and mechanisms of myocardial lipotoxicity in obesity. *J. Intern. Med.* **2018**, *284*, 478–491. [CrossRef] [PubMed]

35. Bostick, B.; Aroor, A.R.; Habibi, J.; Durante, W.; Ma, L.; DeMarco, V.G. Daily exercise prevents diastolic dysfunction and oxidative stress in a female mouse model of western diet induced obesity by maintaining cardiac heme oxygenase-1 levels. *Metabolism* **2017**, *66*, 14–22. [CrossRef] [PubMed]

36. Bostick, B.; Habibi, J.; Ma, L.; Aroor, A.; Rehmer, N.; Hayden, M.R.; Sowers, J.R. Dipeptidyl peptidase inhibition prevents diastolic dysfunction and reduces myocardial fibrosis in a Mouse model of Western diet induced obesity. *Metabolism* **2014**, *63*, 1000–1011. [CrossRef] [PubMed]

37. Jeckel, K.M.; Veeramachaneni, D.N.R.; Chicco, A.J.; Chapman, P.L.; Mulligan, C.M.; Hegarty, J.R. Docosahexaenoic acid supplementation does not improve Western diet-induced cardiomyopathy in rats. *PLoS ONE* **2012**, *7*, e51994. [CrossRef] [PubMed]

38. Hecker, P.A.; Mapanga, R.F.; Kimar, C.P.; Ribeiro, R.F.; Brown, B.H.; O'Connell, K.A.; Cox, J.W.; Shekar, K.C.; Asemu, G.; Essop, M.F.; et al. Effects of glucose-6-phosphate dehydrogenase deficiency on the metabolic and cardiac responses to obesogenic or high-fructose diets. *Am. J. Physiol. Endocrinol. Metab.* **2012**, *303*, E959–E972. [CrossRef]

39. Nguyen, S.; Shao, D.; Tomasi, L.C.; Braun, A.; de Mattos, A.B.M.; Choi, Y.S.; Villet, O.; Roe, N.; Halterman, C.R.; Tian, R.; et al. The effects of fatty acid composition on cardiac hypertrophy and function in mouse models of diet-induced obesity. *J. Nutr. Biochem.* **2017**, *46*, 137–142. [CrossRef]

40. Medford, H.M.; Chatham, J.C.; Marsh, S.A. Chronic ingestion of a Western diet increases O-linked-β-N-acetylglucosamine (O-GlcNAc) protein modification in the rat heart. *Life Sci.* **2012**, *90*, 883–888. [CrossRef]

41. Marsh, S.A.; Dell'Italia, L.J.; Chatham, J.C. Interaction of diet and diabetes on cardiovascular function in rats. *Am. J. Physiol. Circ. Physiol.* **2009**, *296*, H282–H292. [CrossRef]

42. Qin, L.; Zhao, Y.; Zhang, B.; Li, Y. Amentoflavone improves cardiovascular dysfunction and metabolic abnormalities in high fructose and fat diet-fed rats. *Food Funct.* **2018**, *9*, 243–252. [CrossRef]

43. Poudyal, H.; Campbell, F.; Brown, L. Olive leaf extract attenuates cardiac, hepatic, and metabolic changes in high carbohydrate-, high fat-fed rats. *J. Nutr.* **2010**, *140*, 946–953. [CrossRef]

44. Ferron, A.; Francisqueti, F.; Minatel, I.; Silva, C.; Bazan, S.; Kitawara, K.; Garcia, J.L.; Corrêa, C.R.; Moreto, F.; Ferreira, A.L.A.; et al. Association between Cardiac Remodeling and Metabolic Alteration in an Experimental Model of Obesity Induced by Western Diet. *Nutrients* **2018**, *10*, 1675. [CrossRef] [PubMed]

45. Iyer, A.; Brown, L. Fermented wheat germ extract (avemar) in the treatment of cardiac remodeling and metabolic symptoms in rats. *Evid. Based Complement. Alternat. Med.* **2011**, *2011*, 508957. [CrossRef] [PubMed]

46. Mirtschink, P.; Jang, C.; Arany, Z.; Krek, W. Fructose metabolism, cardiometabolic risk, and the epidemic of coronary artery disease. *Eur. Heart J.* **2018**, *39*, 2497–2505. [CrossRef] [PubMed]

Nutrients **2020**, *12*, 68

47. Bouchard-Thomassin, A.-A.; Lachance, D.; Drolet, M.-C.; Couet, J.; Arsenault, M. A high-fructose diet worsens eccentric left ventricular hypertrophy in experimental volume overload. *Am. J. Physiol. Heart Circ. Physiol.* **2011**, *300*, H125–H134. [CrossRef] [PubMed]

48. Liu, L.; Huang, X.; Gao, J.; Guo, Y.; Di, Y.; Sun, S. Improved endogenous epoxyeicosatrienoic acid production mends heart function via increased PGC 1α-mitochondrial functions in metabolic syndrome. *J. Pharmacol. Sci.* **2018**, *138*, 138–145. [CrossRef]

49. Lian, Y.-G.; Zhao, H.-Y.; Wang, S.-J.; Xu, Q.-L.; Xia, X.-J. NLRP4 is an essential negative regulator of fructose-induced cardiac injury in vitro and in vivo. *Biomed. Pharmacother.* **2017**, *91*, 590–601. [CrossRef]

50. Wu, X.; Pan, B.; Wang, Y.; Liu, L.; Huang, X.; Tian, J. The protective role of low-concentration alcohol in high-fructose induced adverse cardiovascular events in mice. *Biochem. Biophys. Res. Commun.* **2018**, *495*, 1403–1410. [CrossRef]

51. Farah, D.; Nunes, J.; Sartori, M.; Dias, D.D.; Sirvente, R.; Silva, M.B.; Fiorino, P.; Morris, M.; Llesuy, S.; Farah, V.; et al. Exercise Training Prevents Cardiovascular Derangements Induced by Fructose Overload in Developing Rats. *PLoS ONE* **2016**, *11*, e0167291. [CrossRef]

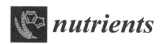

Article

Effects of Whey Protein Supplementation on Aortic Stiffness, Cerebral Blood Flow, and Cognitive Function in Community-Dwelling Older Adults: Findings from the ANCHORS A-WHEY Clinical Trial

Wesley K. Lefferts, Jacqueline A. Augustine, Nicole L. Spartano, William E. Hughes, Matthew C. Babcock, Brigid K. Heenan and Kevin S. Heffernan *

Human Performance Laboratory, Department of Exercise Science, Syracuse University, Syracuse, NY 13244, USA; wleffert@uic.edu (W.K.L.); jacqueline.augustin@cortland.edu (J.A.A.); spartano@bu.edu (N.L.S.); whughes@mcw.edu (W.E.H.); Matthew.Babcock@CUAnschutz.EDU (M.C.B.); brigid.heenan@gmail.com (B.K.H.)
* Correspondence: ksheffer@syr.edu; Tel.: +1-315-443-9801

Received: 20 March 2020; Accepted: 8 April 2020; Published: 10 April 2020

Abstract: ANCHORS A-WHEY was a 12-week randomized controlled trial (RCT) designed to examine the effect of whey protein on large artery stiffness, cerebrovascular responses to cognitive activity and cognitive function in older adults. Methods: 99 older adults (mean ± SD; age 67 ± 6 years, BMI 27.2 ± 4.7kg/m^2, 45% female) were randomly assigned to 50g/daily of whey protein isolate (WPI) or an iso-caloric carbohydrate (CHO) control for 12 weeks (NCT01956994). Aortic stiffness was determined as carotid-femoral pulse wave velocity (cfPWV). Aortic hemodynamic load was assessed as the product of aortic systolic blood pressure and heart rate (Ao SBP × HR). Cerebrovascular response to cognitive activity was assessed as change in middle-cerebral artery (MCA) blood velocity pulsatility index (PI) during a cognitive perturbation (Stroop task). Cognitive function was assessed using a computerized neurocognitive battery. Results: cfPWV increased slightly in CHO and significantly decreased in WPI ($p < 0.05$). Ao SBP × HR was unaltered in CHO but decreased significantly in WPI ($p < 0.05$). Although emotion recognition selectively improved with WPI ($p < 0.05$), WPI had no effect on other domains of cognitive function or MCA PI response to cognitive activity ($p > 0.05$ for all). Conclusions: Compared to CHO, WPI supplementation results in favorable reductions in aortic stiffness and aortic hemodynamic load with limited effects on cognitive function and cerebrovascular function in community-dwelling older adults.

Keywords: vascular stiffness; blood pressure; whey protein isolate; older adults

---

1. Introduction

Vascular dysfunction is a phenotypic expression of human aging that contributes to increases in cardiovascular and cerebrovascular disease prevalence in older adults [1]. With advancing age, central elastic arteries become stiffer, owing to numerous structural and functional aberrations [2]. This stiffening impairs the inherent buffering capacity of the large central arteries and increases blood pressure (BP) and blood flow pulsatility. Arterial stiffness and subsequent increases in central hemodynamic pulsatility are associated with several pathologies of aging including hypertension, left ventricular hypertrophy and heart failure, renal dysfunction, and retinal damage [2]. Moreover, increased arterial stiffness and central hemodynamic pulsatility are independent predictors of cardiovascular and cerebrovascular events and mortality [3,4].

While prolonging life is an important public health goal, preserving the capacity to live and function independently is equally significant [5]. Identifying proven interventions that can prevent disability is a major public health challenge. Cognition is an important contributing factor to overall functional ability and quality of life with advancing age [6,7]. The brain is a high flow target organ that is particularly sensitive to excessive hemodynamic pulsatility, with central hemodynamic pulsatility potentially infiltrating and damaging the delicate cerebral microvasculature. Numerous studies note relationships between central artery stiffness, pulsatile hemodynamics, cerebrovascular pulsatility, and cognitive function [8–10]. Arterial stiffness and cerebral pulsatility also predict cognitive decline with advancing age and incident dementia [11,12]. As such, the American Heart Association and the American Stroke Association acknowledge the importance of arterial stiffness as a significant factor governing cognitive impairment with aging and disease, advocating early intervention to postpone or prevent onset of vascular cognitive impairment [13].

Interventions that improve vascular function may in turn have favorable effects on cognitive function. Combining nutrition with pharmacology has given rise to nutraceuticals: foods and/or dietary supplements with bioactive properties leading to possible physiological and health benefits. Whey protein is one such nutraceutical with the potential to improve both cardiovascular and cognitive health [14,15]. Whey protein comprises approximately 20% of the protein in milk. Milk proteins like whey may be one of the mechanisms partially responsible for associations between higher dairy consumption and reduced risk for incident hypertension [16], reduced arterial stiffness [17] and improved cognitive function [18]. Indeed, whey protein is encrypted with angiotensin converting enzyme (ACE) inhibitory peptides (i.e., lactokinins) [19] and is a notable source of l-arginine, the precursor for nitric oxide. Acute whey protein intake is associated with improved vascular endothelial function [20] and cognitive function [21] while longer term (12 weeks) consumption has been shown to improve endothelial function, lower brachial blood pressure and lower central hemodynamic load (assessed as augmentation index or blood pressure attributable to global wave reflections) [22,23]. Considering arterial stiffness may represent a novel modifiable target for cognitive impairment in older adults, whey protein supplementation could serve as a beneficial nutraceutical strategy to stave both cardiovascular and cognitive decline in older adults.

The Aging, Neurocognitive, and Cardiovascular Health Outcomes Research Study: Add Whey (ANCHORS A-WHEY) was a double-blind, placebo controlled, randomized controlled trial designed to compare the effects of whey protein isolate (WPI) supplementation to a carbohydrate (CHO) control on large artery stiffness (aortic and carotid), central blood pressure pulsatility, cerebrovascular response to cognitive activity, and cognitive function in community-dwelling older adults. We hypothesized that compared to CHO, WPI would: (1) lower large artery stiffness and central blood pressure pulsatility; (2) improve the cerebrovascular response to cognitive activity; (3) improve cognitive function.

2. Methods

This study was approved by the Institutional Review Board of Syracuse University and all participants were required to provide written informed consent prior to study initiation. One-hundred and twenty-two men and women between 60–85 years of age voluntarily participated in this study. Participants were recruited from the community via local newspaper and radio advertisements. Exclusion criteria included self-reported history of stroke, Alzheimer's disease, neurological disease of any kind, smoking, head trauma (i.e., concussion/loss of consciousness within the past 6 months), diabetes mellitus, pulmonary disease, severe arrhythmia, peripheral artery disease, renal disease, habitual consumption of whey protein supplements, and laboratory measured severe obesity (body mass index $\geq$35 kg/m^2), high depressive symptomology (score >18), cognitive impairment (Montreal Cognitive Assessment score <24), and color blindness. This study was registered at ClinicalTrials.gov (NCT01956994).

Participants were randomized to supplement their regular, daily diet with 50 g of WPI (NOW food brands whey protein isolate) or 50 g of carbohydrate (NOW Foods Brand Carbogain, maltodextrin) as an iso-caloric control condition. The randomization scheme was generated by the study coordinator using an online resource (randomization.com). Participants were instructed to consume two servings of 25 g (50 g/day) for 12 weeks. This dosage and study length were chosen based on a previous study noting changes in blood pressure and vascular function with similar dosages and similar length interventions [23]. Both supplements were approximately 100 kcals per serving and had <0.5 g fat per serving. Supplements were distributed in powder form in pre-measured packets. Both supplements were Vanilla flavored and similar in color and composition to ensure both participants and research study personnel were blinded to condition. Participants were instructed to maintain their habitual physical activity and diet during the intervention trial but refrain from consuming additional protein supplements. Supplements were given in 3-week supply. Participants returned to the Human Performance Lab every 3-weeks to receive a new supply, complete a urine test to assess global kidney function (urinary protein, glucose, ketones, leukocytes, nitrite, pH, specific gravity and P:C ratio) and return empty packets as a qualitative assessment of compliance.

2.1. Study Design

At the study onset, participants reported to the Human Performance Laboratory for two separate visits. Each visit occurred first thing in the morning (0600-0900) after an overnight fast. For the consent and initial screening visit, participants completed a health history questionnaire, visual acuity and Ishihara color-blindness tests, basic body anthropometrics (height, weight and waist circumference), and depressive symptomology (Center for Epidemiologic Studies Depression Scale (CES-D)) and global cognitive function assessment (Montreal Cognitive Assessment (MOCA)). Additional assessments included body composition via air displacement plethysmography (BodPod; COSMED, Concord, CA), urinalysis to assess the presence/absence of glucose, protein and ketones, and creatinine levels in the urine (Clinitek Status+ Analyzer, Siemans, IL), and fasting glucose and lipid levels via finger stick (Cholestech LDX). Participants were familiarized with all instrumentation and vascular-hemodynamic measures. Participants also completed a 6m walk test to assess gait speed as a measure of global physical function.

Participants returned to the Human Performance Lab approximately 7 days after the initial screening visit for vascular and hemodynamic data acquisition. Vascular-hemodynamic testing occurred in a quiet, dimly lit, temperature-controlled laboratory during the morning hours following an overnight fast. Participants were instructed to abstain from vigorous exercise and caffeine/alcohol consumption for ≥ 12 h before testing. Participants did not refrain from taking essential medication. Participants were once again familiarized with all instrumentation and vascular-hemodynamic measures. Following familiarization, participants were instrumented and rested in the supine position for 15 min. Participants remained supine for all hemodynamic measures. Baseline measures were then collected for blood pressure (brachial and aortic), blood flow velocity (carotid and cerebral), and large artery stiffness (carotid and aortic). Select hemodynamic measures were then reassessed (in duplicate) during a 4-min cognitive perturbation protocol to assess cerebrovascular responses to cognitive activity (described below). Finally, participants completed a 30-min computerized cognitive testing battery. All aforementioned measures were again completed following the 12-week intervention in a single visit in the morning (within 48 h of consuming the last dose of WPI/CHO).

2.2. Brachial Blood Pressure

Blood pressures were measured using a validated, automated oscillometric cuff (EW3109, Panasonic Electric Works, Secaucus, NJ, USA). Blood pressure readings were taken in duplicate, with additional readings acquired if values differed by >5 mmHg. Mean and pulse pressure were calculated as 1/3 systolic pressure + 2/3 diastolic pressure, and systolic pressure – diastolic pressure, respectively.

2.3. Aortic Stiffness and Blood Pressure

Pressure waveforms from the right carotid and right femoral arteries were acquired via applanation tonometry. Following palpation of the carotid artery pulse and femoral artery pulse, the distance (in mm) between the carotid artery pulse site and suprasternal notch and femoral artery pulse site and suprasternal notch was obtained with a tape measure. Aortic path length (transit distance) was estimated as suprasternal notch-carotid distance subtracted from the suprasternal notch-femoral distance. Carotid-femoral pulse wave velocity (cfPWV) was calculated as the transit distance/transit time. All measures followed current professional consensus recommendations [2].

Applanation tonometry was also used to capture two 10-s epochs of radial artery pressure waveforms (Millar Instruments, Houston, TX, USA). A single composite central aortic pressure waveform was reconstructed from the aforementioned radial artery pressure waveforms using a generalized validated transfer function, (SphygmoCor, AtCor Medical, Sydney, NSW, Australia). The synthesized aortic pressure waveforms were calibrated to brachial mean and diastolic pressure as mean and diastolic pressure are assumed to be somewhat stable throughout the systemic circulation. Augmentation index (AIx) was calculated as the ratio of amplitude of the pressure wave above its systolic shoulder to the total pulse pressure expressed as a percentage $((P_2 - P_1)/PP \times 100)$. AIx was also expressed relative to a standardized heart rate as AIx@75. Aortic rate pressure product was calculated as aortic systolic pressure x heart rate and taken as a measure of central hemodynamic load. Measures were made in duplicate and averaged values used for subsequent analyses. If AIx differed between measures by >5% suggesting a difference in pulse wave contour, a third measure was taken and the average of the 2 closest measures used for analyses.

2.4. Carotid Blood Flow and Stiffness

The left common carotid artery (CCA) was imaged 5–7 cm below the carotid bulb using Doppler ultrasound (ProSound α7, Aloka, Tokyo, Japan) and 7.5–10.0 mHz linear-array probe. The distance between the near wall and far wall lumen-intima interface was continuously traced with eTracking software and used to assess maximum (systolic) and minimum (diastolic) CCA diameters (determined from simultaneous ECG gating from a single lead modified CM5 configuration). Blood velocity waveforms were measured using range gated color Doppler signals averaged along the Doppler beam. Insonation angles were maintained at ≤60° all measures, with sample volume manually adjusted to encompass the entire vessel. CCA pulsatility index (PI) was calculated using semi-automated flow tracing software as $(V_s - V_d)/V_m$, where vs. is the peak systolic velocity, V_d diastolic velocity and V_m the mean velocity.

CCA β-stiffness was determined as $\ln(P_{max}/P_{min})/(D_{max} - D_{min})/D_{min})$, where P and D correspond to carotid pressure and diameter, respectively, and Max and Min refer to the maximum (systolic) and minimum (diastolic) values during the cardiac cycle. Carotid pressure was simultaneously obtained from the right carotid artery via applanation tonometry from a 10 s epoch (SphygmoCor, AtCor Medical, Sydney, NSW, Australia). Carotid pressure waveforms were calibrated in the same manner as the synthesized aortic pressure waveform, described above.

CCA wave intensity was calculated using time derivatives of blood pressure (P) and velocity (U), where wave intensity = (dP/dt × dU/dt); thus the area under the dP/dt × dU/dt curve represents the energy transfer of the wave. According to WIA, W_1 characterizes a forward compression wave generated by left ventricular contraction that accelerates flow and increases pressure; the negative area (NA) occurring after W_1 is a backward travelling compression wave (wave reflection) that decelerates flow but augments pressure. CCA WIA was measured to provide insight into cerebrovascular function as changes in NA in the CCA are thought to be due to wave reflections from cerebral origin [24] and changes in CCA WIA predict cognitive decline in later-life [25].

2.5. Cerebral Blood Flow Velocity

Left middle cerebral artery (MCA) blood velocity was measured using a 2-mHz transcranial Doppler ultrasound probe (DWL Doppler Box-X, Compumedics, Germany) applied to the temporal window. Mean MCA blood velocity and PI were measured at depths of 45–60 mm, as has been commonly reported for MCA measurements. Mean velocity was calculated from the velocity spectrum envelope using a standard algorithm implemented on the instrument with use of a fast Fourier transform. MCA pulsatility index was calculated with automated flow tracing software using the same equation as defined previously for CCA PI.

2.6. Cerebrovascular Response to Cognitive Activity

Participants remained supine while a specialized wall mount suspended a 42-inch flat screen television horizontally over the participant. The television interfaced with a laptop (Dell) and remote response clicker to run a 4-min customized color-word interference Stroop task (E-Prime 2.0, Psychology Software Tools Inc., Sharpsburg, PA, USA). A detailed description of this protocol may be found here [26,27]. This cognitive task has been used previously to assess cardiovascular responses and neural activation to cognitive stimuli during fMRI [28]. Brachial blood pressure, CCA diameter and MCA blood velocity were each measured in duplicate during the Stroop task. We operationally defined cerebrovascular responses to cognitive activity as the change from rest to Stroop for: (1) CCA diameter; (2) MCA mean velocity; (3) and MCA PI. Change in CCA diameter during mental stress has previously been used as a measure of carotid endothelial function [29]. Additionally, change in MCA PI during mental stress has previously been used as a measure of neurovascular coupling and been shown to predict cognitive performance in older adults [30].

2.7. Computerized Cognitive Function Battery

All participants completed a comprehensive computerized neurocognitive battery that interrogated numerous cognitive domains including executive function, attention, information processing, response speed/sensorimotor function, impulsivity, memory, and emotion recognition (social cognition). For a detailed description of the tasks, please see our previous work [31].

2.8. Physical Activity

Physical activity was assessed qualitatively via the short form International Physical Activity Questionnaire (IPAQ), and quantitatively via accelerometry (ActiGraph GT3X+ accelerometer; ActiGraph LLC, Pensacola, FL, USA) in a subset of participants (WPI $n = 34$, CHO $n = 32$). This was done to ensure no seasonal changes in physical activity across the duration of the intervention as a potential confounder of vascular and cognitive function. Accelerometers were worn on the waist (directly below the right mid-axillary line) for 7 consecutive days. Data from the GT3X+ device were downloaded using the low frequency filter from the ActiLife software (version 6.13, ActiGraph LLC, Pensacola, FL, USA). Participants needed to acquire a minimum of 4 days of wear data with at least 10 h of awake wear time per day to be included in data analysis [32]. Raw accelerometer data was converted to counts and summed over a 60 sec epoch for days that accrued at least 10 h of awake wear time. Furthermore, periods of non-wear were defined as consecutive blocks of at least 60 min of 0 activity counts, including up to 2 consecutive minutes of activity counts less than 100, in line with the National Health and Nutrition Examination Survey (NHANES) criteria [32]. A cut point of 2020 activity counts/min was used to determine the amount of time in minutes spent at a physical activity level of moderate-to-vigorous intensity (MVPA) [32].

2.9. Statistical Approach

2.9.1. Sample Size Estimation

Sample size estimates were based on the anticipated differences and standard deviation in large artery stiffness between the WPI and CHO group since we hypothesized that all changes in cerebral and cognitive function would stem from changes in large artery stiffness. Samples sizes were estimated by using R.V. Lenth's Java Applets for Power and Sample Size (retrieved April 9, 2012, from http://www.stat.uiowa.edu/~{}rlenth/Power). Sample sizes were calculated to give 80% power for an α 0.05 level, two-sided test. Studies note an approximate 20%–30% reduction in large artery stiffness (increase in compliance) following various pharmacological, dietary and other lifestyle interventions of similar length [33–37]. This yields an effect size f as ranging from approximately 0.35–0.49. Thus, for a power of 0.8 with an alpha set at 0.05 for a two tailed test, approximately 30–40 participants per group would be needed to detect a similarly-sized main effect in central artery stiffness. Based on the sample size estimates from our primary outcomes, an estimated drop-out rate of ~10%, and poor transcranial Doppler windows in ~10% of older adults precluding measurement of MCA flow velocity, we enrolled 120 participants with the goal of 40 subjects per group completing this RCT to detect significant changes in desired outcomes.

2.9.2. Statistical Analyses

All data are reported as mean ± standard deviation with statistical significance established a priori as $p < 0.05$. Data normality was assessed quantitatively using the Shapiro-Wilk test, with non-normal data logarithmically transformed to meet normality assumptions. Descriptive characteristics between WPI and CHO groups were compared using independent T-tests for continuous variables and χ^2 tests for categorical data.

The effects of 12-week supplementation with WPI compared to CHO on using vascular and secondary outcomes (body weight, lipids, physical activity) were examined using a 2×2 (2 group × 2 time) repeated measures ANOVA. Any significant group by time interactions were further explored using Bonferroni corrected post-hoc tests. Cognitive performance outcomes were non-normally distributed and unable to be successfully transformed to meet normality assumptions. Cognitive function and physical activity (IPAQ, MVPA) metrics were thus analyzed via Mann–Whitney U-tests to test the effect of group (WPI vs. CHO), and group by time interaction (change in cognitive function metric post-pre for WPI vs. CHO), with Wilcoxon signed-rank tests used to test the effect of time (baseline vs. 12 weeks). All significant non-parametric analyses were adjusted for multiple comparisons via Bonferroni correction, since these analyses could not be run simultaneously. Composite Z-scores were computed for each cognitive construct by summing z-scores for each performance metric (e.g., accuracy, reaction time, learning rate, etc.) on a given task. All reaction times and error-based performance metric Z-scores were reverse scored so that positive values indicated better performance. The effects of the intervention on the detailed metrics of cognitive function that were used to compute these composite z-scores are displayed in the Supplemental Results (Tables S1–S3). Effect sizes for our main effects are presented with their corresponding *p*-values and expressed as partial eta squared (η^2) and Z/√n for ANOVA and non-parametric analyses, respectively.

3. Results

Sample characteristics. Of the 122 adults originally recruited, 7 were lost to follow up prior to randomization, 16 dropped out of the trial, and 99 completed the 12-week intervention (Figure 1, $n = 53$ WPI, $n = 46$ CHO). Among the individuals who finished the trial (98% non-Hispanic white), WPI and CHO groups did not have statistically different (1) distribution of males and females, (2) prevalence of hypertension, dyslipidemia, asthma, and family history of CVD, (3) education status, and (4) depression (CES-D) and global cognitive function (MOCA) at baseline (Table 1).

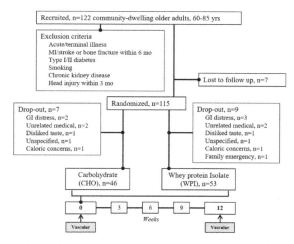

Figure 1. Participant exclusion criteria and recruitment/enrollment flow chart. MI, myocardial infarction; mo, months; yrs, years; GI, gastrointestinal.

Table 1. Descriptive characteristics (*n* (%), unless otherwise noted).

	WPI *n* = 53	CHO *n* = 46	*p* Value	df
Female Sex	26(49.1)	19(41.3)	0.54	98
Asthma	1(1.9)	0(0.0)	1.00	98
Hypertension	23(43.4)	17(37.0)	0.54	98
Dyslipidemia	23(43.4)	28(60.9)	0.11	98
Fam Hx CVD	32(60.4)	28(62.2)	1.00	98
Handedness			0.25	98
Right	42(79.2)	40(87.0)		
Left	9(17.0)	3(6.5)		
Ambidextrous	2(3.8)	3(6.5)		
Education			0.08	98
High School	5(9.4)	1(2.2)		
Some college	8(15.1)	3(6.5)		
2-yr Degree	3(5.7)	1(2.2)		
College	12(22.6)	21(45.7)		
Graduate degree	25(47.2)	20(43.5)		
Age (years) ^	69 ± 7	67 ± 6	0.25	98
Height (m) ^	1.67 ± 0.13	1.68 ± 0.10	0.95	98
CESD Score ^	7 ± 6	7 ± 8	0.89	95
MOCA Score ^	27 ± 2	27 ± 2	0.70	98

^ mean ± SD. WPI, whey protein isolate; CHO, carbohydrate; Fam Hx CVD, Family history of cardiovascular disease; CESD, Center for Epidemiological Studies Depression; MOCA, Montreal Cognitive Assessment; df, degrees of freedom.

3.1. Intervention Effect on Anthropometrics and Secondary Outcomes

A main effect of time was observed for 6m walk, with participants walking slower at 12 weeks compared to baseline (*p* < 0.05; Table 2). A group-by-time interaction revealed BMI significantly increased from baseline to 12 weeks in the CHO group, with no mean changes observed for WPI. This effect was driven by a trend for increased body weight at 12 weeks in the CHO group compared to baseline (interaction effect *p* = 0.051). There were no significant main effects or interactions detected for blood lipids or glucose.

Table 2. Changes in anthropometrics, blood lipids, mobility, and global cognition from baseline to 12 weeks in WPI vs. CHO (mean ± SD).

| | WPI | | CHO | | Effects, p-Value (Partial η²) | | | |
	Baseline	12 weeks	Baseline	12 weeks	Group	Time	Group × Time	df
Weight (kg)	78.2 ± 16.3	78.1 ± 16.3	76.3 ± 14.5	77.3 ± 15.0	0.67(0.00)	0.18(0.02)	0.051(0.04)	98
BMI (kg/m²)	27.9 ± 5.6	27.8 ± 5.6	27.0 ± 3.9	27.4 ± 4.1 *	0.65(0.00)	0.18(0.02)	**0.04(0.04)**	98
Body fat (%)	30.9 ± 12.3	29.8 ± 13.3	29.4 ± 9.9	29.8 ± 10.7	0.76(0.00)	0.51(0.01)	0.14(0.02)	93
Waist Circ (cm)	96.6 ± 13.2	96.1 ± 13.8	95.8 ± 12.0	96.3 ± 12.5	0.91(0.00)	0.97(0.00)	0.32(0.01)	94
Total cholesterol (mg/dL)	189 ± 34	184 ± 36	182 ± 33	183 ± 34	0.51(0.01)	0.41(0.01)	0.20(0.02)	93
HDL (mg/dL)	60 ± 22	58 ± 21	57 ± 19	55 ± 19	0.53(0.00)	0.11(0.03)	0.82(0.00)	92
LDL (mg/dL)	105 ± 30	103 ± 34	98 ± 27	101 ± 26	0.39(0.01)	0.80(0.00)	0.36(0.01)	83
Triglycerides (mg/dL)	112 ± 46	107 ± 48	129 ± 78	133 ± 57	0.08(0.03)	0.70(0.00)	0.11(0.03)	91
Glucose (mg/dL)	94 ± 14	95 ± 15	92 ± 11	94 ± 11	0.43(0.01)	0.09(0.03)	0.53(0.00)	93
6 m Walk (s)	4.72 ± 0.64	4.78 ± 0.72	4.59 ± 0.64	4.86 ± 0.71	0.80(0.00)	**<0.01(0.08)**	0.07(0.04)	88
IPAQ ^	3065 ± 3023	2602 ± 2552	4597 ± 4009	4367 ± 4314	0.15(0.22)	0.32(0.18)	0.99(0.02)	78
MVPA (min/d) ^	23.2 ± 19.3	19.2 ± 15.8	26.0 ± 27.6	30.9 ± 34.0	0.99(0.08)	0.99(0.04)	0.13(0.25)	65

^ Non-parametric analyses with Bonferroni correction, effect sizes calculated as $Z/\sqrt{n}$. WPI, whey protein isolate; CHO, carbohydrate; BMI, body mass index; HDL, high density lipoprotein; LDL, low density lipoprotein; IPAQ, international physical activity questionnaire; MVPA, moderate-to-vigorous physical activity. * $p < 0.05$ vs. Baseline. Bold highlights statistically significant effects.

Table 3. Changes in blood pressure and central hemodynamics from baseline to 12 weeks in WPI vs. CHO (mean ± SD).

| | WPI | | CHO | | Effects, p-Value (Partial η²) | | | |
	Baseline	12 weeks	Baseline	12 weeks	Group	Time	Group × Time	df
Brachial								
Systolic pressure (mmHg)	125 ± 13	123 ± 12	127 ± 11	128 ± 12	0.10(0.03)	0.42(0.01)	0.13(0.02)	96
Diastolic pressure (mmHg)	79 ± 8	76 ± 7	79 ± 5	78 ± 6	0.30(0.01)	**<0.01(0.09)**	0.20(0.02)	96
Pulse pressure (mmHg)	46 ± 9	46 ± 9	48 ± 8	49 ± 9	0.13(0.02)	0.28(0.01)	0.28(0.01)	96
Mean pressure (mmHg)	94 ± 9	92 ± 8	95 ± 7	95 ± 7	0.12(0.03)	**0.03(0.05)**	0.13(0.02)	96
Aorta								
Augmentation index 75	24 ± 10	23 ± 11	25 ± 9	25 ± 8	0.25(0.01)	0.50(0.01)	0.52(0.00)	96
Systolic pressure (mmHg)	115 ± 13	112 ± 12	117 ± 11	119 ± 12	**0.04(0.04)**	0.48(0.00)	0.09(0.03)	97
Pulse pressure (mmHg)	35 ± 10	35 ± 7	37 ± 8	39 ± 10	0.39(0.01)	0.24(0.01)	0.26(0.01)	97
Heart rate (b/min)	60 ± 8	56 ± 8 *	57 ± 9	56 ± 9	0.73(0.00)	**<0.001(0.13)**	**<0.01(0.07)**	96
Cf-PWV/MAP (m/s/mmHg ×10²)	10.7 ± 3.1	10.5 ± 3.0	10.0 ± 2.3	10.6 ± 2.8 *		0.46(0.01)	**0.03(0.05)**	95

WPI, whey protein isolate; CHO, carbohydrate; Cf-PWV/MAP, carotid femoral pulse wave velocity relative to mean arterial pressure; * $p < 0.05$ vs. Baseline. Bold highlights statistically significant effects.

Table 4. Cerebrovascular hemodynamics at rest and in response to cognitive activity (ΔStroop) at baseline and 12 weeks in WPI vs. CHO (mean ± SD).

	WPI		CHO		Effects, *p*-Value (Partial η^2)			
	Baseline	12 weeks	Baseline	12 weeks	Group	Time	Group × Time	df
Common Carotid Artery								
Pulsatility index	1.37 ± 0.24	1.40 ± 0.30	1.40 ± 0.28	1.41 ± 0.29	0.77(0.00)	0.34(0.01)	0.84(0.00)	96
β-stiffness	8.5 ± 4.3	8.5 ± 3.8	8.0 ± 2.5	9.3 ± 5.0	0.39(0.01)	0.45(0.01)	0.16(0.02)	94
W1 (mmHg/m/s³)	7.1 ± 4.7	7.2 ± 4.1	7.2 ± 4.2	7.6 ± 6.6	0.84(0.00)	0.91(0.00)	0.75(0.00)	93
NA (mmHg/m/s²)	22.9 ± 11.6	24.5 ± 14.4	25.2 ± 16.6	26.0 ± 23.8	0.80(0.00)	0.80(0.00)	0.34(0.01)	93
Mean Diameter (mm)	5.92 ± 0.62	5.88 ± 0.63	5.86 ± 0.65	5.86 ± 0.67	0.48(0.01)	0.55(0.00)	0.48(0.01)	96
ΔDiameter (mm)	+0.11 ± 0.15	+0.17 ± 0.15	+0.10 ± 0.20	+0.13 ± 0.13	0.08(0.03)	0.31(0.01)	0.57(0.00)	95
IMT (mm)	0.66 ± 0.10	0.68 ± 0.12	0.67 ± 0.14	0.67 ± 0.14	0.80(0.00)	0.24(0.01)	0.09(0.03)	96
Mean velocity (cm/s)	54 ± 12	52 ± 14	53 ± 15	51 ± 14	0.85(0.00)	**<0.01(0.09)**	0.65(0.00)	92
Middle Cerebral Artery								
Mean velocity (cm/s)	54 ± 12	52 ± 14	53 ± 15	51 ± 14	0.85(0.00)	**<0.01(0.09)**	0.65(0.00)	93
ΔMean velocity (cm/s)	+5 ± 7	+4 ± 5	+5 ± 6	+5 ± 5	0.38(0.01)	0.36(0.01)	0.57(0.00)	92
Pulsatility index	0.86 ± 0.15	0.88 ± 0.18	0.87 ± 0.13	0.88 ± 0.18	0.79(0.00)	0.67(0.00)	0.62(0.00)	93
ΔPulsatility index	+0.00 ± 0.06	-0.02 ± 0.05	-0.00 ± 0.05	-0.01 ± 0.05	0.70(0.00)	**0.02(0.06)**	0.42(0.01)	92
Conductance (cm/s/mmHg ×10²)	58.0 ± 15.2	57.2 ± 17.0	55.6 ± 16.8	54.5 ± 17.1	0.54(0.00)	0.13(0.02)	0.77(0.00)	93
ΔConductance (cm/s/mmHg × 10²)	+0.2 ± 6.0	-0.9 ± 6.6	+0.2 ± 6.5	+0.4 ± 5.6	0.51(0.01)	0.60(0.00)	0.41(0.01)	90

WPI, whey protein isolate; CHO, carbohydrate; IMT, intima media thickness; NA, negative area; Δdenotes change in variable from rest to during cognitive Stroop perturbation. Bold highlights statistically significant effects.

Table 5. Composite Z-scores across cognitive function domains in WPI vs. CHO at baseline and 12 weeks (mean ± SD).

		WPI		CHO		Effects, *p*-Value (z/sqrt(*n*))			
Domain/Construct	Task	Baseline	12 weeks	Baseline	12 weeks	Group	Time	Group × Time	df
Executive function	Maze	-0.34 ± 2.80	0.34 ± 2.14	-0.29 ± 2.08	0.74 ± 2.62	0.99(0.07)	**<0.01(0.33)**	0.99(0.08)	93
Impulsivity	Go-no-go	-0.23 ± 1.65	0.28 ± 1.16	-0.12 ± 1.54	0.18 ± 1.12	0.99(0.04)	0.05(0.25)	0.77(0.12)	92
Emotion Identification	Recognition	-0.14 ± 1.15	0.43 ± 1.37*	-0.15 ± 1.98	-0.11 ± 2.06	0.87(0.11)	**<0.01(0.31)**	**0.04(0.25)**	96
Memory	Recall	0.30 ± 5.76	0.66 ± 5.25	-0.21 ± 5.29	-0.43 ± 6.40	0.53(0.14)	0.99(0.05)	0.36(0.16)	94
Information Processing	Interference	0.85 ± 4.73	2.30 ± 3.62	-0.06 ± 5.75	0.62 ± 5.19	0.98(0.46)	**0.04(0.27)**	0.92(0.11)	81
Attention	CPT	0.02 ± 2.05	0.03 ± 1.82	-0.10 ± 2.34	0.28 ± 1.56	0.99(0.04)	0.79(0.11)	0.77(0.12)	95
Working memory	Digit span	0.23 ± 1.65	0.27 ± 1.93	-0.38 ± 2.23	0.00 ± 1.71	0.52(0.09)	0.99(0.09)	0.99(0.05)	87

WPI, whey protein isolate; CHO, carbohydrate; CPT, continuous performance test; * *p* < 0.05 vs. Baseline. Bold highlights statistically significant effects.

3.2. Intervention Effect on Blood Pressure and Central Hemodynamics

The main effects of time were detected for brachial diastolic and mean pressure, with reductions at 12 weeks compared to baseline in both WPI and CHO ($p < 0.05$; Table 3). Significant group-by-time interactions were found for heart rate, aortic RPP, aortic stiffness (cfPWV), and aortic stiffness corrected for mean pressure ($p < 0.05$). Heart rate, aortic RPP (Figure 2B, Baseline: WPI 6965 ± 1088, CHO 6805 ± 1212; 12-week: WPI 6610 ± 1081, CHO 6794 ± 1191 mmHg/min), and aortic stiffness (Figure 2A, Baseline: WPI 10.1 ± 2.9, CHO 9.6 ± 2.5; 12-week: WPI 9.6 ± 2.7, CHO 10.1 ± 2.9 m/s) significantly decreased from baseline to 12 weeks in WPI, but not in CHO ($p < 0.05$). When expressed relative to mean pressure, aortic stiffness was unaltered in WPI but increased from baseline to 12 weeks in CHO ($p < 0.05$). No significant main effects or interactions were detected for pulse pressure, augmentation index, or aortic systolic pressure.

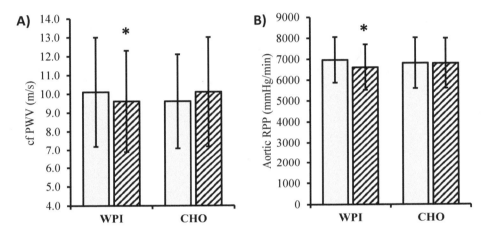

Figure 2. Changes in (**A**) aortic stiffness (cf PWV) and (**B**) aortic rate pressure product (RPP) from baseline to 12 weeks in WPI (whey protein isolate) vs. CHO (carbohydrate) (mean ± SD). Effects, *p*-value (partial η^2). * $p < 0.05$ vs. baseline. (A) Group 0.88(0.00); time 0.88(0.00); G × T **0.01(0.00)**; df 96. (B) Group 0.96(0.00); time **0.03(0.05)**; G × T **0.04(0.04)**; df 94. Bold highlights statistically significant effects.

3.3. Intervention Effect on Cerebrovascular Hemodynamics

The main effects of time were detected for CCA and MCA mean blood velocity which decreased from baseline to 12 weeks in both WPI and CHO groups ($p < 0.05$; Table 4). No main effects were detected; however, for changes in MCA mean velocity relative to mean arterial pressure (i.e., MCA conductance). No significant main effects or interactions were detected for CCA and MCA pulsatility index, CCA forward or reflected wave intensity, and CCA diameter during the intervention.

3.4. Intervention Effect on Cerebrovascular Response to Cognitive Activity

A main effect of time was detected for changes in MCA pulsatility during the Stroop task, which decreased more at 12 weeks compared to baseline in WPI and CHO ($p < 0.05$; Table 4). No main effects or interactions were observed for changes in CCA diameter, MCA mean velocity, or MCA conductance.

3.5. Intervention Effect on Cognitive Function

The main effects of time were observed for executive function and information processing composite scores, both of which increased (improved) from baseline to 12 weeks ($p < 0.05$; Table 5). A significant group-by-time interaction was detected for the emotion identification composite score which improved from baseline to 12 weeks in WPI but not CHO ($p < 0.05$). No significant main effects or interactions were detected for working memory, attention, memory, or impulsivity composite scores.

4. Discussion

This study used a double-blind, randomized controlled trial to compare the effects of WPI versus CHO (control) on large artery stiffness, central blood pressure, cerebral responses to cognitive activity, and cognitive function in community dwelling older adults. Our results indicate that compared to 12 weeks of CHO supplementation, WPI supplementation resulted in modest reductions in aortic stiffness and central hemodynamic load (assessed as the product of aortic systolic pressure and heart rate). WPI had no effect on carotid vascular properties, cerebrovascular response to cognitive activity, and limited effects on cognitive function. Taken together, these data suggest that compared to CHO supplementation, WPI may favorably alter cardiovascular function in older adults but does not have a substantial impact on cerebrovascular or neurocognitive function.

We noted reductions in aortic stiffness, assessed via gold-standard cfPWV, following 12 weeks of WPI compared to CHO. Our study adds to a growing literature noting favorable vascular effects of whey protein [23] with two RCTs discovering improved endothelial function with WPI in prehypertensive adults [22,38]. Aortic stiffness has been identified as a therapeutic target [13] owing to its ability to predict cardiovascular (CV) events and mortality [3,4], and offer insight into residual CVD risk [39]. The reduction in aortic stiffness with WPI may be partially driven by reductions in mean pressure. When expressed relative to blood pressure (cf PWV/MAP), we noted a slight increase in cfPWV in the CHO condition. This increase in arterial stiffness may be due to the effects of aging over the 12-week period, detrimental vascular effects of CHO, or both (i.e., CHO augmented age-associated increases in cfPWV and hastened vascular aging). WPI prevented increases in cfPWV/MAP seen with CHO. Even modest reductions in aortic stiffness are of physiological interest and clinically relevant. The effect of WPI on reducing aortic stiffness observed herein (~ −0.5 m/s) may help reduce CVD risk, particularly when compared with CHO (~ +0.5 m/s). A difference in aortic stiffness of 1.0 m/s is associated with a 15% reduction in CVD risk [3].

We observed significant reductions in aortic rate pressure product, a measure of central hemodynamic load with WPI compared to CHO. Rate pressure product is a mechanical hemodynamic parameter often used as proxy of cardiac oxygen consumption [40]. Aortic rate pressure product also quantifies the mechanical load experienced by the aorta (i.e., cycles of stretch) that contributes to aortic stiffening over time. Reductions in aortic rate pressure product herein appear driven by significant reductions in heart rate and modest reductions in aortic systolic pressure in the WPI versus CHO group. The unrelenting cyclic stress exerted by each cardiac contraction against the aortic walls amplifies oxidative stress and contributes to the fatigue and fracture of elastin [41], resulting in greater reliance on stiffer collagen fibers for wall load bearing. Indeed, a higher heart rate is associated with increased large artery stiffness [42]. Moreover, a higher resting heart rate is associated with accelerated progression of aortic stiffness over time [43]. Heart rate itself has been identified as an indicator and underappreciated risk factor for cardiovascular disease risk [44,45]. In addition to aforementioned links to large artery stiffening, elevated heart rate has been linked to inflammation, microalbuminuria, endothelial dysfunction, detrimental vascular remodeling and atherosclerosis [42]. Heart rate reduction has been shown in experimental (animal) studies to lower oxidative stress, restore endothelial function, and inhibit atherogenesis [42]. Reducing aortic rate pressure product via reductions in heart rate may thus help slow the progression of aortic stiffening over time by reducing cycles of stretch. Lower heart rate may also impact aortic stiffness via effects on mean (distension) pressure as a longer cardiac cycle with lower heart rate equates to more time spent in diastole. Overall, our findings suggest that compared to CHO, the heart rate-lowering effect of WPI in older adults may have a favorable effect on aortic stiffness and in turn CVD risk.

Given the significant association between increased heart rate and cardiovascular mortality, heart rate has been considered a potential therapeutic target [46]. Pharmacological means of lowering heart rate has been shown to reduce mortality in clinical populations [47] although this is not a universal finding across pharmacological agents. A meta-analysis of >68,000 patients suggests that lowering heart rate with Beta-blockers is associated with increased mortality risk in hypertensives [48]. This may be because the lowering heart rate with Beta-blockers is associated with increased pressure from wave reflections [49,50]. Heart rate is inversely related to pressure from wave reflections, such that lower heart rates are associated with increased pressure from wave reflections [51]. This inverse association may be stronger in older adults with higher aortic stiffness, such that a smaller decrease in heart rate may induce a larger increase in pressure from wave reflections [52]. Separate from cardiovascular effects of aortic stiffness, increased pressure from wave reflections increases cardiac afterload and is associated with numerous morbidities and mortality [3]. It is important to underscore that reductions in heart rate within the WPI group occurred without concomitant changes in global wave reflections, as augmentation index was unaltered. Reductions in HR with WPI may be related to ACE-inhibitory properties [53] but more research will be needed to further explore the potential mechanism. Thus, unlike what may be seen with select medications [54], WPI may be able to lower heart rate in older adults without having a detrimental impact on central hemodynamic load.

We noted no effects of WPI compared to CHO on carotid artery stiffness and subsequent cerebrovascular hemodynamics. Although the carotid artery and aorta are both considered central elastic arteries, they "age" at slightly different rates, are influenced differently by traditional CVD risk factors, and are differentially associated with target organ damage and cerebrovascular risk [55–57]. In the context of higher blood pressure, the aorta may stiffen more than the carotid artery, suggesting the higher sensitivity of the aorta to the effects of aging [57]. It is possible that each artery may respond differently to dietary manipulation and that the aorta may be more sensitive to supplementation with WPI compared to the carotid artery. When performing secondary exploratory analyses, central hemodynamic load (RPP) was associated with cfPWV at baseline ($r = 0.38$, $p = 0.001$) and 12 weeks ($r = 0.25$, $p = 0.015$) and change in RPP across the intervention was associated with change in cfPWV ($r = 0.38$, $p = 0.007$). Conversely, central hemodynamic load (RPP) was not associated with carotid stiffness at baseline ($r = 0.09$, $p = 0.39$) and 12 weeks ($r = -0.04$, $p = 0.71$), and change in RPP across the intervention was not associated with change in carotid stiffness ($r = 0.09$, $p = 0.40$). The carotid artery may be more resilient to the effects of hemodynamic load. Overall, our findings suggest that although lowering central hemodynamic load with WPI may have a favorable effect on aortic stiffness compared to CHO, this does not translate to a similar favorable effect on carotid artery stiffness.

Cerebrovascular and cognitive function was generally unaltered with WPI compared to CHO. We did observe a select improvement in emotion identification among the WPI group compared to CHO, which is linked to general cognition and may play an integral role in the organization of information processing [58]. Despite this modest effect, we noted no further significant group differences in executive function, memory/working memory, attention, impulsivity, or information processing. The latter findings are consistent with a recent meta-analysis suggesting that milk and dairy intake may not improve cognitive function in older adults [59], and an RCT noting that WPI specifically may not impact cognitive function [60]. Overall, it is possible that the common carotid artery serves as an extra-cranial "gatekeeper", either buffering entry of hemodynamic pulsatility to the brain or facilitating transmission of excess pulsatile energy [61]. Thus, by not affecting carotid artery stiffness, WPI may have been ineffective in further impacting cerebrovascular response to cognitive activity and cognitive function itself.

We chose maltodextrin as our control, given its similar appearance and energy yield to WPI and we view this as a delimitation. Maltodextrin is the most commonly used control reported in this area of scholarship. Maltodextrin may not be an inert placebo and could have influenced some outcome measures. Although maltodextrin is a polysaccharide and complex CHO, when compared to WPI, maltodextrin has a higher glycemic index [62] which in theory could have a detrimental effect on glycemic control and thus vascular function. As mentioned previously, our findings should be interpreted in the context that noted interactions (cfPWV) could have been driven partially by a) direct detrimental effects of CHO on vascular function and thus aortic stiffness, and/or b) CHO amplifying vascular aging. We believe this unlikely as a recent ancillary study from the large multicenter Protein Supplementation Trial noted specifically that although maltodextrin supplementation (45 g/daily for 18 months) increases glycemic load, it does not have a detrimental effect on systemic inflammation or insulin resistance [63]. Moreover, maltodextrin does not have detrimental effects on vascular endothelial function measured as brachial flow-mediated dilation or circulating biomarkers of vascular endothelial inflammation [22,38]. Our study noted no detrimental effects of maltodextrin on blood pressure, heart rate or other cardiometabolic parameters (e.g., fasting glucose and triglycerides), all notable determinants of change in PWV over time [64–66]. Thus while maltodextrin is not a completely "inert placebo", it does not appear to have effects on many of the more prominent determinants of vascular stiffness (i.e., systemic inflammation, vascular inflammation, vascular endothelial function, blood pressure, heart rate, insulin resistance).

We did not control participants' dietary intake, and this may be viewed as a study limitation. The majority of previous studies comparing WPI to CHO have found expected changes in macronutrient composition when comparing supplement groups (i.e., higher dietary protein composition and lower CHO in the WPI group and higher dietary CHO composition with lower protein in the CHO group) [22,38,67–69]. Interestingly, although changes in macronutrients occur as expected, older adults may decrease ad libitum caloric intake resulting in an iso-caloric total energy state across the intervention period [70]. Increased intake of one macronutrient results in a decreased intake of at least one of the other macronutrients under isocaloric conditions [71]. Thus, we cannot distinguish the effects of increased protein consumption from the effects of possible decreased carbohydrate consumption in the WPI group. WPI may have a slightly greater effect on satiety resulting in an anorexigenic response compared to maltodextrin [62], and a slightly greater reduction in total caloric intake across the intervention compared to CHO [72]. Our results would support these observations as there was no significant change in body mass in the WPI group but a small nonsignificant increase (~1 kg) in the CHO group. Of overall importance for the interpretation of our findings, statistically adjusting for change in BMI did not have an effect on group differences in cfPWV thus it is unlikely that the ~1kg increase in body mass in the CHO group was responsible for noted group differences in aortic stiffness.

Additional limitations should be noted. Our participants were well-educated with ~75% completing college and an additional ~40% completing a graduate degree. Education may increase cognitive reserve and be related to a more enriched environment later in life, preserving cognitive flexibility [73]. As such, our participants were a higher functioning group with less room for cognitive improvement. Our study population comprised 98% non-Hispanic white adults. There are known racial differences in large artery stiffness [74] and the blood pressure response to ACE-inhibitors [75]. Additional research exploring the impact of WPI on cardiovascular health in non-Hispanic black/African American adults and Hispanic adults is warranted. Finally, our strict exclusion criteria may limit the generalizability of our findings to other populations of older adults (e.g., diabetics).

5. Conclusions

In conclusion, WPI has a modest but favorable effect on aortic stiffness and central hemodynamic load (appraised as the product of heart rate and central systolic blood pressure) in community-dwelling older adults when compared to a CHO control. WPI may not affect carotid artery stiffness or cerebrovascular response to cognitive activity, and appears to have limited effects on cognitive function among older adults. Although a logical extension of our findings would suggest WPI has potential as a nutritional strategy to help manage age-associated increases in aortic stiffness, further studies utilizing longer intervention periods and alternative control conditions will be needed to corroborate our findings.

Supplementary Materials: The following are available online at http://www.mdpi.com/2072-6643/12/4/1054/s1, Table S1: Memory, impulsivity, emotion identification, and response speed at baseline and 12 weeks in WPI and CHO groups (mean ± SD), Table S2: Working memory, and attention and concentration at baseline and 12 weeks in

Whey and Carbohydrate groups (mean ± SD), Table S3: Information processing efficiency and executive function at baseline and 12 weeks in Whey and Carbohydrate groups (mean ± SD).

Author Contributions: Conceptualization, K.S.H.; Data curation, W.K.L., J.A.A., N.L.S., W.E.H., M.C.B., B.K.H. and K.S.H.; Formal analysis, W.K.L. and K.S.H.; Funding acquisition, K.S.H.; Investigation, W.K.L., J.A.A., W.E.H., M.C.B., B.K.H. and K.S.H.; Methodology, N.L.S. and K.S.H.; Project administration, J.A.A., N.L.S., B.K.H. and K.S.H.; Resources, B.K.H. and K.S.H.; Supervision, K.S.H.; Writing—original draft, W.K.L., J.A.A., N.L.S., W.E.H., M.C.B., B.K.H. and K.S.H.; Writing—review and editing, W.K.L., J.A.A., N.L.S., W.E.H., M.C.B., B.K.H. and K.S.H. All authors have read and agreed to the published version of the manuscript.

Funding: Findings from the ANCHORS A-WHEY Clinical Trial. Funding for this study provided by: The Dairy Management Inc, (Dairy Research Institute) Grant1154 (Principle Investigator Heffernan) and NIH NIA P30 AG0344645 05 (Project Director Heffernan). Whey protein isolate and carbohydrate (Carbogain) were donated by NOW supplements (Bloomingdale IL).

Acknowledgments: We thank all participants for graciously giving their time. We thank Tiago Barreira for assistance processing accelerometer data.

Conflicts of Interest: This study was funded by The Dairy Management Inc, (Dairy Research Institute) Grant1154 (Principle Investigator Heffernan) and NIH NIA P30 AG0344645 05 (Project Director Heffernan). Whey protein isolate and carbohydrate (Carbogain) were donated by NOW supplements (Bloomingdale IL).

References

1. Najjar, S.S.; Scuteri, A.; Lakatta, E.G. Arterial aging: Is it an immutable cardiovascular risk factor? *Hypertension* **2005**, *46*, 454–462. [CrossRef] [PubMed]
2. Townsend, R.R.; Wilkinson, I.B.; Schiffrin, E.L.; Avolio, A.P.; Chirinos, J.A.; Cockcroft, J.R.; Heffernan, K.S.; Lakatta, E.G.; McEniery, C.M.; Mitchell, G.F.; et al. Recommendations for Improving and Standardizing Vascular Research on Arterial Stiffness: A Scientific Statement from the American Heart Association. *Hypertension* **2015**, *66*, 698–722. [CrossRef] [PubMed]
3. Vlachopoulos, C.; Aznaouridis, K.; Stefanadis, C. Prediction of cardiovascular events and all-cause mortality with arterial stiffness: A systematic review and meta-analysis. *J. Am. Coll. Cardiol.* **2010**, *55*, 1318–1327. [CrossRef] [PubMed]
4. Vlachopoulos, C.; Aznaouridis, K.; O'Rourke, M.F.; Safar, M.E.; Baou, K.; Stefanadis, C. Prediction of cardiovascular events and all-cause mortality with central haemodynamics: A systematic review and meta-analysis. *Eur. Heart J.* **2010**, *31*, 1865–1871. [CrossRef]
5. Katz, S.; Branch, L.G.; Branson, M.H.; Papsidero, J.A.; Beck, J.C.; Greer, D.S. Active life expectancy. *N. Engl. J. Med.* **1983**, *309*, 1218–1224. [CrossRef]
6. Castro-Lionard, K.; Thomas-Anterion, C.; Crawford-Achour, E.; Rouch, I.; Trombert-Paviot, B.; Barthelemy, J.C.; Laurent, B.; Roche, F.; Gonthier, R. Can maintaining cognitive function at 65 years old predict successful ageing 6 years later? The PROOF study. *Age Ageing* **2011**, *40*, 259–265. [CrossRef]
7. Gaugler, J.E.; Yu, F.; Krichbaum, K.; Wyman, J.F. Predictors of nursing home admission for persons with dementia. *Med. Care* **2009**, *47*, 191–198. [CrossRef]
8. Pase, M.P.; Herbert, A.; Grima, N.A.; Pipingas, A.; O'Rourke, M.F. Arterial stiffness as a cause of cognitive decline and dementia: A systematic review and meta-analysis. *Intern. Med. J.* **2011**. [CrossRef]
9. Van Sloten, T.T.; Protogerou, A.D.; Henry, R.M.; Schram, M.T.; Launer, L.J.; Stehouwer, C.D. Association between arterial stiffness, cerebral small vessel disease and cognitive impairment: A systematic review and meta-analysis. *Neurosci. Biobehav. Rev.* **2015**, *53*, 121–130. [CrossRef]
10. Alvarez-Bueno, C.; Cunha, P.G.; Martinez-Vizcaino, V.; Pozuelo-Carrascosa, D.P.; Visier-Alfonso, M.E.; Jimenez-Lopez, E.; Cavero-Redondo, I. Arterial Stiffness and Cognition Among Adults: A Systematic Review and Meta-Analysis of Observational and Longitudinal Studies. *J. Am. Heart Assoc.* **2020**, *9*, e014621. [CrossRef]
11. Scuteri, A.; Tesauro, M.; Appolloni, S.; Preziosi, F.; Brancati, A.M.; Volpe, M. Arterial stiffness as an independent predictor of longitudinal changes in cognitive function in the older individual. *J. Hypertens* **2007**, *25*, 1035–1040. [CrossRef]
12. Chung, C.P.; Lee, H.Y.; Lin, P.C.; Wang, P.N. Cerebral Artery Pulsatility is Associated with Cognitive Impairment and Predicts Dementia in Individuals with Subjective Memory Decline or Mild Cognitive Impairment. *J. Alzheimer's Dis. JAD* **2017**, *60*, 625–632. [CrossRef] [PubMed]

13. Gorelick, P.B.; Scuteri, A.; Black, S.E.; Decarli, C.; Greenberg, S.M.; Iadecola, C.; Launer, L.J.; Laurent, S.; Lopez, O.L.; Nyenhuis, D.; et al. Vascular contributions to cognitive impairment and dementia: A statement for healthcare professionals from the american heart association/american stroke association. *Stroke* **2011**, *42*, 2672–2713. [CrossRef] [PubMed]

14. Camfield, D.A.; Owen, L.; Scholey, A.B.; Pipingas, A.; Stough, C. Dairy constituents and neurocognitive health in ageing. *Br. J. Nutr.* **2011**, *106*, 159–174. [CrossRef] [PubMed]

15. Patel, S. Emerging trends in nutraceutical applications of whey protein and its derivatives. *J. Food Sci. Technol.* **2015**, *52*, 6847–6858. [CrossRef] [PubMed]

16. Soedamah-Muthu, S.S.; Verberne, L.D.; Ding, E.L.; Engberink, M.F.; Geleijnse, J.M. Dairy consumption and incidence of hypertension: A dose-response meta-analysis of prospective cohort studies. *Hypertension* **2012**, *60*, 1131–1137. [CrossRef] [PubMed]

17. Crichton, G.E.; Elias, M.F.; Dore, G.A.; Abhayaratna, W.P.; Robbins, M.A. Relations between dairy food intake and arterial stiffness: Pulse wave velocity and pulse pressure. *Hypertension* **2012**, *59*, 1044–1051. [CrossRef]

18. Crichton, G.E.; Elias, M.F.; Dore, G.A.; Robbins, M.A. Relation between dairy food intake and cognitive function: The Maine-Syracuse Longitudinal Study. *Int. Dairy J.* **2012**, *22*, 15–23. [CrossRef]

19. FitzGerald, R.J.; Murray, B.A.; Walsh, D.J. Hypotensive peptides from milk proteins. *J. Nutr.* **2004**, *134*, 980S–988S. [CrossRef]

20. Ballard, K.D.; Kupchak, B.R.; Volk, B.M.; Mah, E.; Shkreta, A.; Liptak, C.; Ptolemy, A.S.; Kellogg, M.S.; Bruno, R.S.; Seip, R.L.; et al. Acute effects of ingestion of a novel whey-derived extract on vascular endothelial function in overweight, middle-aged men and women. *Br. J. Nutr.* **2012**, 1–12. [CrossRef]

21. Markus, C.R.; Olivier, B.; de Haan, E.H. Whey protein rich in alpha-lactalbumin increases the ratio of plasma tryptophan to the sum of the other large neutral amino acids and improves cognitive performance in stress-vulnerable subjects. *Am. J. Clin. Nutr.* **2002**, *75*, 1051–1056. [CrossRef] [PubMed]

22. Fekete, A.A.; Giromini, C.; Chatzidiakou, Y.; Givens, D.I.; Lovegrove, J.A. Whey protein lowers blood pressure and improves endothelial function and lipid biomarkers in adults with prehypertension and mild hypertension: Results from the chronic Whey2Go randomized controlled trial. *Am. J. Clin. Nutr.* **2016**, *104*, 1534–1544. [CrossRef] [PubMed]

23. Pal, S.; Ellis, V. The chronic effects of whey proteins on blood pressure, vascular function, and inflammatory markers in overweight individuals. *Obesity* **2010**, *18*, 1354–1359. [CrossRef] [PubMed]

24. Bleasdale, R.A.; Mumford, C.E.; Campbell, R.I.; Fraser, A.G.; Jones, C.J.; Frenneaux, M.P. Wave intensity analysis from the common carotid artery: A new noninvasive index of cerebral vasomotor tone. *Heart Vessel.* **2003**, *18*, 202–206. [CrossRef]

25. Chiesa, S.T.; Masi, S.; Shipley, M.J.; Ellins, E.A.; Fraser, A.G.; Hughes, A.D.; Patel, R.S.; Khir, A.W.; Halcox, J.P.; Singh-Manoux, A.; et al. Carotid artery wave intensity in mid- to late-life predicts cognitive decline: The Whitehall II study. *Eur. Heart J.* **2019**, *40*, 2300–2309. [CrossRef]

26. Heffernan, K.S.; Spartano, N.L.; Augustine, J.A.; Lefferts, W.K.; Hughes, W.E.; Mitchell, G.F.; Jorgensen, R.S.; Gump, B.B. Carotid artery stiffness and hemodynamic pulsatility during cognitive engagement in healthy adults: A pilot investigation. *Am. J. Hypertens.* **2015**, *28*, 615–622. [CrossRef]

27. Lefferts, W.K.; DeBlois, J.P.; Barreira, T.V.; Heffernan, K.S. Neurovascular Coupling during Cognitive Activity in Adults with Controlled Hypertension. *J. Appl. Physiol.* **2018**. [CrossRef]

28. Sheu, L.K.; Jennings, J.R.; Gianaros, P.J. Test-retest reliability of an fMRI paradigm for studies of cardiovascular reactivity. *Psychophysiology* **2012**, *49*, 873–884. [CrossRef]

29. Naqvi, T.Z.; Hyuhn, H.K. Cerebrovascular mental stress reactivity is impaired in hypertension. *Cardiovasc. Ultrasound* **2009**, *7*, 32. [CrossRef]

30. Heffernan, K.S.; Augustine, J.A.; Lefferts, W.K.; Spartano, N.L.; Hughes, W.E.; Jorgensen, R.S.; Gump, B.B. Arterial stiffness and cerebral hemodynamic pulsatility during cognitive engagement in younger and older adults. *Exp. Gerontol.* **2018**, *101*, 54–62. [CrossRef]

31. Lefferts, W.K.; Hughes, W.E.; White, C.N.; Brutsaert, T.D.; Heffernan, K.S. Effect of acute nitrate supplementation on neurovascular coupling and cognitive performance in hypoxia. *Appl. Physiol. Nutr. Metab* **2016**, *41*, 133–141. [CrossRef]

32. Troiano, R.P.; Berrigan, D.; Dodd, K.W.; Masse, L.C.; Tilert, T.; McDowell, M. Physical activity in the United States measured by accelerometer. *Med. Sci. Sports Exerc.* **2008**, *40*, 181–188. [CrossRef] [PubMed]

33. Ratchford, E.V.; Gutierrez, J.; Lorenzo, D.; McClendon, M.S.; Della-Morte, D.; DeRosa, J.T.; Elkind, M.S.; Sacco, R.L.; Rundek, T. Short-term effect of atorvastatin on carotid artery elasticity: A pilot study. *Stroke* **2011**, *42*, 3460–3464. [CrossRef] [PubMed]

34. Lunder, M.; Janic, M.; Habjan, S.; Sabovic, M. Subtherapeutic, low-dose fluvastatin improves functional and morphological arterial wall properties in apparently healthy, middle-aged males—A pilot study. *Atherosclerosis* **2011**, *215*, 446–451. [CrossRef]

35. Gates, P.E.; Tanaka, H.; Hiatt, W.R.; Seals, D.R. Dietary sodium restriction rapidly improves large elastic artery compliance in older adults with systolic hypertension. *Hypertension* **2004**, *44*, 35–41. [CrossRef]

36. Moreau, K.L.; Donato, A.J.; Seals, D.R.; DeSouza, C.A.; Tanaka, H. Regular exercise, hormone replacement therapy and the age-related decline in carotid arterial compliance in healthy women. *Cardiovasc. Res.* **2003**, *57*, 861–868. [CrossRef]

37. Balkestein, E.J.; van Aggel-Leijssen, D.P.; van Baak, M.A.; Struijker-Boudier, H.A.; Van Bortel, L.M. The effect of weight loss with or without exercise training on large artery compliance in healthy obese men. *J. Hypertens.* **1999**, *17*, 1831–1835. [CrossRef]

38. Yang, J.; Wang, H.P.; Tong, X.; Li, Z.N.; Xu, J.Y.; Zhou, L.; Zhou, B.Y.; Qin, L.Q. Effect of whey protein on blood pressure in pre- and mildly hypertensive adults: A randomized controlled study. *Food Sci. Nutr.* **2019**, *7*, 1857–1864. [CrossRef]

39. Niiranen, T.J.; Kalesan, B.; Hamburg, N.M.; Benjamin, E.J.; Mitchell, G.F.; Vasan, R.S. Relative Contributions of Arterial Stiffness and Hypertension to Cardiovascular Disease: The Framingham Heart Study. *J. Am. Heart Assoc.* **2016**, *5*. [CrossRef]

40. Westerhof, N. Cardiac work and efficiency. *Cardiovasc. Res.* **2000**, *48*, 4–7. [CrossRef]

41. O'Rourke, M.F.; Hashimoto, J. Mechanical factors in arterial aging: A clinical perspective. *J. Am. Coll. Cardiol.* **2007**, *50*, 1–13. [CrossRef]

42. Custodis, F.; Schirmer, S.H.; Baumhakel, M.; Heusch, G.; Bohm, M.; Laufs, U. Vascular pathophysiology in response to increased heart rate. *J. Am. Coll. Cardiol.* **2010**, *56*, 1973–1983. [CrossRef]

43. Benetos, A.; Adamopoulos, C.; Bureau, J.M.; Temmar, M.; Labat, C.; Bean, K.; Thomas, F.; Pannier, B.; Asmar, R.; Zureik, M.; et al. Determinants of accelerated progression of arterial stiffness in normotensive subjects and in treated hypertensive subjects over a 6-year period. *Circulation* **2002**, *105*, 1202–1207. [CrossRef]

44. Aune, D.; Sen, A.; o'Hartaigh, B.; Janszky, I.; Romundstad, P.R.; Tonstad, S.; Vatten, L.J. Resting heart rate and the risk of cardiovascular disease, total cancer, and all-cause mortality—A systematic review and dose-response meta-analysis of prospective studies. *Nutr. Metab. Cardiovasc. Dis. NMCD* **2017**, *27*, 504–517. [CrossRef]

45. Bohm, M.; Reil, J.C.; Deedwania, P.; Kim, J.B.; Borer, J.S. Resting heart rate: Risk indicator and emerging risk factor in cardiovascular disease. *Am. J. Med.* **2015**, *128*, 219–228. [CrossRef]

46. Oliva, F.; Sormani, P.; Contri, R.; Campana, C.; Carubelli, V.; Ciro, A.; Morandi, F.; Di Tano, G.; Mortara, A.; Senni, M.; et al. Heart rate as a prognostic marker and therapeutic target in acute and chronic heart failure. *Int. J. Cardiol.* **2018**, *253*, 97–104. [CrossRef]

47. Dobre, D.; Borer, J.S.; Fox, K.; Swedberg, K.; Adams, K.F.; Cleland, J.G.; Cohen-Solal, A.; Gheorghiade, M.; Gueyffier, F.; O'Connor, C.M.; et al. Heart rate: A prognostic factor and therapeutic target in chronic heart failure. The distinct roles of drugs with heart rate-lowering properties. *Eur. J. Heart Fail.* **2014**, *16*, 76–85. [CrossRef]

48. Bangalore, S.; Sawhney, S.; Messerli, F.H. Relation of beta-blocker-induced heart rate lowering and cardioprotection in hypertension. *J. Am. Coll. Cardiol.* **2008**, *52*, 1482–1489. [CrossRef]

49. Olafiranye, O.; Qureshi, G.; Salciccioli, L.; Weber, M.; Lazar, J.M. Association of beta-blocker use with increased aortic wave reflection. *J. Am. Soc. Hypertens. JASH* **2008**, *2*, 64–69. [CrossRef]

50. Manisty, C.H.; Zambanini, A.; Parker, K.H.; Davies, J.E.; Francis, D.P.; Mayet, J.; Mc, G.T.S.A.; Hughes, A.D. Differences in the magnitude of wave reflection account for differential effects of amlodipine- versus atenolol-based regimens on central blood pressure: An Anglo-Scandinavian Cardiac Outcome Trial substudy. *Hypertension* **2009**, *54*, 724–730. [CrossRef] [PubMed]

51. Wilkinson, I.B.; MacCallum, H.; Flint, L.; Cockcroft, J.R.; Newby, D.E.; Webb, D.J. The influence of heart rate on augmentation index and central arterial pressure in humans. *J. Physiol.* **2000**, *525*, 263–270. [CrossRef]

52. Papaioannou, T.G.; Vlachopoulos, C.V.; Alexopoulos, N.A.; Dima, I.; Pietri, P.G.; Protogerou, A.D.; Vyssoulis, G.G.; Stefanadis, C.I. The effect of heart rate on wave reflections may be determined by the level of aortic stiffness: Clinical and technical implications. *Am. J. Hypertens.* **2008**, *21*, 334–340. [CrossRef]

53. Pierdomenico, S.D.; Bucci, A.; Lapenna, D.; Cuccurullo, F.; Mezzetti, A. Heart rate in hypertensive patients treated with ACE inhibitors and long-acting dihydropyridine calcium antagonists. *J. Cardiovasc. Pharmacol.* **2002**, *40*, 288–295. [CrossRef]

54. Hohneck, A.L.; Fries, P.; Stroder, J.; Schneider, G.; Wagenpfeil, S.; Schirmer, S.H.; Bohm, M.; Laufs, U.; Custodis, F. Effects of heart rate reduction with ivabradine on vascular stiffness and endothelial function in chronic stable coronary artery disease. *J. Hypertens.* **2019**, *37*, 1023–1031. [CrossRef]

55. Bruno, R.M.; Cartoni, G.; Stea, F.; Armenia, S.; Bianchini, E.; Buralli, S.; Giannarelli, C.; Taddei, S.; Ghiadoni, L. Carotid and aortic stiffness in essential hypertension and their relation with target organ damage: The CATOD study. *J. Hypertens.* **2017**, *35*, 310–318. [CrossRef]

56. Van Sloten, T.T.; Sedaghat, S.; Laurent, S.; London, G.M.; Pannier, B.; Ikram, M.A.; Kavousi, M.; Mattace-Raso, F.; Franco, O.H.; Boutouyrie, P.; et al. Carotid stiffness is associated with incident stroke: A systematic review and individual participant data·meta-analysis. *J. Am. Coll. Cardiol.* **2015**, *66*, 2116–2125. [CrossRef]

57. Paini, A.; Boutouyrie, P.; Calvet, D.; Tropeano, A.I.; Laloux, B.; Laurent, S. Carotid and aortic stiffness: Determinants of discrepancies. *Hypertension* **2006**, *47*, 371–376. [CrossRef]

58. Mathersul, D.; Palmer, D.M.; Gur, R.C.; Gur, R.E.; Cooper, N.; Gordon, E.; Williams, L.M. Explicit identification and implicit recognition of facial emotions: II. Core domains and relationships with general cognition. *J. Clin. Exp. Neuropsychol.* **2009**, *31*, 278–291. [CrossRef]

59. Lee, J.; Fu, Z.; Chung, M.; Jang, D.J.; Lee, H.J. Role of milk and dairy intake in cognitive function in older adults: A systematic review and meta-analysis. *Nutr. J.* **2018**, *17*, 82. [CrossRef]

60. Zajac, I.T.; Herreen, D.; Bastiaans, K.; Dhillon, V.S.; Fenech, M. The Effect of Whey and Soy Protein Isolates on Cognitive Function in Older Australians with Low Vitamin B12: A Randomised Controlled Crossover Trial. *Nutrients* **2018**, *11*, 19. [CrossRef]

61. Heffernan, K.S. Carotid artery stiffness and cognitive function in adults with and without type 2 diabetes: Extracranial contribution to an intracranial problem? *Atherosclerosis* **2016**, *253*, 268–269. [CrossRef] [PubMed]

62. Rigamonti, A.E.; Leoncini, R.; Casnici, C.; Marelli, O.; Col, A.; Tamini, S.; Lucchetti, E.; Cicolini, S.; Abbruzzese, L.; Cella, S.G.; et al. Whey Proteins Reduce Appetite, Stimulate Anorexigenic Gastrointestinal Peptides and Improve Glucometabolic Homeostasis in Young Obese Women. *Nutrients* **2019**, *11*, 247. [CrossRef] [PubMed]

63. Stojkovic, V.; Simpson, C.A.; Sullivan, R.R.; Cusano, A.M.; Kerstetter, J.E.; Kenny, A.M.; Insogna, K.L.; Bihuniak, J.D. The Effect of Dietary Glycemic Properties on Markers of Inflammation, Insulin Resistance, and Body Composition in Postmenopausal American Women: An Ancillary Study from a Multicenter Protein Supplementation Trial. *Nutrients* **2017**, *9*, 484. [CrossRef] [PubMed]

64. Tomiyama, H.; Hashimoto, H.; Tanaka, H.; Matsumoto, C.; Odaira, M.; Yamada, J.; Yoshida, M.; Shiina, K.; Nagata, M.; Yamashina, A. Synergistic relationship between changes in the pulse wave velocity and changes in the heart rate in middle-aged Japanese adults: A prospective study. *J. Hypertens.* **2010**, *28*, 687–694. [CrossRef]

65. Jae, S.Y.; Heffernan, K.S.; Yoon, E.S.; Park, S.H.; Choi, Y.H.; Fernhall, B.; Park, J.B. Pulsatile stress, inflammation and change in arterial stiffness. *J. Atheroscler. Thromb.* **2012**, *19*, 1035–1042. [CrossRef]

66. McEniery, C.M.; Wilkinson, I.B.; Johansen, N.B.; Witte, D.R.; Singh-Manoux, A.; Kivimaki, M.; Tabak, A.G.; Brunner, E.J.; Shipley, M.J. Nondiabetic Glucometabolic Status and Progression of Aortic Stiffness: The Whitehall II Study. *Diabetes Care* **2017**, *40*, 599–606. [CrossRef]

67. Zhu, K.; Meng, X.; Kerr, D.A.; Devine, A.; Solah, V.; Binns, C.W.; Prince, R.L. The effects of a two-year randomized, controlled trial of whey protein supplementation on bone structure, IGF-1, and urinary calcium excretion in older postmenopausal women. *J. Bone Miner. Res.* **2011**, *26*, 2298–2306. [CrossRef]

68. Chale, A.; Cloutier, G.J.; Hau, C.; Phillips, E.M.; Dallal, G.E.; Fielding, R.A. Efficacy of whey protein supplementation on resistance exercise-induced changes in lean mass, muscle strength, and physical function in mobility-limited older adults. *J. Gerontol. Ser. A Biol. Sci. Med Sci.* **2013**, *68*, 682–690. [CrossRef]

69. Sattler, F.R.; Rajicic, N.; Mulligan, K.; Yarasheski, K.E.; Koletar, S.L.; Zolopa, A.; Alston Smith, B.; Zackin, R.; Bistrian, B. Evaluation of high-protein supplementation in weight-stable HIV-positive subjects with a history of weight loss: A randomized, double-blind, multicenter trial. *Am. J. Clin. Nutr.* **2008**, *88*, 1313–1321. [CrossRef]

70. Fiatarone, M.A.; O'Neill, E.F.; Ryan, N.D.; Clements, K.M.; Solares, G.R.; Nelson, M.E.; Roberts, S.B.; Kehayias, J.J.; Lipsitz, L.A.; Evans, W.J. Exercise training and nutritional supplementation for physical frailty in very elderly people. *N. Engl. J. Med.* **1994**, *330*, 1769–1775. [CrossRef]

71. Altorf-van der Kuil, W.; Engberink, M.F.; Brink, E.J.; van Baak, M.A.; Bakker, S.J.; Navis, G.; van't Veer, P.; Geleijnse, J.M. Dietary protein and blood pressure: A systematic review. *PLoS ONE* **2010**, *5*, e12102. [CrossRef]

72. Kerstetter, J.E.; Bihuniak, J.D.; Brindisi, J.; Sullivan, R.R.; Mangano, K.M.; Larocque, S.; Kotler, B.M.; Simpson, C.A.; Cusano, A.M.; Gaffney-Stomberg, E.; et al. The Effect of a Whey Protein Supplement on Bone Mass in Older Caucasian Adults. *J. Clin. Endocrinol. Metab.* **2015**, *100*, 2214–2222. [CrossRef]

73. Roldan-Tapia, M.D.; Canovas, R.; Leon, I.; Garcia-Garcia, J. Cognitive Vulnerability in Aging May Be Modulated by Education and Reserve in Healthy People. *Front. Aging Neurosci.* **2017**, *9*, 340. [CrossRef]

74. Heffernan, K.S.; Jae, S.Y.; Wilund, K.R.; Woods, J.A.; Fernhall, B. Racial differences in central blood pressure and vascular function in young men. *Am. J. Physiol. Heart Circ. Physiol.* **2008**, *295*, H2380–H2387. [CrossRef]

75. Exner, D.V.; Dries, D.L.; Domanski, M.J.; Cohn, J.N. Lesser response to angiotensin-converting-enzyme inhibitor therapy in black as compared with white patients with left ventricular dysfunction. *N. Engl. J. Med.* **2001**, *344*, 1351–1357. [CrossRef]

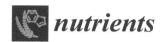

Review

Dietary Factors and Risks of Cardiovascular Diseases: An Umbrella Review

Kridsada Chareonrungrueangchai [1], Keerati Wongkawinwoot [1], Thunyarat Anothaisintawee [1,2,*] and Sirimon Reutrakul [3]

[1] Department of Family Medicine, Faculty of Medicine, Ramathibodi Hospital, Mahidol University, Praram VI Road, Rachathevee, Bangkok 10400, Thailand; thonsmn@gmail.com (K.C.); miupang3456@gmail.com (K.W.)

[2] Department of Clinical Epidemiology and Biostatistics, Ramathibodi Hospital, Mahidol University, Praram VI Road, Rachathevee, Bangkok 10400, Thailand

[3] Division of Endocrinology, Diabetes and Metabolism, University of Illinois College of Medicine at Chicago, 835 S Wolcott, Ste E625, Chicago, IL 60612, USA; sreutrak@uic.edu

* Correspondence: thunyarat.ano@mahidol.ac.th; Tel.: +662-2011406; Fax: +662-2011486

Received: 20 March 2020; Accepted: 9 April 2020; Published: 15 April 2020

Abstract: Unhealthy diet is a significant risk factor for cardiovascular diseases (CVD). Therefore, this umbrella review aims to comprehensively review the effects of dietary factors, including dietary patterns, food groups, and nutrients on CVD risks. Medline and Scopus databases were searched through March 2020. Systematic reviews with meta-analyses (SRMA) of randomized controlled trials (RCTs) or observational studies measuring the effects of dietary factors on CVD risks were eligible. Fifty-four SRMAs, including 35 SRMAs of observational studies, 10 SRMAs of RCTs, and 9 SRMAs of combined RCT and observational studies, were included for review. Findings from the SRMAs of RCTs suggest the significant benefit of Mediterranean and high-quality diets for lowering CVD risk, with pooled risk ratios (RRs) ranging from 0.55 (95%CI: 0.39–0.76) to 0.64 (95%CI: 0.53–0.79) and 0.70 (95%CI: 0.57–0.87), respectively. For food nutrients, two SRMAs of RCTs found that high intake of n-3 polyunsaturated fatty acid (PUFA) significantly reduced CVD risks, with pooled RRs ranging from 0.89 (95%CI: 0.82, 0.98) to 0.90 (95%CI: 0.85–0.96), while evidence of efficacy of n-6 PUFA and combined n-3 and n-6 PUFA were inconsistent. Moreover, results from the SRMAs of RCTs did not find a significant benefit of a low-salt diet and low total fat intake for CVD prevention. For food groups, results from the SRMAs of cohort studies suggest that high intakes of legumes, nuts, and chocolate, as well as a vegetarian diet significantly reduced the risk of coronary heart disease, with pooled RRs of 0.90 (95%CI: 0.84–0.97), 0.68 (95%CI: 0.59–0.78), 0.90 (95%CI: 0.82–0.97), and 0.71 (95%CI: 0.57–0.87), respectively. Healthy dietary patterns had a significant benefit for CVD prevention. With the substitutional and synergistic interactions between different food groups and nutrients, dietary recommendations for CVD prevention should be focused more on healthy dietary patterns than single food groups or nutrients.

Keywords: dietary factor; cardiovascular disease; umbrella review

1. Introduction

Cardiovascular diseases (CVD), today's leading causes of death, accounts for one third of all mortality worldwide [1]. In the past decade, CVD mortalities have increased globally by 12.5% [2]. One significant risk factor of CVD is an unhealthy diet, which is also related to other CVD risk factors, such as hypertension, diabetes mellitus (DM), and obesity [3,4]. Therefore, encouraging healthy diet adherence is important in decreasing CVD morbidity and mortality.

CVD dietary factors is usually classified into three main types: dietary patterns (e.g., the Mediterranean diet and the Dietary Approaches to Stop Hypertension (DASH) diet), food groups (e.g., fruits, vegetables, nuts, whole grains, and legumes), and food nutrients (e.g., sodium, saturated fat, and monounsaturated fat). However, most evidence has focused on dietary fats, due to the established relationship between serum cholesterol level and CVD risks. Previous evidence on the association between dietary fat intake and CVD prevention is inconsistent and is still being debated. For instance, in 2017 the American Heart Association (AHA) recommended lowering saturated fat intake and replacing it with unsaturated fat, especially polyunsaturated fatty acids (PUFA), for CVD prevention [5]. However, some systematic reviews and meta-analyses (SRMA) of randomized controlled trials (RCT) did not show a significant benefit of PUFA for reducing CVD risks [6,7], and the findings from an 18-country cohort study also concluded that "total fat and types of fat were not associated with CVD" [8]. Similarly, findings from SRMAs [9–12] of the effects of other dietary factors, such as vegetables, fruits, and fibers on CVD risks were conflicting, demonstrating the complexity of the link between diets and CVD pathogenesis.

Humans usually have dietary patterns that are a combination of multiple diets composed of multiple nutrients that have synergistic interactions. Hence, to understand the association between diets and CVD risk, we must consider all nutrients, food groups, and dietary patterns, as well as the interrelationship between them. Many SRMAs measuring the effects of dietary factors and CVD risks have been published over the past decade [6,7,9–12]. However, findings from these SRMAs are mostly conflicting. Therefore, to comprehensively summarize the effects of dietary factors on CVD risks, the strength, precision, and potential bias of the findings from previous SRMAs should be explored.

An umbrella review is tertiary research that provides a comprehensive overview of evidence from SRMAs [13]. Hence, this type of review can reveal the strength and precision of the effect estimates and explore the potential bias of previous SRMAs. Therefore, this umbrella review aims to comprehensively review the evidence regarding the effects of nutrients, food groups, and dietary patterns on CVD risks. The effects of each dietary factors on subtypes of CVD, including coronary heart disease (CHD), stroke, CVD mortality, and all-cause mortality were also explored. Moreover, the potential bias and the consistency of evidence from the previous SRMAs of RCTs and observational studies were investigated.

2. Materials and Methods

This umbrella review was conducted according to the preferred reporting items for systematic reviews and meta-analyses (PRISMA) guidelines [14]. The review protocol was registered in PROSPERO (CRD42018105292).

2.1. Literature Search and Study Selection

Medline and Scopus databases were searched from their inceptions to March 2020 to identify the relevant studies. Search terms and strategies of each database are presented in the Appendix S1. Two reviewers (K.C. and K.W.) independently selected the studies. Disagreement between two reviewers were decided by consensus with the third party (T.A.). Systematic reviews with meta-analyses of observational studies or RCTs were eligible, if they met the following criteria; (1) the study's participants were from the general population or were people with high risks for CVD; (2) interested interventions or exposures were dietary factors; (3) the outcomes of interest were CVD, or all-cause mortality; and (4) the pooled risk ratios (RR) or odds ratios (OR), in accordance with their 95% confidence intervals (CI) for dietary factors/diet interventions and outcomes, were reported. Studies were excluded if they included only CVD patients as participants.

2.2. Data Extraction

The following information was extracted from each SRMA: (1) characteristics of eligible SRMAs, including first authors, year of publication, country of corresponding authors, sources of funding support, conflict of interest (COI), types of participants, interested exposures, interventions, comparisons, outcomes, and numbers of primary studies included in SRMA; (2) results of meta-analysis, including pooled RRs or ORs, and their 95%CIs for high versus low, as well as dose response meta-analyses, degree of heterogeneity, and publication bias. The data of primary studies included in each SRMA (i.e., mean age and total numbers of study's participants, percentage male, and study settings) were also extracted. Two reviewers (K.C. and K.W.) extracted the data, and the data were validated by the third reviewer (T.A.).

2.3. Methodological Quality Assessment

The methodological quality of included SRMAs were assessed using the Assessing the Methodological Quality of Systematic Review (AMSTAR) 2. AMSTAR 2 has 16 items in total, including reporting review questions according to Population, Intervention, Comparator, Outcome, protocol registration, study selection, literature search, data extraction, risk of bias assessment, sources of funding, methods of meta-analysis, using risk of bias assessment for data analysis and interpretation, reporting of heterogeneity, publication bias, and conflict of interest. The items were classified as critical and non-critical domains. Overall confidence in the results of the SRMA was rated as high, moderate, low, or critically low confidence, if the SRMA answered "yes" in 0–1 items of a non-critical domain, >1 items in a non-critical domain, 1 item in a critical flaw domain with/without a non-critical domain, or >1 items in a critical flaw domain with/without non-critical domain, respectively.

2.4. Dietary Factors or Interventions

Dietary factors were classified as (1) dietary patterns, (2) food groups, and (3) food nutrients. Dietary patterns referred to the combination of different foods, beverages, and nutrients, and the frequency with which they are routinely consumed [15], such as the Mediterranean diet, the DASH diet, a high quality diet as measured by Healthy Eating Index (HEI) or Alternate Healthy Eating Index (AHEI) scores, or a diet with a low glycemic index. Each food group is defined as a compilation of foods with similar nutritional properties; the food groups were divided into (1) dairy products; (2) fruits; (3) vegetables; (4) meat; (5) grains, beans, and legumes; (6) oils; (7) confections (e.g., sugar-sweetened beverages and chocolate); and (8) coffee. Nutrients, such as protein, fat, carbohydrates, fiber, vitamins, and minerals, are chemical compounds that are used by human bodies to preserve health [16].

Diet interventions referred to any modification or treatment on an individual's diet with a prepared goal [17]. These interventions could be provided by diet supplements or education only.

2.5. Outcomes of Interest

The outcomes of interest were all-cause mortality and cardiovascular diseases. Cardiovascular diseases were defined as cardiovascular mortality; coronary heart diseases (CHD), including acute myocardial infarction (MI); stable and unstable angina; and cerebrovascular disease (CVA), including hemorrhagic and ischemic strokes.

2.6. Data Analysis

Characteristics of included SRMAs were described qualitatively. The pooled effect size of each dietary factor and interventions for each CVD outcome were summarized qualitatively. Heterogeneity between studies and publication bias for each pooling were also presented. Pooled effect sizes of each dietary factor are presented in forest plots, since we could not include the results from all included studies. If there were more than one systematic review and meta-analyses that investigated the effect size of the similar type of dietary factor, pooled risk ratios from SRMAs of RCTs with the highest quality from AMSTAR 2 were selected to present in the forest plots. If there were no SRMAs of RCTs, pooled risk ratios from SRMAs of observational studies with the highest quality according to AMSTAR 2 were selected to present in the forest plots instead.

3. Results

The results of study selection and reasons for exclusion are presented in Figure 1. Fifty-four SRMAs met the inclusion criteria and were eligible for review. Characteristics of included SRMAs are presented in Tables S1 and S2. Almost all SRMAs (48/54) were published after the year 2010. Eighteen SRMAs (33.33%) were conducted in European countries, followed by Asian countries (31.48%), the United Kingdom (16.67%), and the United States (7.41%). Two, three, and one SRMAs were conducted in East Asia, Australia and New Zealand, and South America, respectively. Six SRMAs had a COI with food industries, forty-one SRMAs reported no COI, and four SRMAs did not state anything about a COI. Thirty-five SRMAs (65%) included only observational studies, 10 SRMAs (19%) included only RCTs, and nine SRMAs (17%) included both observational studies and RCTs. In addition, 15, 10, 14, and 5 SRMAs featured dietary patterns, food groups, food nutrients, and both food groups and nutrients, respectively. Lastly, seven, two, and one SRMAs featured diet interventions in food nutrients, dietary patterns, and both food nutrients and dietary patterns, respectively [17].

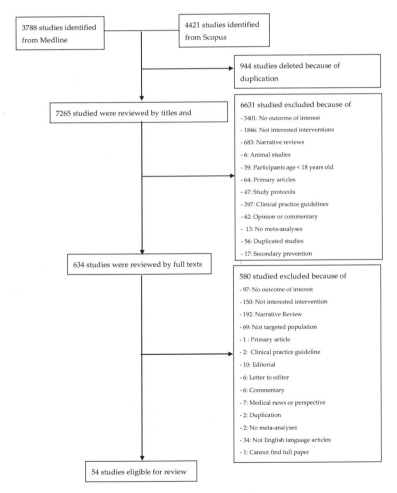

Figure 1. Flow chart of study selection.

3.1. Dietary Patterns

A total of 18 SMRAs, (13 SRMAs of observational studies, two SRMAs of RCTs and observational studies, and three SRMAs of RCTs) assessed the effects of dietary patterns and CVD risks. For SRMAs of observational studies, dietary patterns were Mediterranean diet (eight SRMAs), DASH diet (three SRMAs), diets with high HEI and AHEI scores (two SRMAs), HEI/AHEI and cardiovascular health (CVH) scores (one SRMA), and Diet Inflammatory Index (DII) scores (one SRMA). For SRMAs of RCTs, the interventions were prescribing a Mediterranean diet (one SRMA) [18] and modifying diet quality by lowering the consumption of carbohydrates, fat, and calories, and increasing the consumption of fish, vegetables, complex carbohydrates, and fiber (two SRMA) [17,19]. Most of the SRMAs (16/18) considered the general population as the study's participants, while two included only high-risk populations (e.g., patients with obesity, hypertension, and DM). The mean age and percentage of male participants ranged from 18 to 104 years, and 0% to 100%, respectively (see Table S1). The effects of each dietary pattern are described in Figure 2A–D and Table S3.

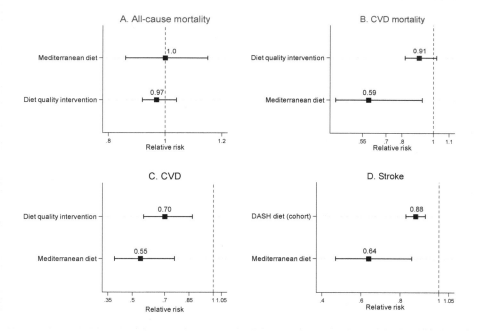

Figure 2. Pooled risk ratios of dietary patterns and the risk of all-cause (**A**) and cardiovascular mortality (**B**), cardiovascular disease (**C**), and stroke (**D**). Results are from systematic reviews and meta-analyses of randomized controlled trials, except for that of the Dietary Approaches to Stop Hypertension (DASH) diet, which is from observational studies. (CVD, cardiovascular diseases)

3.1.1. Mediterranean Diet

For all-cause mortality, two SRMAs of observational studies [20,21] found that adherence to Mediterranean diet significantly decreased risk of all-cause mortality in the general population, with a pooled RR ranging from 0.91 (95%CI: 0.89–0.94) to 0.92 (95%CI: 0.90–0.94). However, a finding from an SRMA of RCTs [18] suggested a non-significant benefit of the Mediterranean diet in reducing all-cause mortality in high-risk populations (pooled RR = 1.00; 95%CI: 0.86–1.15; see Figure 2A).

For CVD mortality, both SRMAs of observational studies and RCTs [20,22] found a significant benefit of the Mediterranean diet in decreasing CVD mortality in the general population, with pooled RRs ranging from 0.59 to 0.91 (see Figure 2B), while the SRMA of RCTs [18] found no significant effect in high-risk populations (pooled RR = 0.90; 95%CI: 0.72–1.11; see Table S3).

Four [18,22–24], three [18,22,24], and six [18,22,24–27] SRMAs reported the outcomes as CVD, CHD, and stroke, respectively. Both the SRMAs of observational studies and RCTs found the significant benefit of a Mediterranean diet in reducing the risk of CVD (pooled RRs ranging from 0.55 to 0.81), CHD (pooled RRs ranging from 0.65 to 0.72), and stroke (pooled RRs ranging from 0.64 to 0.84) in both general and high-risk populations (see Figure 2C–D).

3.1.2. DASH Diet

Three SRMAs of observational studies [28–30] assessed the effect of a DASH diet on CVD risk. These SRMAs found that high adherence to a DASH diet significantly decreased the risk of CHD (pooled RRs ranging from 0.79 (95%CI: 0.71–0.88) to 0.95 (95%CI: 0.94–0.97)) and stroke (pooled RRs ranging from 0.81 (95%CI: 0.72–0.92) and 0.88 (95%CI: 0.83–0.93; see Figure 2D and Table S3).

3.1.3. Diet Quality

Diet quality was measured by HEI/AHEI (two SRMAs) [31,32], HEI/AHEI and CVH (one SRMA) [33], and DII (one SRMA) [34] scores. The effects of diet quality on CVD risk are presented in Table S3. High HEI/AHEI and CVH scores reflect the high quality of diet, whereas high DII scores reveal a poor-quality diet. Participants of all SRMAs were the general population. All three SRMAs of observational studies have consistent findings that consuming diets with high HEI/AHEI and CVH scores significantly decreased the risk of all-cause mortality (pooled RRs ranging from 0.54 to 0.78), CVD mortality (pooled RRs ranging from 0.30 to 0.77), and CVD (pooled RR = 0.78). However, diets with a high DII score showed a significantly increased risk of CVD (pooled RR = 1.35; 95%CI: 1.11–1.63) and CVD mortality (pooled RR = 1.37; 95%CI: 1.11–1.70; see Table S3).

Evidence from the SRMA of RCTs suggests that increasing high-quality diet consumption in the high-risk population significantly decreased CVD risk [19] (pooled RR = 0.70; 95%CI: 0.57–0.87; see Figure 2C). However, there was no significant effect of increasing high-quality diet consumption in lowering all-cause (pooled RR = 0.97; 95%CI: 0.92–1.04) and CVD mortality (pooled RR = 0.91; 95%CI: 0.82–1.02) in the general population [17] (see Figure 2A–B).

3.2. *Food Groups*

A total of 14 SRMAs (10 SRMAs of observational studies and four SRMAs of both observational studies and RCTs) assessed the effects of food groups on CVD risks. The food groups considered were (1) fruits and vegetables; (2) nuts, whole grains, and legumes; (3) fish; (4) a vegetarian diet; (5) olive oil; (6) chocolate; (7) coffee; and (8) green tea. Participants of all 14 SRMAs were from the general population. Mean age, male percentage, and total number of participants ranged from 20 to 100 years, 0% to 100%, and 51 to 454,775, respectively. The effects of each food group are presented in Figure 3 and Table S3.

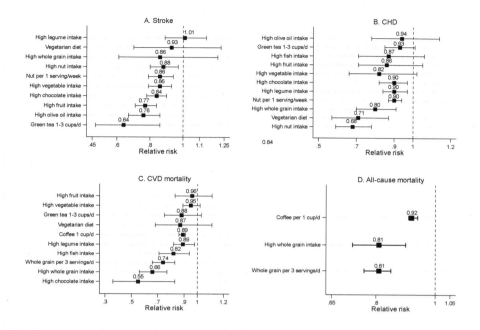

Figure 3. Pooled risk ratios of food groups and risk of stroke (**A**), coronary heart disease (**B**), cardiovascular mortality (**C**), and all-cause mortality(**D**). Results are from systematic reviews and meta-analyses of observational studies. (CHD, coronary heart disease)

3.2.1. Fruits and Vegetables

Three SRMAs of observational studies assessed the association between fruit and vegetable intake and CVD risks [10–12]. High fruit and vegetables intake significantly decreased the risk of stroke (pooled RR ranging from 0.77 (95%CI: 0.71–0.84) to 0.86 (95%CI: 0.79–0.93)) [11] (Figure 3A), but did not decrease the risk of CHD (pooled RR ranging from 0.82 (95%CI: 0.66–1.02) to 0.86 (95%CI: 0.71–1.05)) [10] (Figure 3B), and CVD mortality (pooled RRs ranging from 0.95 (95%CI: 0.89–1.02) to 0.96 (95%CI: 0.83–1.11) [12] (Figure 3C).

3.2.2. Vegetarian Diet

One SRMA of observational studies investigated the association between vegetarian diet and CVD risks [35]. High adherence to vegetarian diet significantly lowered the CHD risk, with a pooled RR of 0.71 and 95%CI: 0.57–0.87 (Figure 3B), but did not lower CVD mortality (pooled RR = 0.87; 95%CI: 0.68–1.11) and risk of stroke (pooled RR = 0.93; 95%CI: 0.70–1.23; see Figure 3A,C).

3.2.3. Nuts, Whole Grains, and Legumes

Two SRMAs each of observational studies assessed the effect of nuts [36,37], legumes [12,38], and whole grains [39,40]. Both high vs. low and dose response analyses of nut intake demonstrated a significantly beneficial effect on the risk of CHD, with pooled RRs ranging from 0.68 (95%CI: 0.59–0.78) to 0.90 (95%CI: 0.87–0.94) [37] (Figure 3B), and stroke, with pooled RRs ranging from 0.86 (95%CI: 0.79–0.94) to 0.88 (95%CI: 0.80–0.97) [36] (Figure 3A). Both high vs. low and dose response analyses of whole grain intake indicated a significant effect in lowering all-cause (pooled RRs ranging from 0.81 (95%CI: 0.76–0.85) to 0.87 (95%CI: 0.84–0.90)) and CVD mortality (pooled RRs ranging from 0.66

(95%CI: 0.56–0.67) to 0.81 (95%CI: 0.74–0.89)) [39,40] (see Figure 3C,D). In addition, a high intake of whole grain significantly decreased risk of CHD, with a pooled RR of 0.80 (95%CI: 0.70–0.91), but did not reduce risk of stroke (pooled RR = 0.86; 95%CI: 0.61–1.21). High legume intake also significantly reduced CVD mortality (pooled RR = 0.89; 95%CI: 0.82–0.98) [12] and CHD risk (pooled RR = 0.90; 95%CI: 0.84–0.97) [38] (see Figure 3B,C), but not risk of stroke (pooled RR = 1.01; 95%CI: 0.89–1.14) [38] (see Figure 3A).

3.2.4. Fish

Two SRMAs of observational studies assessed the association between fish intake and CVD risks [6,41], and found that high fish intake significantly reduced CVD mortality, with pooled RRs ranging from 0.75 (95%CI: 0.62–0.92) to 0.82 (95%CI: 0.71, 0.94; see Figure 3C). However, the results of CHD risk were inconsistent between the two SRMAs, as Whelton et al. [41] show a significant benefit of high fish intake (pooled RR = 0.83; 95%CI: 0.69–0.99), while Skeaff et al.'s results [6] are non-significant (pooled RR = 0.87; 95%CI: 0.71–1.06).

3.2.5. Olive Oil

Findings from one SRMA of observational studies and RCTs indicate that high olive oil consumption [42] significantly decreases the risk of stroke (pooled RR = 0.76; 95%CI: 0.67–0.86; see Figure 3A). There was no significant effect of olive oil on CHD risk (pooled RR = 0.94; 95%CI: 0.78–1.14; see Figure 3B).

3.2.6. Chocolate

Two SRMAs of observational studies investigated the association between chocolate consumption and CVD risks [43,44]. The results demonstrate that high chocolate consumption significantly decreased the risk of CHD (pooled RRs ranging from 0.71 (95%CI: 0.56–0.92) to 0.90 (95%CI: 0.82–0.97)), stroke (pooled RRs ranging from 0.79 (95%CI: 0.70–0.87) to 0.84 (95%CI: 0.78–0.90)), and CVD mortality (pooled RR = 0.55 (95%CI: 0.36–0.83; see Figure 3A–C).

3.2.7. Coffee and Green Tea

One SRMA of observational studies found that drinking one cup of coffee per day significantly reduced all-cause and CVD mortality, with pooled RRs of 0.92 (95%CI: 0.91–0.94) and 0.89 (95%CI: 0.86–0.91), respectively [45] (see Figure 3C,D). For green tea, consuming 1–3 cups of green tea per day significantly lowers the risk of stroke (pooled RR = 0.64 (95%CI: 0.47–0.86), while the risk of CVD, all-cause, and CVD mortality were not significantly different between green tea intake and non-intake [46].

3.3. Food Nutrients

Sixteen SRMAs of observational studies, seven SRMAs of RCTs, and one SRMA of combined observational studies and RCTs investigated the effect of food nutrients on CVD risk in the general population. Mean age, percentage male, and total number of study's participants ranged from 20–89 years, 0–100%, and 16–388,229, respectively. Most SRMAs studied fat intake (11/24), followed by fiber (5/20), sodium (3/20), flavonoid (3/20), potassium (1/20), and calcium intakes (1/20). Effect of each food nutrients are presented in Figures 4 and 5, and Table S3.

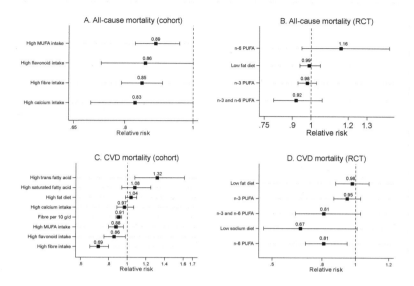

Figure 4. Pooled risk ratios of food nutrients and risk of all-cause and cardiovascular disease mortality. Results are from systematic reviews and meta-analyses of observational studies for (**A**) and (**C**), and systematic reviews and meta-analyses of randomized controlled trials (RCTs) for (**B**) and (**D**).

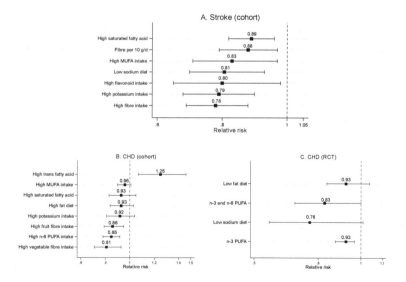

Figure 5. Pooled risk ratios for food nutrients and the risk of stroke and coronary heart disease. Results are from systematic reviews and meta-analyses of observational studies for (**A**) and (**B**), and systematic reviews and meta-analyses of RCTs for (**C**).

3.3.1. Fat Intake

Fat intake was classified as (1) total fat intake, (2) saturated fatty acid (SFA), (3) MUFA, (4) n-3 PUFA, (5) n-6 PUFA, and (6) trans fatty acid (TFA). For total fat intake, the results from SRMAs of observational studies found that a high total fat intake did not significantly increase risk of CVD mortality (pooled RRs ranging from 0.94 (95%CI: 0.74–1.18) to 1.04 (95%CI: 0.98–1.10)) [6,47] (Figure 4C) and CHD (pooled RR = 0.93; 95%CI: 0.84–1.03) [6] (Figure 5B). Evidence from SRMAs of RCTs also indicated that modification of the amount of total fat intake did not significantly decrease risk of all-cause mortality (pooled RRs ranging from 0.98 (95%CI: 0.86–1.12) to 0.99 (95%CI: 0.94–1.05)) [48,49] (Figure 4B), CVD mortality (pooled RRs ranging from 0.91 (95%CI: 0.77–1.07) to 1.00 (95%CI: 0.80–1.24)) [6,48,49], or CHD (pooled RR = 0.93 (95%CI: 0.84–1.04) [6] (Figure 5C) in the general population.

Findings from two SRMAs of observational studies showed that high SFA intake was not significantly associated with risk of CVD mortality [6,47] and CHD [6] (see Figures 4B and 5B). However, one SRMA of observational studies found that a high SFA intake was significantly associated with lower risk of ischemic stroke (pooled RR = 0.89; 95%CI: 0.82–0.96) [50] (see Figure 5A).

One meta-analysis of cohort studies assessed the association between high trans-fat intake and CVD risk, and found that high trans-fat intake significantly increased the risk of CVD mortality (pooled RR = 1.32; 95%CI: 1.08–1.61; Figure 4C) and CHD (pooled RR = 1.25; 95%CI: 1.07–1.46; Figure 5B).

Findings from one SRMA of observational studies suggest that high MUFA intake significantly decreased the risk of all-cause mortality (pooled RR = 0.89; 95%CI: 0.83–0.96) (Figure 4A) and stroke (pooled RR = 0.83; 95%CI: 0.71–0.97) (Figure 5A). However, the effects of MUFA on CVD mortality were inconsistent between two SRMAs. Schwingshackl et al. show that high MUFA intake significantly reduced the risk of CVD mortality (pooled RR = 0.88; 95%CI: 0.80–0.96) [51], while Skeaff et al. show a non-significant effect (pooled RR = 0.85; 95%CI: 0.60–1.20) [6]. However, both SRMAs found that high MUFA intake did not significantly reduce CHD risk (see Figure 5B).

PUFA is classified as n-3 PUFA, n-6 PUFA, and combined n-3 and n-6 PUFA. Three SRMAs of RCTs assessed the effect of n-3 PUFA on CVD risk. Two SRMAs found that n-3 PUFA significantly lowered the risk of CVD (pooled RR ranging from 0.89 (95%CI: 0.82-0.98) to 0.90 (95%CI: 0.85-0.96)) [6,52], while one SRMA found a non-significant effect of n-3 PUFA (pooled RR = 0.99; 95%CI: 0.94-1.04) [53]. However, all-cause mortality rate was not significantly different between n-3 PUFA and placebo groups [52] (see Figure 4B). The findings about the effect of n-3 PUFA on CVD mortality were inconsistent between these two SRMAs, as the results of Delgado-Lista et al. suggest a significant benefit (pooled RR = 0.91; 95%CI: 0.83–0.99) [52], while results of Skeaff et al. [6] and Abdelhamid et al. [53] indicated a non-significant effect (pooled RRs ranging from = 0.88; 95%CI: 0.76–1.01 to 0.99; 95%CI: 0.94–1.04). In addition, the results from Abdelhamid et al. indicated that n-3 PUFA significantly decreased the risk of CHD, but the benefit of n-3 PUFA was not seen for stroke prevention.

One meta-analysis of RCTs indicated a non-significant benefit of n-6 PUFA for the prevention of all-cause mortality (Figure 4A), while there were inconsistent findings for the outcomes on CVD mortality and CHD risk. One meta-analysis of RCTs found that high n-6 PUFA intake significantly decreased the risk of CVD mortality (pooled RR = 0.81; 95%CI: 0.70–0.95) [54], while another meta-analysis of RCT found a non-significant effect (pooled RR = 1.17; 95%CI: 0.82–1.68) [7]. Two meta-analyses of cohort studies assessing the effect of n-6 PUFA on the risk of CHD also show conflicting results, with Farvid et al. suggesting the significant benefit of high n-6 intake for prevention of CHD (pooled RR = 0.81; 95%CI: 0.70–0.95) [54], and Skeaff et al. demonstrating a non-significant benefit (pooled RR = 1.05; 95%CI: 0.92–1.20) [6]. For combined n-3 and n-6 PUFA, the results from two SRMAs of RCTs [6,7] indicate that high PUFA intake was not significantly associated with CHD risk, all-cause, and CVD mortality.

3.3.2. Fiber

Five SRMAs of observational studies assessed the association between fiber intake and CVD risk. Both high vs. low and dose response analyses from all SRMAs suggest that high fiber intake significantly reduced the risk of all-cause mortality (pooled RR = 0.85; 95%CI: 0.79–0.91), CVD mortality (pooled RRs ranging from 0.69 (95%CI: 0.60–0.81) to 0.91 (95%CI: 0.88–0.94); Figure 4C) [12,40], stroke (pooled RRs ranging from 0.78 (95%CI: 0.69–0.88) to 0.88 (95%CI: 0.79–0.97); Figure 5A) [9,40,55], and CHD (pooled RRs ranging from 0.76 (95%CI: 0.69–0.83) to 0.86 (95%CI: 0.79–0.95); Figure 5B) [10,40].

3.3.3. Sodium

One SRMA of RCTs, one SRMA of cohort studies, and one SRMA of observational studies and RCTs found that low sodium intake did not significantly reduce risk of CVD, all-cause mortality, and CVD mortality [56,57]; however, meta-analysis of cohort studies suggested that low sodium intake could significantly decrease the risk of stroke, with pooled RRs ranging from of 0.81 (95%CI: 0.70–0.93) to 0.94; 95%CI: 0.90–0.98 [57,58] (see Figure 5A).

3.3.4. Flavonoid

Two SRMAs of observational studies found that the risk of CVD mortality and stroke in people having a high flavonoid intake was significantly lower than those with a low intake, with pooled RRs of 0.86 (95%CI: 0.75–0.98; Figure 4C) and 0.80 (95%CI: 0.65–0.98; Figure 5A) [59,60]. However, the risk of all-cause mortality was not significantly different between the two groups [59] (see Figure 4A).

One SRMA of observational studies assessed the effect of anthocyanins, which are a subtype of flavonoid, on CVD risk [61]. This SRMA found that a high intake of anthocyanins significantly decreased the risk of CVD mortality and CHD, with pooled RRs of 0.92 (95%CI: 0.87–0.97) and 0.91 (95%CI: 0.83–0.99), respectively (see Table S3). However, the risk of stroke did not significantly decrease in people with a high intake of anthocyanins.

3.3.5. Potassium

One SRMA of observational studies assessed the association between potassium intake and CVD risk [62]. High potassium intake significantly decreased the risk of stroke (pooled RR = 0.79; 95%CI: 0.68–0.90; Figure 5A), while risk of CHD was not significantly different between high and low potassium intake (pooled RR = 0.92; 95%CI: 0.81–1.04; Figure 5B).

3.3.6. Calcium

One meta-analysis of cohort studies assessed the effect of high calcium intake and CVD mortality [63], and found that a high calcium intake from diet and supplements did not significantly reduce the risk of all-cause mortality (pooled RR = 0.83; 95%CI: 0.70–1.00) or CVD mortality (pooled RR = 0.97; 95%CI: 0.89–1.07) (see Figure 4A,C).

3.4. Methodological Quality Assessment

Results of quality assessment are presented in Table S4. Forty-eight out of 54 studies were classified as critically low confidence, five studies were classified as low confidence, and one study was classified as high confidence, according to AMSTAR-2 criteria. All of the studies having critically low confidence did not registered the review protocols, and most of those studies (90%) did not provide a list of excluded studies and reasons for exclusion. Around 50% of included studies did not consider the results of the risk of bias assessment in individual studies when interpreted, nor discussed the results. Most of the studies (51/54) used more than two databases for searching relevant studies, but only nine studies searched in databases for grey literatures. Most of the studies used appropriated methods of meta-analysis (52/54) and reported publication bias (45/54).

4. Discussion

This umbrella review provides a comprehensive summary of evidence about the effect of dietary factors on the risk of CVD. Evidence from RCTs and observational studies confirms the benefit of healthy dietary patterns, especially the Mediterranean diet, for the prevention of CVD, but the benefit for lowering all-cause and CVD mortality were inconsistent. The DASH diet also exhibited the ability to prevent CVD, but was only supported by observational studies.

A high intake of whole grains, legumes, fish, chocolate, and drinking one cup of coffee per day significantly decreased the risk of CVD mortality; a high intake of legumes, nuts, and chocolate, as well as a vegetarian diet could reduce risk of CHD. In addition, high intakes of vegetables and fruits, olive oil, and nuts, as well as dinking 1–3 cups of green tea per day significantly lowered risk of stroke. Evidence from RCTs and observational studies found that total fat intake was not associated with all-cause and CVD mortality, or the risk of CVD. However, high TFA intake significantly increased the risk of CVD and CVD mortality. Evidence from RCTs indicated consistent and inconsistent benefits of n-3 PUFA and n-6 PUFA for CVD prevention, respectively. Observational studies suggest the benefit of SFA for lowering stroke risk, and MUFA for lowering all-cause mortality and risk of stroke. In addition, evidence from observational studies also linked high fiber to CVD prevention and flavonoids to lowering CVD mortality. High potassium and low sodium intake also reduced the risk of stroke.

Our results, found from both RCTs and observational studies, suggest the significant benefit of healthy dietary patterns, especially the Mediterranean diet, for prevention of CVD. These findings correspond with the 2019 American College of Cardiology/American Heart Association (ACC/AHA) guidelines, which recommends healthy dietary patterns for lowering CVD [64]. Common characteristics of healthy diet patterns include a lower intake of red and processed meats, refined carbohydrates, sugar-sweetened beverages, and whole-fat dairy products; a higher consumption of fruits, vegetables, whole grains, nuts, and legumes; and a moderate consumption of alcohol. These dietary patterns are not nutrient-oriented, but rather consider a combination of multiple food groups. This approach provides several advantages. Firstly, people eat foods, not nutrients. Therefore, providing recommendation by dietary patterns is more practical in both public health and routine clinical practices than by nutrient alone [65]. Secondly, single-nutrient recommendations usually fail to consider substitutional effects and food replacement. For instance, our study found no benefit of a low-fat diet for CVD prevention, which may have resulted from the excess intake of other high-risk foods, such as refined carbohydrates and sugar to substitute the energy from fat [66,67]. Since the effect of foods on health depends on both synergistic and antagonistic interactions between multiple nutrients [68], nutrient orientation in generating dietary recommendations is not appropriate for CVD prevention.

The Mediterranean diet, among all healthy dietary patterns, has been the primary focus of previous studies. Several SRMAs of RCTs consistently found that the Mediterranean diet significantly decreased CVD mortality, CHD, and stroke risk. The key features of Mediterranean diet are a low intake of meat, with very low consumption of red and processed meat; a high intake of vegetables, fruits, nuts, legumes, cereals; and moderate intake of alcohol [69], all of which food groups had differing effects in CVD prevention. For instance, our review found that high intake of nuts, whole grains, and legumes, with a moderate intake of fish (2–4 servings/week) significantly decreased CVD mortality and CVD risk. Fish contains long-chain n-3 PUFAs that have a beneficial effect on CVD outcomes. Findings from SRs of RCTs support the hypothesis that prescribing supplement of n-3 PUFAs significantly reduces CVD risk. In addition, a recent RCT found that icosapent ethyl significantly decreases CVD risk beyond cholesterol-lowering therapy, and now has been approved by the U.S. Food and Drug Administration (FDA) for CVD prevention in high-risk patients [70].

Olive oil and extra-virgin olive oil are major sources of fat in the Mediterranean diet. Bioactive polyphenols—agents postulated to prevent CVD [71]—are only found in extra-virgin olive oil but not in common olive oil, which could explain the lack of the link between olive oil and CHD prevention in our review. In contrast, previous RCTs have suggested the significant benefit of extra-virgin olive oil in Mediterranean diet [72]. Hence, recommendation of olive oil for CVD prevention should focus on extra-virgin olive oil rather than common olive oil. Apart from bioactive polyphenols, the cardioprotective property of olive oil may come from its high content of MUFA [73]. However, results from our review show inconsistent evidence of the benefits of MUFA for CVD prevention.

Evidence of dietary patterns have usually focused on western diets, such as the Mediterranean and DASH diets. However, diets in other regions are different from those in Western countries, and it is not practical to recommend Western dietary patterns to other regions, e.g., Asian countries. Recently, the Japan Collaborative Cohort study that evaluated the effect of high Japanese food scores (i.e., high of consumption of rice, miso soup, seaweeds, pickles, green and yellow vegetables, fish, and green tea, and low consumption of beef, pork, and coffee) found that adherence to a Japanese food score may have benefits for CVD prevention [74]. However, more evidence is needed to confirm the benefits of Japanese food and other Asian dietary patterns on CVD prevention. Recommendations of dietary patterns should take into account the food culture of each region.

SRMAs of cohort studies found no benefit of high vegetable and fruit intake, which is recommended in Mediterranean and other healthy diet patterns, on CVD outcomes. However, SRMAs of observational studies found significant benefits in high dietary fiber intake for lowering CVD mortality and CVD risk. These conflicting results might have resulted from dietary fiber consisting of vegetables, fruits, nuts, whole grains, and legumes. However, nuts, whole grains, and legumes consist of not only fiber, but also of plant protein, unsaturated fats, minerals, and phytochemicals that might be attributable for their CVD-prevention properties [75]. Evidence of CVD dietary risk factors have mainly focused on fat, which is divided into total fat intake and subtypes of fatty acids, such as saturated fat, MUFA, and n-3 and n-6 PUFA. Inconsistent results according to different outcomes were found for each subtype of fat. For instance, high saturated fat intake did not significantly increase risk of CHD and CVD mortality, but was significantly associated with lower stroke risk. Moreover, n-3 PUFA substantially decreased CVD risk, but did not decrease all-cause and CVD mortality risk. Evidence of n-6 PUFAs were conflicting for CVD mortality and CHD. Guidelines from ACC/AHD year 2019 recommends replacing saturated fat with dietary MUFA and PUFA to reduce CVD risk [64]. However, this guideline does not state clearly the type of PUFA that is beneficial for CVD prevention.

Studies regarding some food groups and nutrients, such as vegetables, fruits, a vegetarian diet, olive oil, flavonoids, green tea, and potassium also had inconsistent findings, according to CVD outcomes. These might have resulted from the complex relationship between dietary and other lifestyle factors (e.g., physical activity), which might have confounded the findings of the previous studies.

Strengths and Limitations

This is the first umbrella review that comprehensively reviews the evidence of diets and CVD outcomes. We considered the effect of all dietary patterns, food groups, and nutrients, according to all types of CVD outcomes, including all-cause mortality, CVD mortality, CVD, CHD, and stroke. Only systematic reviews and meta-analyses, which are in the top hierarchy of evidence, were included in the review. The quality of systematic reviews and meta-analyses were assessed using AMSTAR 2. However, our study has some limitations. Firstly, the quality of most included SRMAs were critically low. Moreover, evidence of food groups and some nutrients were from SRMAs of observational studies having more bias and confounding effects than SRMAs of RCTs. Therefore, the results from those SRMAs should be interpreted with caution. In addition, the results from the included SRMAs were qualitatively analyzed, and dietary effects on CVD outcomes cannot be exactly quantified.

5. Conclusions

Healthy dietary patterns, such as the Mediterranean diet, have significant beneficial effects on CVD risk. A high intake of food groups and nutrients like nuts, whole grains, legumes, and dietary fiber, and moderate intake of fish also acts to prevent CVD, while a high intake of trans fatty acids significantly increased CVD risk. With the substitutional and synergistic interactions between different food groups and nutrients, dietary recommendations for CVD prevention should be focused more on healthy dietary patterns than single food groups or nutrients.

Supplementary Materials: The following are available online at http://www.mdpi.com/2072-6643/12/4/1088/s1, Appendix S1: Search terms and search strategies from Medline and Scopus databases. Table S1: Characteristics of included systematic reviews and meta-analyses. Table S2: Details of diet intervention and dietary factors. Table S3: Pooled risk ratios of dietary factors, according to outcomes. Table S4: Results of methodological quality assessment.

Author Contributions: Conceptualization, T.A. and K.C.; methodology, K.C., K.W., and T.A.; formal analysis, K.C. and T.A.; investigation, T.A.; writing—original draft preparation, K.C. and T.A.; writing—review and editing, T.A. and S.R.; supervision, T.A. and S.R.; funding acquisition, T.A. All authors have read and agreed to the published version of the manuscript.

Funding: This study was funded by the Prince Mahidol Award Foundation, Thai Health Promotion Foundation, and International Decision Support Initiative. The Health Intervention and Technology Assessment Program (HITAP) is funded by the Thailand Research Fund (TRF) under a grant for senior research scholar (RTA5980011). HITAP's International Unit is supported by the International Decision Support Initiative (iDSI), which is funded by the Bill and Melinda Gates Foundation, the United Kingdom's Department for International Development, and the Rockefeller Foundation.

Acknowledgments: We would like to express our special thanks of gratitude to Sasin Thamakaison, who helped us in editing the English language of the manuscript.

Conflicts of Interest: The authors declare no conflict of interest. The funders had no role in the design of the study; in the collection, analyses, or interpretation of data; in the writing of the manuscript, or in the decision to publish the results.

References

1. Roth, G.A.; Johnson, C.; Abajobir, A.; Abd-Allah, F.; Abera, S.F.; Abyu, G.; Ahmed, M.; Aksut, B.; Alam, T.; Alam, K.; et al. Global, Regional, and National Burden of Cardiovascular Diseases for 10 Causes, 1990 to 2015. *J. Am. Coll. Cardiol.* **2017**, *70*, 1–25. [CrossRef]

2. Wang, H.; Naghavi, M.; Allen, C.; Barber, R.M.; Bhutta, Z.A.; Carter, A.; Casey, D.C.; Charlson, F.J.; Chen, A.Z.; Coates, M.M.; et al. Global, regional, and national life expectancy, all-cause mortality, and cause-specific mortality for 249 causes of death, 1980–2015: A systematic analysis for the Global Burden of Disease Study 2015. *Lancet* **2016**, *388*, 1459–1544. [CrossRef]

3. Yusuf, S.; Hawken, S.; Ounpuu, S.; Dans, T.; Avezum, A.; Lanas, F.; McQueen, M.; Budaj, A.; Pais, P.; Varigos, J.; et al. Effect of potentially modifiable risk factors associated with myocardial infarction in 52 countries (the INTERHEART study): Case-control study. *Lancet* **2004**, *364*, 937–952. [CrossRef]

4. O'Donnell, M.J.; Chin, S.L.; Rangarajan, S.; Xavier, D.; Liu, L.; Zhang, H.; Rao-Melacini, P.; Zhang, X.; Pais, P.; Agapay, S.; et al. Global and regional effects of potentially modifiable risk factors associated with acute stroke in 32 countries (INTERSTROKE): A case-control study. *Lancet* **2016**, *388*, 761–775. [CrossRef]

5. Sacks, F.M.; Lichtenstein, A.H.; Wu, J.H.Y.; Appel, L.J.; Creager, M.A.; Kris-Etherton, P.M.; Miller, M.; Rimm, E.B.; Rudel, L.L.; Robinson, J.G.; et al. Dietary Fats and Cardiovascular Disease: A Presidential Advisory From the American Heart Association. *Circulation* **2017**, *136*, e1–e23. [CrossRef] [PubMed]

6. Skeaff, C.M.; Miller, J. Dietary fat and coronary heart disease: Summary of evidence from prospective cohort and randomised controlled trials. *Ann. Nutr. Metab.* **2009**, *55*, 173–201. [CrossRef] [PubMed]

7. Ramsden, C.E.; Hibbeln, J.R.; Majchrzak, S.F.; Davis, J.M. N-6 Fatty acid-specific and mixed polyunsaturate dietary interventions have different effects on CHD risk: A meta-analysis of randomised controlled trials. *Br. J. Nutr.* **2010**, *104*, 1586–1600. [CrossRef]

8. Dehghan, M.; Mente, A.; Zhang, X.; Swaminathan, S.; Li, W.; Mohan, V.; Iqbal, R.; Kumar, R.; Wentzel-Viljoen, E.; Rosengren, A.; et al. Associations of fats and carbohydrate intake with cardiovascular disease and mortality in 18 countries from five continents (PURE): A prospective cohort study. *Lancet* **2017**, *390*, 2050–2062. [CrossRef]

9. Chen, G.C.; Lv, D.B.; Pang, Z.; Dong, J.Y.; Liu, Q.F. Dietary fiber intake and stroke risk: A meta-analysis of prospective cohort studies. *Eur. J. Clin. Nutr.* **2013**, *67*, 96–100. [CrossRef]

10. Law, M.R.; Morris, J.K. By how much does fruit and vegetable consumption reduce the risk of ischaemic heart disease? *Eur. J. Clin. Nutr.* **1998**, *52*, 549–556. [CrossRef]

11. Hu, D.; Huang, J.; Wang, Y.; Zhang, D.; Qu, Y. Fruits and vegetables consumption and risk of stroke: A meta-analysis of prospective cohort studies. *Stroke* **2014**, *45*, 1613–1619. [CrossRef] [PubMed]

12. Kim, Y.; Je, Y. Dietary fibre intake and mortality from cardiovascular disease and all cancers: A meta-analysis of prospective cohort studies. *Arch. Cardiovasc. Dis.* **2016**, *109*, 39–54. [CrossRef] [PubMed]

13. Aromataris, E.; Fernandez, R.; Godfrey, C.M.; Holly, C.; Khalil, H.; Tungpunkom, P. Summarizing systematic reviews: Methodological development, conduct and reporting of an umbrella review approach. *Int. J. Evid.-Based Healthc.* **2015**, *13*, 132–140. [CrossRef] [PubMed]

14. Moher, D.; Liberati, A.; Tetzlaff, J.; Altman, D.G.; The, P.G. Preferred Reporting Items for Systematic Reviews and Meta-Analyses: The PRISMA Statement. *PLoS Med.* **2009**, *6*, e1000097. [CrossRef] [PubMed]

15. Schulze, M.B.; Martínez-González, M.A.; Fung, T.T.; Lichtenstein, A.H.; Forouhi, N.G. Food based dietary patterns and chronic disease prevention. *BMJ* **2018**, *361*, k2396. [CrossRef]

16. NIH. Definitions of Health Terms: Nutrition. Available online: https://medlineplus.gov/definitions/nutritiondefinitions.html (accessed on 2 April 2020).

17. Studer, M.; Briel, M.; Leimenstoll, B.; Glass, T.R.; Bucher, H.C. Effect of different antilipidemic agents and diets on mortality: A systematic review. *Arch. Intern. Med.* **2005**, *165*, 725–730. [CrossRef] [PubMed]

18. Liyanage, T.; Ninomiya, T.; Wang, A.; Neal, B.; Jun, M.; Wong, M.G.; Jardine, M.; Hillis, G.S.; Perkovic, V. Effects of the Mediterranean Diet on Cardiovascular Outcomes-A Systematic Review and Meta-Analysis. *PLoS ONE* **2016**, *11*, e0159252. [CrossRef]

19. Semlitsch, T.; Jeitler, K.; Berghold, A.; Horvath, K.; Posch, N.; Poggenburg, S.; Siebenhofer, A. Long-term effects of weight-reducing diets in people with hypertension. *Cochrane Database Syst. Rev.* **2016**, *3*, Cd008274. [CrossRef]

20. Sofi, F.; Cesari, F.; Abbate, R.; Gensini, G.F.; Casini, A. Adherence to Mediterranean diet and health status: Meta-analysis. *BMJ* **2008**, *337*, a1344. [CrossRef]

21. Sofi, F.; Abbate, R.; Gensini, G.F.; Casini, A. Accruing evidence on benefits of adherence to the Mediterranean diet on health: An updated systematic review and meta-analysis. *Am. J. Clin. Nutr.* **2010**, *92*, 1189–1196. [CrossRef]

22. Grosso, G.; Marventano, S.; Yang, J.; Micek, A.; Pajak, A.; Scalfi, L.; Galvano, F.; Kales, S.N. A comprehensive meta-analysis on evidence of Mediterranean diet and cardiovascular disease: Are individual components equal? *Crit. Rev. Food Sci. Nutr.* **2017**, *57*, 3218–3232. [CrossRef] [PubMed]

23. Martinez-Gonzalez, M.A.; Bes-Rastrollo, M. Dietary patterns, Mediterranean diet, and cardiovascular disease. *Curr. Opin. Lipidol.* **2014**, *25*, 20–26. [CrossRef] [PubMed]

24. Rosato, V.; Temple, N.J.; La Vecchia, C.; Castellan, G.; Tavani, A.; Guercio, V. Mediterranean diet and cardiovascular disease: A systematic review and meta-analysis of observational studies. *Eur. J. Nutr.* **2019**, *58*, 173–191. [CrossRef] [PubMed]

25. Psaltopoulou, T.; Sergentanis, T.N.; Panagiotakos, D.B.; Sergentanis, I.N.; Kosti, R.; Scarmeas, N. Mediterranean diet, stroke, cognitive impairment, and depression: A meta-analysis. *Ann. Neurol.* **2013**, *74*, 580–591. [CrossRef]

26. Kontogianni, M.D.; Panagiotakos, D.B. Dietary patterns and stroke: A systematic review and re-meta-analysis. *Maturitas* **2014**, *79*, 41–47. [CrossRef]

27. Chen, G.C.; Neelakantan, N.; Martín-Calvo, N.; Koh, W.P.; Yuan, J.M.; Bonaccio, M.; Iacoviello, L.; Martínez-González, M.A.; Qin, L.Q.; van Dam, R.M. Adherence to the Mediterranean diet and risk of stroke and stroke subtypes. *Eur. J. Epidemiol.* **2019**, *34*, 337–349. [CrossRef]

28. Salehi-Abargouei, A.; Maghsoudi, Z.; Shirani, F.; Azadbakht, L. Effects of Dietary Approaches to Stop Hypertension (DASH)-style diet on fatal or nonfatal cardiovascular diseases-Incidence: A systematic review and meta-analysis on observational prospective studies. *Nutrition* **2013**, *29*, 611–618. [CrossRef]

29. Yang, Z.Q.; Yang, Z.; Duan, M.L. Dietary approach to stop hypertension diet and risk of coronary artery disease: A meta-analysis of prospective cohort studies. *Int. J. Food Sci. Nutr.* **2019**, *70*, 668–674. [CrossRef]

30. Feng, Q.; Fan, S.; Wu, Y.; Zhou, D.; Zhao, R.; Liu, M.; Song, Y. Adherence to the dietary approaches to stop hypertension diet and risk of stroke: A meta-analysis of prospective studies. *Medicine* **2018**, *97*. [CrossRef] [PubMed]

31. Onvani, S.; Haghighatdoost, F.; Surkan, P.J.; Larijani, B.; Azadbakht, L. Adherence to the Healthy Eating Index and Alternative Healthy Eating Index dietary patterns and mortality from all causes, cardiovascular disease and cancer: A meta-analysis of observational studies. *J. Hum. Nutr. Diet.* **2017**, *30*, 216–226. [CrossRef] [PubMed]

32. Schwingshackl, L.; Hoffmann, G. Diet quality as assessed by the Healthy Eating Index, the Alternate Healthy Eating Index, the Dietary Approaches to Stop Hypertension score, and health outcomes: A systematic review and meta-analysis of cohort studies. *J. Acad. Nutr. Diet.* **2015**, *115*, 780–800. [CrossRef] [PubMed]

33. Guo, L.; Zhang, S. Association between ideal cardiovascular health metrics and risk of cardiovascular events or mortality: A meta-analysis of prospective studies. *Clin. Cardiol.* **2017**, *40*, 1339–1346. [CrossRef] [PubMed]

34. Shivappa, N.; Godos, J.; Hébert, J.R.; Wirth, M.D.; Piuri, G.; Speciani, A.F.; Grosso, G. Dietary inflammatory index and cardiovascular risk and mortality—A meta-analysis. *Nutrients* **2018**, *10*, 200. [CrossRef] [PubMed]

35. Kwok, C.S.; Umar, S.; Myint, P.K.; Mamas, M.A.; Loke, Y.K. Vegetarian diet, Seventh Day Adventists and risk of cardiovascular mortality: A systematic review and meta-analysis. *Int. J. Cardiol.* **2014**, *176*, 680–686. [CrossRef]

36. Shao, C.; Tang, H.; Zhao, W.; He, J. Nut intake and stroke risk: A dose-response meta-analysis of prospective cohort studies. *Sci. Rep.* **2016**, *6*, 30394. [CrossRef]

37. Weng, Y.Q.; Yao, J.; Guo, M.L.; Qin, Q.J.; Li, P. Association between nut consumption and coronary heart disease: A meta-analysis. *Coron. Artery Dis.* **2016**, *27*, 227–232. [CrossRef]

38. Marventano, S.; Izquierdo Pulido, M.; Sanchez-Gonzalez, C.; Godos, J.; Speciani, A.; Galvano, F.; Grosso, G. Legume consumption and CVD risk: A systematic review and meta-analysis. *Public Health Nutr.* **2017**, *20*, 245–254. [CrossRef]

39. Wei, H.; Gao, Z.; Liang, R.; Li, Z.; Hao, H.; Liu, X. Whole-grain consumption and the risk of all-cause, CVD and cancer mortality: A meta-analysis of prospective cohort studies. *Br. J. Nutr.* **2016**, *116*, 514–525. [CrossRef]

40. Reynolds, A.; Mann, J.; Cummings, J.; Winter, N.; Mete, E.; Te Morenga, L. Carbohydrate quality and human health: A series of systematic reviews and meta-analyses. *Lancet* **2019**, *393*, 434–445. [CrossRef]

41. Whelton, S.P.; He, J.; Whelton, P.K.; Muntner, P. Meta-analysis of observational studies on fish intake and coronary heart disease. *Am. J. Cardiol.* **2004**, *93*, 1119–1123. [CrossRef]

42. Martinez-Gonzalez, M.A.; Dominguez, L.J.; Delgado-Rodriguez, M. Olive oil consumption and risk of CHD and/or stroke: A meta-analysis of case-control, cohort and intervention studies. *Br. J. Nutr.* **2014**, *112*, 248–259. [CrossRef] [PubMed]

43. Yuan, S.; Li, X.; Jin, Y.; Lu, J. Chocolate consumption and risk of coronary heart disease, stroke, and diabetes: A meta-analysis of prospective studies. *Nutrients* **2017**, *9*, 688. [CrossRef]

44. Kwok, C.S.; Boekholdt, S.M.; Lentjes, M.A.; Loke, Y.K.; Luben, R.N.; Yeong, J.K.; Wareham, N.J.; Myint, P.K.; Khaw, K.T. Habitual chocolate consumption and risk of cardiovascular disease among healthy men and women. *Heart* **2015**, *101*, 1279–1287. [CrossRef] [PubMed]

45. Crippa, A.; Discacciati, A.; Larsson, S.C.; Wolk, A.; Orsini, N. Coffee consumption and mortality from all causes, cardiovascular disease, and cancer: A dose-response meta-analysis. *Am. J. Epidemiol.* **2014**, *180*, 763–775. [CrossRef] [PubMed]

46. Pang, J.; Zhang, Z.; Zheng, T.Z.; Bassig, B.A.; Mao, C.; Liu, X.; Zhu, Y.; Shi, K.; Ge, J.; Yang, Y.J.; et al. Green tea consumption and risk of cardiovascular and ischemic related diseases: A meta-analysis. *Int. J. Cardiol.* **2016**, *202*, 967–974. [CrossRef] [PubMed]

47. Harcombe, Z.; Baker, J.S.; Davies, B. Evidence from prospective cohort studies does not support current dietary fat guidelines: A systematic review and meta-analysis. *Br. J. Sports Med.* **2017**, *51*, 1743–1749. [CrossRef]

48. Harcombe, Z.; Baker, J.S.; DiNicolantonio, J.J.; Grace, F.; Davies, B. Evidence from randomised controlled trials does not support current dietary fat guidelines: A systematic review and meta-analysis. *Open Heart* **2016**, *3*, e000409. [CrossRef]

49. Hooper, L.; Summerbell, C.D.; Higgins, J.P.; Thompson, R.L.; Clements, G.; Capps, N.; Davey, S.; Riemersma, R.A.; Ebrahim, S. Reduced or modified dietary fat for preventing cardiovascular disease. *Cochrane Database Syst. Rev.* **2001**, Cd002137. [CrossRef]

50. Muto, M.; Ezaki, O. High dietary saturated fat is associated with a low risk of intracerebral hemorrhage and ischemic stroke in japanese but not in non-Japanese: A review and meta-analysis of prospective cohort studies. *J. Atheroscler. Thromb.* **2018**, *25*, 375–392. [CrossRef]

51. Schwingshackl, L.; Hoffmann, G. Monounsaturated fatty acids, olive oil and health status: A systematic review and meta-analysis of cohort studies. *Lipids Health Dis.* **2014**, *13*, 154. [CrossRef]

52. Delgado-Lista, J.; Perez-Martinez, P.; Lopez-Miranda, J.; Perez-Jimenez, F. Long chain omega-3 fatty acids and cardiovascular disease: A systematic review. *Br. J. Nutr.* **2012**, *107*, S201–S213. [CrossRef] [PubMed]

53. Abdelhamid, A.S.; Brown, T.J.; Brainard, J.S.; Biswas, P.; Thorpe, G.C.; Moore, H.J.; Deane, K.H.; Summerbell, C.D.; Worthington, H.V.; Song, F.; et al. Omega-3 fatty acids for the primary and secondary prevention of cardiovascular disease. *Cochrane Database Syst. Rev.* **2020**, *3*, Cd003177. [CrossRef] [PubMed]

54. Mozaffarian, D.; Micha, R.; Wallace, S. Effects on coronary heart disease of increasing polyunsaturated fat in place of saturated fat: A systematic review and meta-analysis of randomized controlled trials. *PLoS Med.* **2010**, *7*. [CrossRef]

55. Li, M.; Cui, F.; Yang, F.; Huang, X. Association between fiber intake and ischemic stroke risk: A meta-analysis of prospective studies. *Int. J. Clin. Exp. Med.* **2017**, *10*, 4659–4668.

56. Adler, A.J.; Taylor, F.; Martin, N.; Gottlieb, S.; Taylor, R.S.; Ebrahim, S. Reduced dietary salt for the prevention of cardiovascular disease. *Cochrane Database Syst. Rev.* **2014**, Cd009217. [CrossRef] [PubMed]

57. Aburto, N.J.; Ziolkovska, A.; Hooper, L.; Elliott, P.; Cappuccio, F.P.; Meerpohl, J.J. Effect of lower sodium intake on health: Systematic review and meta-analyses. *BMJ* **2013**, *346*, f1326. [CrossRef]

58. Jayedi, A.; Ghomashi, F.; Zargar, M.S.; Shab-Bidar, S. Dietary sodium, sodium-to-potassium ratio, and risk of stroke: A systematic review and nonlinear dose-response meta-analysis. *Clin. Nutr.* **2019**, *38*, 1092–1100. [CrossRef]

59. Kim, Y.; Je, Y. Flavonoid intake and mortality from cardiovascular disease and all causes: A meta-analysis of prospective cohort studies. *Clin. Nutr. ESPEN* **2017**, *20*, 68–77. [CrossRef]

60. Hollman, P.C.; Geelen, A.; Kromhout, D. Dietary flavonol intake may lower stroke risk in men and women. *J. Nutr.* **2010**, *140*, 600–604. [CrossRef]

61. Kimble, R.; Keane, K.M.; Lodge, J.K.; Howatson, G. Dietary intake of anthocyanins and risk of cardiovascular disease: A systematic review and meta-analysis of prospective cohort studies. *Crit. Rev. Food Sci. Nutr.* **2019**, *59*, 3032–3043. [CrossRef]

62. D'Elia, L.; Barba, G.; Cappuccio, F.P.; Strazzullo, P. Potassium intake, stroke, and cardiovascular disease: A meta-analysis of prospective studies. *J. Am. Coll. Cardiol.* **2011**, *57*, 1210–1219. [CrossRef] [PubMed]

63. Wang, X.; Chen, H.; Ouyang, Y.; Liu, J.; Zhao, G.; Bao, W.; Yan, M. Dietary calcium intake and mortality risk from cardiovascular disease and all causes: A meta-analysis of prospective cohort studies. *BMC Med.* **2014**, *12*, 1–10. [CrossRef] [PubMed]

64. Arnett, D.K.; Blumenthal, R.S.; Albert, M.A.; Buroker, A.B.; Goldberger, Z.D.; Hahn, E.J.; Himmelfarb, C.D.; Khera, A.; Lloyd-Jones, D.; McEvoy, J.W.; et al. 2019 ACC/AHA Guideline on the Primary Prevention of Cardiovascular Disease. *J. Am. Coll. Cardiol.* **2019**, *74*, e177. [CrossRef] [PubMed]

65. Cespedes, E.M.; Hu, F.B. Dietary patterns: From nutritional epidemiologic analysis to national guidelines. *Am. J. Clin. Nutr.* **2015**, *101*, 899–900. [CrossRef]

66. Li, Y.; Hruby, A.; Bernstein, A.M.; Ley, S.H.; Wang, D.D.; Chiuve, S.E.; Sampson, L.; Rexrode, K.M.; Rimm, E.B.; Willett, W.C.; et al. Saturated Fats Compared With Unsaturated Fats and Sources of Carbohydrates in Relation to Risk of Coronary Heart Disease: A Prospective Cohort Study. *J. Am. Coll. Cardiol.* **2015**, *66*, 1538–1548. [CrossRef]

67. Yang, Q.; Zhang, Z.; Gregg, E.W.; Flanders, W.D.; Merritt, R.; Hu, F.B. Added sugar intake and cardiovascular diseases mortality among US adults. *JAMA Intern. Med.* **2014**, *174*, 516–524. [CrossRef]

68. Jacobs, D.R.; Tapsell, L.C.; Temple, N.J. Food Synergy: The Key to Balancing the Nutrition Research Effort. *Public Health Rev.* **2011**, *33*, 507–529. [CrossRef]

69. Martinez-Gonzalez, M.A.; Gea, A.; Ruiz-Canela, M. The Mediterranean Diet and Cardiovascular Health. *Circ. Res.* **2019**, *124*, 779–798. [CrossRef]

70. Bhatt, D.L.; Steg, P.G.; Miller, M.; Brinton, E.A.; Jacobson, T.A.; Ketchum, S.B.; Doyle, R.T.; Juliano, R.A.; Jiao, L.; Granowitz, C.; et al. Cardiovascular Risk Reduction with Icosapent Ethyl for Hypertriglyceridemia. *N. Engl. J. Med.* **2018**, *380*, 11–22. [CrossRef]

71. Guo, X.; Tresserra-Rimbau, A.; Estruch, R.; Martinez-Gonzalez, M.A.; Medina-Remon, A.; Castaner, O.; Corella, D.; Salas-Salvado, J.; Lamuela-Raventos, R.M. Effects of Polyphenol, Measured by a Biomarker of Total Polyphenols in Urine, on Cardiovascular Risk Factors After a Long-Term Follow-Up in the PREDIMED Study. *Oxidative Med. Cell. Longev.* **2016**, *2016*, 2572606. [CrossRef]

72. Estruch, R.; Ros, E.; Salas-Salvado, J.; Covas, M.I.; Corella, D.; Aros, F.; Gomez-Gracia, E.; Ruiz-Gutierrez, V.; Fiol, M.; Lapetra, J.; et al. Primary Prevention of Cardiovascular Disease with a Mediterranean Diet Supplemented with Extra-Virgin Olive Oil or Nuts. *N. Engl. J. Med.* **2018**, *378*, e34. [CrossRef] [PubMed]

73. Guasch-Ferre, M.; Hu, F.B.; Martinez-Gonzalez, M.A.; Fito, M.; Bullo, M.; Estruch, R.; Ros, E.; Corella, D.; Recondo, J.; Gomez-Gracia, E.; et al. Olive oil intake and risk of cardiovascular disease and mortality in the PREDIMED Study. *BMC Med.* **2014**, *12*, 78. [CrossRef] [PubMed]

74. Okada, E.; Nakamura, K.; Ukawa, S.; Wakai, K.; Date, C.; Iso, H.; Tamakoshi, A. The Japanese food score and risk of all-cause, CVD and cancer mortality: The Japan Collaborative Cohort Study. *Br. J. Nutr.* **2018**, *120*, 464–471. [CrossRef] [PubMed]

75. Tapsell, L.C.; Neale, E.P.; Satija, A.; Hu, F.B. Foods, Nutrients, and Dietary Patterns: Interconnections and Implications for Dietary Guidelines. *Adv. Nutr.* **2016**, *7*, 445–454. [CrossRef]

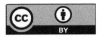

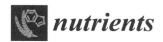

Article

The Effect of Low-Carbohydrate Diet on Macrovascular and Microvascular Endothelial Function is Not Affected by the Provision of Caloric Restriction in Women with Obesity: A Randomized Study

Chueh-Lung Hwang [1], Christine Ranieri [1], Mary R. Szczurek [1], Assem M. Ellythy [1], Ahmed Elokda [2], Abeer M. Mahmoud [1,3] and Shane A. Phillips [1,*]

[1] Department of Physical Therapy, University of Illinois at Chicago, Chicago, IL 60612, USA; clhwang@uic.edu (C.-L.H); christineranieri@gmail.com (C.R.); mszczurek89@gmail.com (M.R.S.); aellyt2@uic.edu (A.M.E.); amahmo4@uic.edu (A.M.M.)

[2] Department of Rehabilitation Sciences, Florida Gulf Coast University, Fort Myers, FL 33965, USA; aelokda@fgcu.edu

[3] Department of Medicine, Division of Endocrinology, Diabetes, and Metabolism, University of Illinois at Chicago, Chicago, IL 60612, USA

* Correspondence: shanep@uic.edu; Tel.: +1-312-355-0277

Received: 18 April 2020; Accepted: 29 May 2020; Published: 2 June 2020

Abstract: Obesity impairs both macro- and microvascular endothelial function due to decreased bioavailability of nitric oxide. Current evidence on the effect of low-carbohydrate (LC) diet on endothelial function is conflicting and confounded by the provision of caloric restriction (CR). We tested the hypothesis that LC without CR diet, but not LC with CR diet, would improve macro- and microvascular endothelial function in women with obesity. Twenty-one healthy women with obesity (age: 33 ± 2 years, body mass index: 33.0 ± 0.6 kg/m^2; mean ± SEM) were randomly assigned to receive either a LC diet (~10% carbohydrate calories) with CR (n = 12; 500 calorie/day deficit) or a LC diet without CR (n = 9) and completed the 6-week diet intervention. After the intervention, macrovascular endothelial function, measured as brachial artery flow-mediated dilation did not change (7.3 ± 0.9% to 8.0 ± 1.1%, p = 0.7). On the other hand, following the LC diet intervention, regardless of CR, blocking nitric oxide production decreased microvascular endothelial function, measured by arteriolar flow-induced dilation ($p \leq 0.02$ for both diets) and the magnitude was more than baseline ($p \leq 0.04$). These data suggest improved NO contributions following the intervention. In conclusion, a 6-week LC diet; regardless of CR, may improve microvascular, but not macrovascular endothelial function, via increasing bioavailability of nitric oxide in women with obesity.

Keywords: low-carbohydrate diet; hypocaloric; isocaloric; women health; obesity; conduit artery; microvasculature; nitric oxide; cardiovascular risks; primary prevention

1. Introduction

Over the past decades, obesity rates are increasing in the United States with more than 1 in 3 adults having obesity [1]. Obesity is associated with several adverse health conditions including hypertension, dyslipidemia, and hyperglycemia [2]. These metabolic abnormalities combined with obesity triple the risks of cardiovascular disease [3], which remains the leading cause of death in the United States [4]. The number of men and women with obesity are similar, but the prevalence of morbid obesity (body mass index, BMI ≥ 40 kg/m^2) among women is reported to be almost twice

Nutrients **2020**, *12*, 1649; doi:10.3390/nu12061649   www.mdpi.com/journal/nutrients

as high as the prevalence among men [1]. Therefore, early intervention for young and middle-aged women is important to decrease the severity of obesity and prevent cardiovascular disease.

The critical site of arteriosclerosis development and the progression to cardiovascular disease is endothelium [5]. Endothelium is a single layer of endothelial cells that form the most inner layer of every blood vessel of the circulation. It synthesizes and releases several vasodilators and vasoconstrictors and plays a key role in controlling vascular tone and maintaining vascular homeostasis. Nitric oxide (NO) is a potent vasodilator synthesized by the endothelium. Decreases in NO bioavailability due to endothelial dysfunction causes impaired endothelium-dependent vasodilation [6]. Assessments of endothelium-dependent vasodilation in peripheral blood vessels have been widely used as surrogate markers of cardiovascular disease risks. The peripheral blood vessels refer to all blood vessels external to the heart and includes the macrovasculature (4 to 25 mm in diameter) and microvasculature (arterioles < 150 μm in diameter). The function and structure of these vasculatures are different: The macrovasculature buffers the increases in blood flow pulsatility, preventing tissue injury, and distributes blood to the body, whereas the microvasculature regulates vascular tone/resistance and blood pressure. In adults with obesity, endothelium-dependent vasodilation in both macro- and micro-vasculature are impaired [7,8].

A low-carbohydrates (LC) diet has been shown to improve glucose control in adults with obesity [9–16]. However, the effect of LC diet on endothelial function in adults with obesity is not clear with conflicting data, showing either no changes [9,10,12–14], increases [17], or even decreases in endothelial function following LC diet [11,15,16]. The conflicting results may be due to the heterogeneity in subject characteristics, LC diet interventions (e.g., % energy restriction, % carbohydrate restriction, fat content, and dietary sources), and experimental designs (e.g., single group or randomized controlled study). One of the potential confounders is the provision of caloric restriction (CR; 20–30% daily energy restriction or 400–800 kcal/day deficit). For studies examining the effect of CR diet without modifications in nutrition components, some found that CR improves both macrovascular and microvascular endothelial function [18–20], while others showed that CR does not have beneficial effects on macrovascular endothelial function [21–23]. In addition, many of the previous studies examining the effect of LC diet focused on macrovascular endothelial function. The effect of LC diet on microvascular endothelial function is lacking and may be different from macrovascular endothelial function [14,24].

Therefore, to isolate the effect of LC diet and its effect on different vasculatures, we conducted a randomized parallel design clinical trial in young and middle-aged women with obesity. We compared the effect of LC diet with vs. without CR on macro- and microvascular endothelial function. We hypothesized that LC without CR diet, but not LC with CR diet, would improve macro- and microvascular endothelial function in this population.

2. Materials and Methods

2.1. Study Design

A prospective randomized parallel design clinical trial was conducted at the Clinical Research Center, at the University of Illinois at Chicago. Subjects were recruited from university campuses and local health clubs via notices posted on bulletin boards and in newsletters. Subjects were also recruited via Craigslist. After informed consent was obtained, participants completed a screening visit to determine qualification using physical examination, self-reported medical history, blood analysis including metabolic panel, lipid profile, insulin, and thyroid function test, and urine pregnancy test. Participants who met the inclusion criteria were enrolled by our research coordinator and were randomized to either a LC with CR diet or LC without CR diet (Figure 1). Macro- and microvascular endothelial function (primary outcomes) as well as cardiovascular risks (secondary outcomes) were assessed before and after the 6-week diet intervention. Data analyses were completed by researchers blinded to the participant diet assignment. Participants were instructed to continue their usual physical activity and received a pedometer (T5E011, Timex Group USA, Inc., Middlebury, CT, USA) to monitor their daily walking activity during the intervention. The average of 7-day step counts was calculated every 2 weeks. Two participants in LC without CR group did not have pedometer record.

The study was approved by the institutional review board of the University of Illinois at Chicago and complied with the Declaration of Helsinki. Written informed consent was obtained from all study participants.

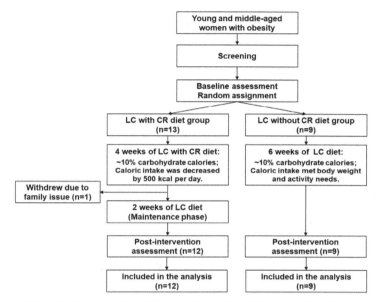

Figure 1. Study flow chart. CR = caloric restriction; LC = low-carbohydrate.

2.2. Study Participants

Apparently healthy women aged between 18 to 50 years, not currently on a diet, and with BMI of 29.0–39.9 kg/m^2 were included in this study. Participants were excluded if they had any one of the following: (1) Inability to give informed consent; (2) no willingness to commit to the LC diet intervention; (3) history of cardiovascular disease or cardiovascular events, diabetes, renal or liver diseases; (4) hypertension (systolic > 160 mmHg and diastolic > 90 mmHg) or use of a antihypertensive drug; (5) history of head injury (past 6 months), seizure disorder, pituitary tumor or thyroid disease; (6) history of gout; (7) glaucoma or adverse reaction to nitroglycerin, lidocaine allergy, or anemia; (8) history of tobacco use (past 6 months), currently abusing alcohol or illicit drugs; (9) a diagnosis of eating disorder, current use of diet pills, history of diet (past 1 month), or current use of antioxidant supplements; (10) prior weight loss surgery (any type); (11) pregnancy (or intend to become pregnant while participating in trial), nursing, or amenorrhea.

2.3. Low-Carbohydrate Diet Intervention

All participants received a custom made individualized 6-week LC diet (10% carbohydrate, 60–62% fat, 28–30% protein). Daily caloric intake was determined by the Mifflin equation for women [25,26] as following: Planned daily caloric intake = Resting energy expenditure (REE) × Physical activity factor, where REE = (10 × body weight (kg)) + (6.25 × body height (cm)) − (5 × age (years)) − 161, and activity factor = 1.2 for sedentary (little or no exercise), 1.375 for lightly active (light exercise, 1–3 days/week), and 1.550 for moderately active (moderate exercise, 3–5 days/week). The factor was determined based on self-reported physical activity. For CR group, participants had a caloric deficit by 500 calories/day less than their calculated values during the first 4 weeks, and then the regular calculated values during the last 2 weeks of the study (Figure 1). The maintenance phase was designed in order to prevent further changes in body weight, which may confound the measurement of endothelial function when individuals are actively losing weight.

To ensure compliance to the diet, all participants were provided the meals for their appropriate diet regime for the entire intervention ranging from 40–51 days until the post-intervention assessments were completed. Meals were delivered to or picked up by participants, 3 times/week. Before the intervention, participants met with the bionutritionist to discuss the diet design. A three-day dietary record was used to determine their usual dietary patterns. In addition, a food preference questionnaire was completed to help plan the diet menus. All meals were prepared by the same bionutritionist, with moderate additions of salt, pepper, dried herbs, and spices for palatability. The major source of protein was from animals. Participants could consume unlimited water and zero-calorie beverages, however, with caffeinated coffee limited to 16 oz/day and diet soda and caffeinated tea limited to 20 oz/day. Participants also received daily multivitamin tablets.

Participants were asked to provide daily food diary and document any deviation from the provided meals. Any leftover food was returned and collected from the participants to ensure accuracy of calculating actual dietary intake. Every 2 weeks, participants met with the bionutritionist to discuss any problems (such as nausea, dizziness, constipation, lethargy, dehydration, bad breath, and loss of appetite) or concerns of adhering to the diet and to test their urine ketone levels. During the week 4, caloric intake was re-calculated for LC with CR diet group and diet modifications were discussed with participants for the final 2 weeks. Dietary intake and nutrients were analyzed using DietMaster Pro V11 (Lifestyles Technologies, Inc., Grants Pass, OR, USA).

2.4. Randomization

The table of random numbers was created by a statistician using a computer-generated random stratified sequence to ensure a balanced ethnic/racial composition within each group. Participants were assigned to the intervention by a staff member who did not know participant's baseline profile.

2.5. Study Procedures

The following procedures were performed in the morning, after a 12-h fast with no caffeine, alcohol, and medication use. Participants were also instructed not to exercise at least 12 h prior to the visits.

2.5.1. Macrovascular Endothelial Function

As previously described [27], flow-mediated dilation (FMD), a measure of endothelium-dependent vasodilation [28], was assessed non-invasively using brachial artery diameter in response to increases in blood flow followed by a transient period of ischemia. Briefly, participants rested in a supine position for at least 15 min, in a quiet, darken, and temperature-controlled room. Imaging of the brachial artery was taken via a 11mHz transducer and the MicroMaxx ultrasound machine (SonoSite, Seattle, WA, USA). The probe was placed ~5 cm above the antecubital fossa of the right arm, abducted ~80 away from the body. Blood flow velocity was determined via a continuous wave Doppler with an insonation of 60. After a 1-min baseline imaging period, Doppler readings of peak flow were recorded for at least 5 s. Then a blood pressure cuff placed on the forearm (distal to the antecubital fossa and right next to the antecubital crease) was inflated to >50 mmHg above supine systolic blood pressure for 5 min. After the cuff release, Doppler readings of peak flow were recorded for the first 10 s. Then, brachial artery was imaged continuously to capture diameter at 30 s, 1 min, 2 min, and 3 min after the cuff release. After 10 min following the release of the cuff, nitroglycerin (NTG)-mediated dilation, independent of endothelial function, was measured as previously described [27]. Briefly, imaging of the brachial artery was taken for 1 min before and for 5 min after the administration of 0.5 mg of NTG sublingually. Along with NTG-mediated dilation, FMD is the gold standard measure of macrovascular endothelial function.

All images were digitally recorded and transferred to Brachial Imager (Medical Imaging, Iowa City, IA, USA) for analyzing the brachial artery diameter. For each baseline and time point, ~75 frames (7.5 frames per second for 10 s) were analyzed to calculate the average of the continuous diameters over the entire cardiac cycle. Both FMD and NTG-mediated dilation were calculated as the percentage of the maximal change after cuff release or NTG administration using the following equation: %change = (peak diameter − baseline diameter)/(baseline diameter) × 100%. The peak flow velocity was measured by analyzing 5 s for baseline and 10 s following the release of the cuff. Shear rate was calculated as blood velocity divided by brachial diameter. To assess NO bioavailability, serum nitrates and nitrites (NOx) levels, a surrogate marker of NO levels, were assessed using commercially available kits following the manufactory guideline (Cayman Chemicals, Ann Arbor, MI, USA).

2.5.2. Microvascular Endothelial Function

As previously described [29], microvascular endothelial function was assessed using flow-induced dilation (FID) in arterioles isolated from subcutaneous adipose tissue of participants. Briefly, participants received subcutaneous fat biopsy with sterile techniques performed by a trained clinician. A small fat biopsy was obtained just underneath the skin of the gluteal region. The skin was locally anesthetized with lidocaine. A small incision (~1 cm) was made to expose the subcutaneous fat and approximately 1 mL of fat tissue was removed by sharp dissection. The incision was closed with Steristrips and covered with a waterproof clear bandage. The fat tissue then was transferred to the HEPES solution (pH= ~7.4 and 4 C). Due to the invasive nature of this procedure, we obtained both baseline and week 6-tissues in a total of 13 participants (LC without CR diet: $n = 5$ and LC with CR diet: $n = 8$).

Adipose arterioles were isolated from the fat tissue and cannulated with glass micropipettes in an organ perfusion chamber. The chamber was circulated with physiological salt solution (pH = ~7.4) using a peristaltic pump and bubbled with air (5% CO_2 and 21% O_2) at a temperature of 37 °C. Following a 30-min pressurization at 60 cm H_2O, arterial diameter was measured at baseline, following a pre-constriction with endothelial-1 (100 to 200 pM), and during intraluminal flow corresponding to pressure gradients of $\Delta10$–$\Delta100$ cm H_2O (5 min each) via an inverted microscope attached to a video monitor and a video-measuring device (model VIA-100; Boeckeler). Vessels were discarded when the pre-constriction with endothelial-1 was less than 30% of baseline diameter. FID at each pressure gradient was calculated as the percentage change using the following equation: %change = (diameter measured for each pressure gradient − pre-constricted diameter by endothelin-1)/(baseline diameter − pre-constricted diameter by endothelin-1) × 100%. At the end of each protocol, endothelium-independent vasodilation was induced by papaverine (10^{-4} M). This protocol was repeated in the presence of the endothelial NO synthase inhibitor (L-NAME, 10^{-4} M) to determine the contribution of NO in FID.

2.5.3. Cardiovascular Risks

Body composition was assessed using a Hologic QDR-4500 fan-beam DXA scanner (Hologic Inc., Bedford, MA, USA). Also measured, were body weight, height (for calculating BMI), and waist and hip circumferences. Venous blood samples were drawn from the arm by trained clinicians into serum tubes and ethylenediaminetetraacetic acid-containing tubes. Fasting blood lipids, insulin, and glucose were analyzed by Alverno Clinical Laboratories (Hammoond, IN, USA). The homeostasis model assessment of insulin resistance (HOMA-IR) was calculated to assess insulin resistance. Seated blood pressure was measured after a 5-min rest using a stethoscope and a blood pressure cuff with a sphygmomanometer. The assessment of cardiovascular risks was repeated at the end of week 4 (except 1 participant in LC with diet and 1 in LC without diet group did not receive blood draw).

2.6. Statistical Analysis

Data are presented as mean ± SEM or n (%). Statistical analyses were performed based on the original diet assignment using IBM SPSS Statistics (Version 24, Chicago, IL, USA). Statistical significance was set at $\alpha = 0.05$. To examine baseline differences between groups (LC with CR diet vs. LC without CR diet), independent *t*-test and $\chi2$ were used for continuous and categorical variables, respectively, except that between-group differences in baseline FID was examined using a two-way (2×5) mixed ANOVA with a between-subject factor (LC with CR diet vs. LC without CR diet) and a within-subject factor (pressure gradients of $\Delta 10$–$\Delta 100$ cm H_2O). To examine dietary intake during the intervention between two groups, independent *t*-test was used. To examine physical activity changes between groups during the intervention, a two-way (2×4) mixed ANOVA was used with group as a between subject factor (LC with CR diet vs. LC without CR diet) and time as a within subject factor (baseline, 2 weeks, 4 weeks, and 6 weeks after the intervention). Main effect of time and group were examined separately if no interaction was found and Bonferroni post hoc pairwise comparisons were performed to examine physical activity between each time point in all participants.

To examine the effect of the LC diet with vs. without CR on macrovascular function and cardiovascular risks, a two-way (2×2) mixed ANOVA was used with group as a between subject factor (LC with CR diet vs. LC without CR diet) and time as a within subject factor (baseline and 6 weeks after the intervention). For cardiovascular risks, the two-way mixed ANOVA was repeated with time as a within subject factor (baseline and 4 weeks after the intervention). When the interaction between the two factors was significant, then Bonferroni post hoc pairwise comparisons were performed. Main effect of time and group were examined separately if no interaction was found.

To examine whether FID changed after the 6-week of intervention within each group (LC without CR diet and LC with CR diet), main effect of time was examined by using a two-way (2×5) repeated-measures ANOVA with two within-subject factors: (1) Timing of measurement: baseline and 6 weeks after the intervention and (2) pressure gradients of $\Delta 10$–$\Delta 100$ cm H_2O. To examine the effect of LNAME on FID at each timepoint (baseline and 6 weeks after the intervention) within each group, main effect of condition (presence or absence of LNAME) was examined by using a two-way repeated-measures ANOVA with two within-subject factors: (1) Presence or absence of LNAME and (2) pressure gradients of $\Delta 10$–$\Delta 100$ cm H_2O.

3. Results

3.1. Dietary Intake and Physical Activity

A total of 21 women (age: 33 ± 2 years and BMI: 33.0 ± 0.6 Kg/m^2) completed the intervention and were included in this study (Figure 1). One participant withdrew from the study due to a death in the family. Overall, participants enjoyed LC diet with good and normal appetite. No serious adverse event was observed. Participants in LC without CR group reported hunger (7.9%), bloating or too much food (3.5%), stomach problems (1.1%), no appetite (0.5%), and nausea (0.2%). In LC with CR group, participants reported hunger (5.9%), loss of appetite or too much food (1.1%), illness or nausea (0.9%), and stomach problems (0.2%).

Caloric intake and dietary composition were not different between groups at baseline (mean for all participants: 2015 ± 101 kcal/day; 44.5 ± 1.4% from carbohydrate, 35.3 ± 2.2% from fat, and 18.4 ± 1.3% from protein; $p \geq 0.4$; Table 1). During the intervention, actual caloric intake in LC without CR group was not different from the baseline value ($p = 0.4$) but less than the planned value ($p = 0.007$; Table 1). The latter caused a lower compliance in LC without CR group vs. LC with CR group (Table 1). However, LC without CR group still consumed more calories than LC with CR group during the 6-week intervention ($p = 0.03$) and no difference was found in the percent energy from carbohydrate, fat, and protein ($p \geq 0.1$; Table 1). Positive urine ketone levels were noted in seven out of the 21 participants at the end of week 2, eight participants at the week 4, and six participants at the week 6 ($p \geq 0.2$ for comparing the number of participants between LC with CR diet vs. LC without CR diet).

Compared to the baseline, physical activity, measured by steps per day, significantly increased in all participants at the end of week 2 and week 4 ($p = 0.01$ for both; Table 1). At the end of week 6, although physical activity was not statistically significant compared to baseline ($p = 0.1$; Table 1), five out of seven participants in LC without CR group (data missing in two participants) and eight out of 12 participants in LC with CR group showed an increase in their daily steps ranging from 368 to 6964 steps/day.

Table 1. Dietary intake and physical activity at baseline and during the 6-week low carbohydrate diet intervention.

	LC without CR Diet (n = 9)	LC with CR Diet (n = 12)	P Between-Groups
Baseline dietary intake			
Caloric intake, kcal/day	1993 ± 109	2032 ± 161	0.9
Carbohydrate, %kcal	45.8 ± 2.4	43.5 ± 1.7	0.4
Fat, %kcal	33.7 ± 3.4	36.6 ± 2.9	0.5
Protein, %kcal	18.3 ± 2.5	18.5 ± 1.3	0.95
Planned/provided diet			
Caloric intake (6 weeks), kcal/day	2328 ± 129	1782 ± 42	<0.0005
Caloric intake (Week 1–4), kcal/day	-	1616 ± 46	-
Caloric intake (Week 5–6), kcal/day	-	2163 ± 57	-
Carbohydrate, %kcal	10		-
Fat, %kcal	60–62		-
Protein, %kcal	28–30		-
Actual dietary intake			
Caloric intake (6 weeks), kcal/day	2090 ± 132	1724 ± 43	0.03
Caloric intake (Week 1–4), kcal/day	-	1596 ± 59	-
Caloric intake (Week 5–6), kcal/day	-	2054 ± 55	-
Compliance, %	89.9 ± 2.9	96.8 ± 1.7 *	0.04
Carbohydrate, %kcal	10.3 ± 0.3	10.9 ± 0.4	0.5
Fat, %kcal	60.4 ± 0.3	59.9 ± 0.3	0.3
Protein, %kcal	29.3 ± 2.8	28.7 ± 0.3	0.1
Dietary fiber, g	24.0 ± 1.7	19.4 ± 1.0 *	0.03
Folate/Folic acid, mcg	141.2 ± 10.7	122.9 ± 7.0	0.2
Vitamin C, mg	80.2 ± 4.8	78.2 ± 3.5	0.8
Sodium, mg	3292 ± 195	2924 ± 86	0.1
Potassium, mg	2184 ± 342	2101 ± 226	0.8
Physical activity-step counts			0.3
Baseline, steps/day	5924 ± 813	5587 ± 702	
Week 2, steps/day	8787 ± 1002	6552 ± 797	
Week 4, steps/day	8622 ± 1251	6943 ± 855	
Week 6, steps/day	7887 ± 1342	6868 ± 835	

Data are mean ± SEM. CR = calories restriction; LC = low carbohydrate. * $p < 0.05$ vs. LC without CR diet.

3.2. Participant Characteristics and Baseline Values

No baseline differences were found between LC without CR and LC with CR groups in participant characteristics and cardiovascular risks ($p \geq 0.1$; Table 2). Baseline FMD, NTG-mediated dilation, and FID were not different between the two groups ($p \geq 0.1$; Table 3 and Figure 2A,B). L-NAME did not change baseline FID in LC without CR group ($p = 0.4$; Figure 2A). In LC with CR group, L-NAME decreased overall baseline FID by 6% ($p = 0.003$; Figure 2B).

Table 2. Participant characteristics and cardiovascular risks in response to the 6-week low carbohydrate diet intervention.

	LC without CR Diet (n = 9)			LC with CR Diet (n = 12)		
	Baseline	Week 4	Week 6	Baseline	Week 4	Week 6
Age, year		33 ± 3			32 ± 2	
Race						
Caucasian, n		4 (44)			5 (42)	
African American, n		3 (33)			4 (33)	
Hispanic, n		1 (11)			2 (17)	
Asian, n		1 (11)			1 (8)	
Body weight, kg [b]	89.1 ± 4.6	85.7 ± 5.2 *	85.6 ± 4.5	90.0 ± 3.8	86.5 ± 3.9 *	87.5 ± 4.3
BMI, kg/m^2 [a,b]	33.5 ± 1.0	32.8 ± 1.1	32.3 ± 0.9	32.6 ± 0.8	31.2 ± 0.9	31.7 ± 0.9
Waist circumference, cm	96.1 ± 3.0	92.7 ± 3.3	92.2 ± 2.9	95.5 ± 2.7	93.6 ± 3.1	93.1 ± 3.2
Waist-to-hip ratio	0.88 ± 0.07	0.84 ± 0.05	0.84 ± 0.04	0.85 ± 0.02	0.81 ± 0.02	0.79 ± 0.03
Body fat, % [b]	44.5 ± 0.7	44.1 ± 1.3	43.4 ± 0.9	43.7 ± 0.9	43.9 ± 1.1	42.5 ± 1.0
SBP, mmHg	115 ± 2	113 ± 3	115 ± 4	118 ± 5	112 ± 4	112 ± 3
DBP, mmHg [b]	70 ± 1	68 ± 3	68 ± 2	72 ± 4	70 ± 3	67 ± 3
Total cholesterol, mg/dL	180 ± 14	194 ± 15	190 ± 14	185 ± 7	181 ± 8	182 ± 7
LDL cholesterol, mg/dL	106 ± 10	121 ± 12	117 ± 12	104 ± 7	110 ± 8	110 ± 7
HDL cholesterol, mg/dL	51 ± 4	56 ± 3	55 ± 3	60 ± 4	56 ± 3	58 ± 3
Triglycerides, mg/Dl [a,b]	116 ± 23	92 ± 15	85 ± 13	104 ± 21	72 ± 6	71 ± 6
Glucose, mg/dL	89 ± 3	93 ± 3	91 ± 4	93 ± 4	89 ± 4	87 ± 3
Insulin, μU/mL	13.9 ± 2.6	12.5 ± 2.4	12.3 ± 1.7	13.5 ± 2.4	10.2 ± 2.2	11.8 ± 3
HOMA-IR	3.0 ± 0.6	3.0 ± 0.6	2.8 ± 0.4	3.2 ± 0.7	2.4 ± 0.6	2.6 ± 0.7

Data are mean ± SEM or n (%). BMI = body mass index; CR = calories restriction; DBP = diastolic blood pressure; HDL = high-density lipoprotein; HOMA-IR = homeostatic model assessment for insulin resistance; LC = low-carbohydrate; LDL = low-density lipoprotein; SBP = systolic blood pressure; * $p < 0.05$ vs. baseline (based on the post-hoc comparison test); [a] $p < 0.05$ for time effect (baseline vs. week 4) in all participants; [b] $p < 0.05$ for time effect (baseline vs. week 6) in all participants.

Table 3. Macrovascular endothelial function in response to the 6-week low carbohydrate diet intervention.

Brachial Artery	LC without CR Diet (n = 9)		LC with CR Diet (n = 12)		P Group × Time	P Group	P Time
	Baseline	Week 6	Baseline	Week 6			
FMD, %	6.5 ± 1.1	5.9 ± 1.5	7.8 ± 1.4	9.6 ± 1.6	0.4	0.1	0.7
Baseline diameter, mm	3.05 ± 0.17	3.15 ± 0.25	3.28 ± 0.15	3.24 ± 0.12	0.4	0.5	0.7
Maximum diameter, mm	3.26 ± 0.19	3.32 ± 0.24	3.52 ± 0.14	3.56 ± 0.14	0.8	0.3	0.4
Peak flow, cm/s	105 ± 12	120 ± 12	94 ± 10	106 ± 10	0.8	0.4	0.08
Peak shear rate,	334 ± 42	373 ± 40	269 ± 27	300 ± 29	0.9	0.1	0.2
NTG-mediated dilation, %	25.8 ± 3.8	24.7 ± 1.9	24.6 ± 2.5	28.5 ± 2.3	0.9	0.99	0.4
Baseline diameter, mm	3.01 ± 0.17	3.01 ± 0.20	3.34 ± 0.14	3.26 ± 0.14	0.6	0.2	0.6
Maximum diameter, mm	3.83 ± 0.21	3.76 ± 0.21	4.11 ± 0.13	4.16 ± 0.13	0.2	0.2	0.8

Data are mean ± SEM. CR = calories restriction; FMD = flow-mediated dilation; LC = low-carbohydrate; NTG = nitroglycerin.

3.3. Effect of LC Diet on Macro- and Micro-Vascular Endothelial Function

After 6 weeks of the intervention, FMD and NTG-mediated dilation remained unchanged ($p \geq 0.4$ for time effect; Table 3). Serum nitrate/nitrite levels did not change following the intervention (14.2 ± 2.0 to 15.5 ± 2.9 μmol; $p = 0.7$ for time effect).

In response to LC without CR diet, overall FID at week 6 significantly increased by 11% vs. baseline ($p = 0.01$ for the time effect). L-NAME decreased the overall FID at week 6 by 20% (Figure 2C) and this change was higher than baseline ($p = 0.04$). In response to LC with CR diet, although FID did not change ($p = 0.1$), L-NAME decreased overall FID at week 6 by 19% (Figure 2D) and this change was higher than baseline ($p = 0.007$).

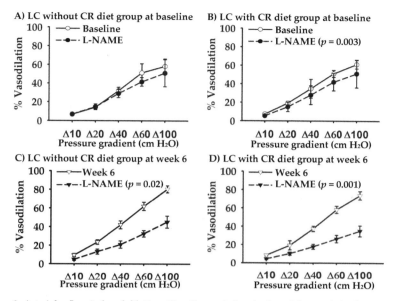

Figure 2. Arteriolar flow-induced dilation at baseline and after the 6-week low-carbohydrate (LC) diet intervention without caloric restriction (CR) diet ($n = 5$) and with CR diet ($n = 8$). Endothelial nitric oxide synthase inhibitor (L-NAME) was used to determine the contribution of nitric oxide in vasodilation.

3.4. Effect of LC Diet on Cardiovascular Risks

At the end of week 4, a significant interaction was noted only in body weight ($p = 0.049$; other outcomes: $p \geq 0.1$). Post hoc pairwise comparisons indicated that body weight significant decreased by 2.6 kg in LC without CR diet ($p = 0.001$) and 3.4 kg in LC with CR diet ($p < 0.0005$; $p = 0.4$ for between-group comparison; Table 2). In addition, BMI and blood triglyceride levels significantly decreased in response to the LC diet regardless of CR ($p \leq 0.009$ for time effect; Table 2). Other outcomes remained unchanged ($p \geq 0.1$ for time effect; Table 2).

After 6 weeks of the intervention, body weight, BMI and % body fat significantly decreased ($p \leq 0.004$ for time effect; $p \geq 0.8$ for interaction effect; Table 2). Diastolic blood pressure and blood triglyceride levels also significantly decreased in response to the LC diet regardless of CR ($p \leq 0.04$ for time effect; $p \geq 0.5$ for interaction effect; Table 2). There was a significant interaction in blood high-density lipoprotein cholesterol levels ($p = 0.03$), however, with no significant post hoc pairwise comparisons noted ($p \geq 0.08$; Table 2). Other outcomes remained unchanged ($p \geq 0.06$ for time effect; $p \geq 0.2$ for interaction effect; Table 2). No significant group effects were found in any outcomes ($p \geq 0.4$).

4. Discussion

This randomized trial is the first study to examine whether the effect of LC diet on both macro- and micro-vascular endothelial function is influenced by the provision of CR in young and middle-aged women with obesity. Our major findings are: (1) Six weeks of LC diet did not change macrovascular endothelial function, measured as brachial artery FMD, regardless of CR; and (2) LC diet without CR increased microvascular endothelial function, measured by arteriolar FID, while following the LC diet, regardless of CR, the magnitude of FID decreased by L-NAME was more than baseline. These findings suggest that the effects of LC diet on macro- and micro-vascular endothelial function are different and the latter benefits from LC diet by improving NO contribution to vasodilation. Furthermore, LC diet decreased cardiovascular risks in women with obesity, as evident by decreases in body weight, BMI, % body fat, diastolic blood pressure, and blood triglyceride levels after the intervention.

Brachial artery FMD reflects the nature of conduit artery or macrovascular endothelial biology. Following a transient period of ischemia (inflating a pressure cuff on the forearm for 5 min, and then deflating it rapidly), blood flow as well as shear stress increase [27]. The latter is considered as a physiological stimulus for inducing the release of NO from endothelium to vascular smooth muscle cells, thus causing vasodilation [27]. Brachial artery FMD is also an independent predictor of cardiovascular disease. For every 1% decrease in FMD, there is a 13% increase in the risks of future cardiovascular events [30]. A recent meta-analysis reported that obesity is associated with a 2% decrease in FMD [7], which may contribute to a 26% increase in cardiovascular disease risks. Therefore, brachial artery FMD is an important therapeutic target in adults with obesity to prevent cardiovascular disease. Previous studies have examined the effect of LC diet on FMD but their findings are either confounded by the provision of CR [9,10,12–17] or based on a single group design [31]. We found that the 6-week LC diet, regardless of CR, did not change FMD in women with obesity. In addition, we found that shear stress (measured as peak shear rate), systemic NO bioavailability (measured as serum NOx levels), and brachial artery smooth muscle function (measured as NTG-mediated dilation) remained unchanged following the intervention. Collectively, these findings suggest that LC diet, at least short-term (6 weeks), does not have effects on macrovascular endothelial function in young and middle-aged women with obesity.

In agreement with our findings, previous studies demonstrated no change [9,10,12–14] or even a decrease [11,15,16] in FMD following a LC diet in adults with obesity. On the other hand, one study found that LC diet improved FMD [17]. The heterogeneity in subject characteristics, LC diet interventions (e.g., % energy restriction, % carbohydrate restriction, nutrient component, and dietary sources), and experimental designs among the published studies makes the comparisons difficult to explain the conflicting results. One factor noted in all three studies showing the deleterious effect of LC diet on FMD is the use of a very low carbohydrate diet combined with CR (≤30 g/day or 4–5% caloric intake from carbohydrate + 25–30% of CR) [11,15,16]. Such modes of LC diets may cause an insufficient intake of important micronutrients such as folate and dietary fiber [11,16], both of which have been shown to provide protective effects on endothelial health [32–34]. In our study, fiber intake was different between the two LC diet groups. However, we did not see significant correlations between the changes in dietary fiber and the changes in endothelial function (data not reported). To our knowledge, only one study demonstrated improvements in FMD following a LC diet [17]. This study included subjects with elevated triglycerides (mean: 211 ± 58 mg/dL). In our study and other studies showing no positive effects on FMD, subjects had lower levels of triglycerides (baseline mean: 72–151 mg/dL) [9–16]. Therefore, LC diet may have benefits on FMD only when macrovascular endothelial dysfunction is associated with elevated triglycerides. Our study and previous studies found that LC diet decreased blood triglycerides [9,10,14,15,17].

Microvascular endothelial function is vital for regulating peripheral vascular tone/resistance and blood pressure. In response to shear stress, the vascular endothelium generates and releases NO, causing vasodilation. Endothelial NO synthase is an enzyme responsible for NO production. In the current study, we measured FID in arterioles isolated from gluteal fat tissues to assess microvascular endothelium-dependent vasodilation. In addition, to determine the contribution of NO in FID, we applied L-NAME, endothelial NO synthase inhibitor, to the arterioles and blocked NO production. At baseline, we found that LNAME decreased overall FID in LC with CR group, but not in LC without CR group. These findings suggest that FID in LC with CR group was NO dependent at baseline, while in LC without CR group, other pathways such as hydrogen peroxide may be responsible for the vasodilation [35]. The different vasodilatory mechanisms between the two groups at baseline may contribute to the different FID responses following the intervention. However, regardless of CR, we found that the 6-week LC diet improved NO contribution or bioavailability in the microcirculation. We did not measure oxidative stress and inflammation, both of which are known as the underlying mechanisms of reduced NO bioavailability. On the other hand, enhanced vasoconstriction, e.g., due to increased generation of cyclo-oxygenase (COX-1)-derived vasoconstrictor metabolites, may also contribute to impaired FID [36,37]. Future studies to further dissect the mechanisms by which LC diet improves microvascular endothelial function in obesity appear warranted.

Our findings suggest that the effect of LC diet may not be the same across the arterial tree. Consistent with this possibility, previous studies demonstrated that a 6-week LC diet (11% caloric intake from carbohydrate) did not change macrovascular but increased microvascular endothelial function [14]. The underlying mechanisms by which LC diet improves microvascular but not macrovascular endothelial function remain to be determined. One possible mechanism is related to the changes in adipose/fat biology or adipokines. Adipokines, such as adiponectin, leptin, resistin, and tumor necrosis factor-alpha, are secreted by fat tissue. Excessive fat, or obesity, is associated with a decrease in adiponectin and/or an increase in leptin, resistin, and tumor necrosis factor-alpha [38]. These changes in adipokines associated with obesity can lead to reduced bioavailability of NO and endothelial dysfunction [38–40]. We isolated arterioles from the subcutaneous adipose tissue of participants. Therefore, such type of arterioles, compared to the brachial artery, may have a direct and immediate effect of changes in adipokine profiles. Previous studies demonstrated that LC diet increased adiponectin [10,41] and decreased leptin [16]. Although we did not measure adipokines in the current study, % body fat decreased following the 6-week LC diet, which may contribute to the improvements in adipokine profiles. On the other hand, interventions longer than 6 weeks may be required to induce adaptations in macrovascular endothelial function.

Following the 6-week LC diet, body weight and BMI decreased in all participants with no differences between the two diet groups and that is unexpected. We defined CR diet as a caloric deficit by 500 calories/day less than the planned caloric intake. We calculated the planned caloric intake for each participant using the Mifflin equation, which considers individual body weight, height, age, and physical activity levels, and has been used in different diet interventions [26,37]. The planned caloric intake should match individual metabolic needs, be similar as their baseline caloric intake, and not induce any body weight changes. In LC without CR group, the planned/calculated caloric intake was higher than the baseline and actual caloric intake during the intervention. We provided meals to study participants, asked them to complete daily food dairy (including their appetite and any comments), and collected any leftover food from them to ensure accuracy of actual dietary intake during the intervention. We cannot exclude the following two possibilities: (1) The baseline caloric intake was underestimated by using a self-reported food diary, and (2) the planned caloric intake was overestimated by using the Mifflin equation due to self-reported physical activity factor. However, LC without CR group consumed overall calories more than LC with CR group during the 6-week intervention. Higher CR with longer intervention length may be required to induce more changes in body weight, other cardiovascular risk factors, and endothelial function. In addition, the maintenance phase in LC with CR diet may contribute to the non-significant differences between the two groups. Physical activity may influence our findings. Surprisingly, in our study, physical activity, measured as step counts per day from pedometer, increased similarly in all participants. The use of a pedometer to monitor physical activity is feasible and user-friendly. In addition, pedometers provide participants instant feedback and reinforcement of physical activity. However, we did not obtain data regarding physical activity duration, intensity, and type other than walking. Future studies can measure physical activity by using accelerometers along with physical activity logs.

Several strengths and limitations are noted in our study. We employed a randomized parallel design to isolate the effect of LC diet from CR. We excluded subjects who had no willingness to commit to the LC diet intervention. We provided meals with daily monitoring and regular meeting with bionutritionist. Therefore, our study has high compliance (~90% or higher) and low dropout ($n = 1$ unrelated to the study) and we were able to control dietary intake at every meal. In addition, we did not see any serious adverse events and the most common problem reported by the participants is hunger (6–8%), which is expected in diet interventions. Overall, the LC diet was well-tolerated. Although we did not report the reasons and number of subjects who were screened but did not meet inclusion/exclusion criteria, our study design and diet intervention may impact the recruitment rate, leading to a small and uneven sample size for each group. A block randomization can be used to ensure equal number of subjects assigned to each diet group. We assessed both macro- and microvascular endothelial function to provide comprehensive evidence of the vascular effects of LC diet. None of our participants were taking oral contraceptives. Two participants in LC with CR group had a diagnosis of polycystic ovary syndrome. When we excluded the two participants from analysis, similar results were observed. Due to the intervention length (6 weeks), we did not control the menstrual cycle phase between baseline and post-intervention visits. For brachial artery FMD, we were not able to measure flow velocity and diameter simultaneously and this was a limitation of our technology. Instead of using an in vivo measurement of microvascular function, an ex vivo model of arterioles allowed us to dissect the mechanisms of changes in NO contributions following the LC diet, without the presence of neurohormonal factors.

We focused on healthy young and middle-aged women with obesity. The severity of obesity is higher in women than men. Therefore, early intervention for women with obesity is essential to prevent the progression of obesity and the development of cardiovascular disease. Our findings may not be generalizable to men, other age groups, and disease populations, and even healthy individuals with normal body weight. In healthy young men whose BMI less than 30 kg/m^2, a one-week LC without CR diet (~10% caloric intake from carbohydrate) significantly decreased brachial artery FMD [31]. However, our findings still provide clinically important implications. Our LC diet was well-tolerated and improved bioavailability of NO in microvasculature, and thus microvascular endothelial function in women with obesity. Microvascular endothelial function drives the development of several cardiovascular diseases including hypertension [42]. Therefore, a long-term LC diet may be beneficial in controlling blood pressure and decreases risks for cardiovascular disease in women with obesity.

5. Conclusions

In conclusion, our findings suggest that the effect of LC diet on macro- and micro-vascular function is not influenced by the provision of CR in young and middle-aged women with obesity. A 6-week LC diet, regardless of CR, may improve microvascular, but not macrovascular, endothelial function via increased bioavailability of NO. Our findings may provide clinical implications of LC diet to decrease risks of cardiovascular disease associated with obesity.

Author Contributions: Conceptualization, C.-L.H. and S.A.P.; methodology, C.-L.H., A.E. and S.A.P.; validation, C.-L.H. and S.A.P.; formal analysis, C.-L.H. and S.A.P.; investigation, C.-L.H., C.R., A.M.M., M.R.S., A.M.E., A.E. and S.A.P.; resources, S.A.P.; data curation, C.-L.H., C.R., M.R.S., A.M.M., A.M.E., A.E. and S.A.P.; writing—original draft preparation, C.-L.H. and S.A.P.; writing—review and editing, C.-L.H., C.R., A.M.M., M.R.S., A.M.E., A.E. and S.A.P.; supervision, S.A.P.; project administration, S.A.P.; funding acquisition, S.A.P. All authors have read and agreed to the published version of the manuscript.

Funding: This research was funded by the National Heart, Lung, and Blood Institute (NHLBI), grants HL095701 (S.A.P.), and the American Heart Association, grant 20POST35120466 (C.-L.H.). The project described was supported by the National Center for Advancing Translational Sciences, National Institutes of Health, through Grant UL1TR002003.

Acknowledgments: We thank the participants for their time and participation. We acknowledge the significant support from Maryann Holtcamp, MS, APN and the rest of the staff at the Center for Clinical and Translational Science.

Conflicts of Interest: The authors declare no conflict of interest. The content is solely the responsibility of the authors and does not necessarily represent the official views of the National Institutes of Health and the American Heart Association.

References

1. *With Special Feature on Mortality*; Health, United States: Hyattsville, MD, USA, 2017.
2. Heymsfield, S.B.; Wadden, T.A. Mechanisms, Pathophysiology, and Management of Obesity. *N. Engl. J. Med.* **2017**, *376*, 254–266. [CrossRef]

3. Fan, J.; Song, Y.; Chen, Y.; Hui, R.; Zhang, W. Combined effect of obesity and cardio-metabolic abnormality on the risk of cardiovascular disease: A meta-analysis of prospective cohort studies. *Int J. Cardiol.* **2013**, *168*, 4761–4768. [CrossRef]

4. Benjamin, E.J.; Muntner, P.; Alonso, A.; Bittencourt, M.S.; Callaway, C.W.; Carson, A.P.; Chamberlain, A.M.; Chang, A.R.; Cheng, S.; Das, S.R.; et al. Heart Disease and Stroke Statistics-2019 Update: A Report From the American Heart Association. *Circulation* **2019**, *139*, e56–e528. [CrossRef]

5. Bonetti, P.O.; Lerman, L.O.; Lerman, A. Endothelial dysfunction: A marker of atherosclerotic risk. *Arterioscler Thromb. Vasc. Biol.* **2003**, *23*, 168–175. [CrossRef]

6. Vanhoutte, P.M.; Zhao, Y.; Xu, A.; Leung, S.W. Thirty Years of Saying NO: Sources, Fate, Actions, and Misfortunes of the Endothelium-Derived Vasodilator Mediator. *Circ. Res.* **2016**, *119*, 375–396. [CrossRef]

7. Ne, J.Y.A.; Cai, T.Y.; Celermajer, D.S.; Caterson, I.D.; Gill, T.; Lee, C.M.Y.; Skilton, M.R. Obesity, arterial function and arterial structure - a systematic review and meta-analysis. *Obes. Sci. Pract.* **2017**, *3*, 171–184. [CrossRef]

8. Virdis, A.; Masi, S.; Colucci, R.; Chiriaco, M.; Uliana, M.; Puxeddu, I.; Bernardini, N.; Blandizzi, C.; Taddei, S. Microvascular Endothelial Dysfunction in Patients with Obesity. *Curr. Hypertens. Rep.* **2019**, *21*, 32. [CrossRef]

9. Keogh, J.B.; Brinkworth, G.D.; Clifton, P.M. Effects of weight loss on a low-carbohydrate diet on flow-mediated dilatation, adhesion molecules and adiponectin. *Br. J. Nutr.* **2007**, *98*, 852–859. [CrossRef]

10. Keogh, J.B.; Brinkworth, G.D.; Noakes, M.; Belobrajdic, D.P.; Buckley, J.D.; Clifton, P.M. Effects of weight loss from a very-low-carbohydrate diet on endothelial function and markers of cardiovascular disease risk in subjects with abdominal obesity. *Am. J. Clin. Nutr.* **2008**, *87*, 567–576. [CrossRef]

11. Wycherley, T.P.; Brinkworth, G.D.; Keogh, J.B.; Noakes, M.; Buckley, J.D.; Clifton, P.M. Long-term effects of weight loss with a very low carbohydrate and low fat diet on vascular function in overweight and obese patients. *J. Intern. Med.* **2010**, *267*, 452–461. [CrossRef]

12. Wycherley, T.P.; Thompson, C.H.; Buckley, J.D.; Luscombe-Marsh, N.D.; Noakes, M.; Wittert, G.A.; Brinkworth, G.D. Long-term effects of weight loss with a very-low carbohydrate, low saturated fat diet on flow mediated dilatation in patients with type 2 diabetes: A randomised controlled trial. *Atherosclerosis* **2016**, *252*, 28–31. [CrossRef]

13. Buscemi, S.; Verga, S.; Tranchina, M.R.; Cottone, S.; Cerasola, G. Effects of hypocaloric very-low-carbohydrate diet vs. Mediterranean diet on endothelial function in obese women*. *Eur. J. Clin. Invest.* **2009**, *39*, 339–347. [CrossRef]

14. Ballard, K.D.; Quann, E.E.; Kupchak, B.R.; Volk, B.M.; Kawiecki, D.M.; Fernandez, M.L.; Seip, R.L.; Maresh, C.M.; Kraemer, W.J.; Volek, J.S. Dietary carbohydrate restriction improves insulin sensitivity, blood pressure, microvascular function, and cellular adhesion markers in individuals taking statins. *Nutr. Res.* **2013**, *33*, 905–912. [CrossRef]

15. Phillips, S.A.; Jurva, J.W.; Syed, A.Q.; Syed, A.Q.; Kulinski, J.P.; Pleuss, J.; Hoffmann, R.G.; Gutterman, D.D. Benefit of low-fat over low-carbohydrate diet on endothelial health in obesity. *Hypertension* **2008**, *51*, 376–382. [CrossRef]

16. Varady, K.A.; Bhutani, S.; Klempel, M.C.; Phillips, S.A. Improvements in vascular health by a low-fat diet, but not a high-fat diet, are mediated by changes in adipocyte biology. *Nutr. J.* **2011**, *10*, 8. [CrossRef]

17. Volek, J.S.; Ballard, K.D.; Silvestre, R.; Judelson, D.A.; Quann, E.E.; Forsythe, C.E.; Fernandez, M.L.; Kraemer, W.J. Effects of dietary carbohydrate restriction versus low-fat diet on flow-mediated dilation. *Metabolism* **2009**, *58*, 1769–1777. [CrossRef]

18. Raitakari, M.; Ilvonen, T.; Ahotupa, M.; Lehtimaki, T.; Harmoinen, A.; Suominen, P.; Elo, J.; Hartiala, J.; Raitakari, O.T. Weight reduction with very-low-caloric diet and endothelial function in overweight adults: Role of plasma glucose. *Arterioscler Thromb. Vasc. Biol.* **2004**, *24*, 124–128. [CrossRef]

19. Pierce, G.L.; Beske, S.D.; Lawson, B.R.; Southall, K.L.; Benay, F.J.; Donato, A.J.; Seals, D.R. Weight loss alone improves conduit and resistance artery endothelial function in young and older overweight/obese adults. *Hypertension* **2008**, *52*, 72–79. [CrossRef]

20. Sasaki, S.; Higashi, Y.; Nakagawa, K.; Kimura, M.; Noma, K.; Sasaki, S.; Hara, K.; Matsuura, H.; Goto, C.; Oshima, T.; et al. A low-calorie diet improves endothelium-dependent vasodilation in obese patients with essential hypertension. *Am. J. Hypertens.* **2002**, *15*, 302–309. [CrossRef]

21. Dengel, D.R.; Kelly, A.S.; Olson, T.P.; Kaiser, D.R.; Dengel, J.L.; Bank, A.J. Effects of weight loss on insulin sensitivity and arterial stiffness in overweight adults. *Metabolism* **2006**, *55*, 907–911. [CrossRef]

22. Brook, R.D.; Bard, R.L.; Glazewski, L.; Kehrer, C.; Bodary, P.F.; Eitzman, D.L.; Rajagopalan, S. Effect of short-term weight loss on the metabolic syndrome and conduit vascular endothelial function in overweight adults. *Am. J. Cardiol.* **2004**, *93*, 1012–1016. [CrossRef] [PubMed]

23. Wycherley, T.P.; Brinkworth, G.D.; Noakes, M.; Buckley, J.D.; Clifton, P.M. Effect of caloric restriction with and without exercise training on oxidative stress and endothelial function in obese subjects with type 2 diabetes. *Diabetes. Obes. Metab.* **2008**, *10*, 1062–1073. [CrossRef] [PubMed]

24. Focardi, M.; Dick, G.M.; Picchi, A.; Zhang, C.; Chilian, W.M. Restoration of coronary endothelial function in obese Zucker rats by a low-carbohydrate diet. *Am. J. Physiol. Heart. Circ. Physiol.* **2007**, *292*, H2093–H2099. [CrossRef] [PubMed]

25. Mifflin, M.D.; St Jeor, S.T.; Hill, L.A.; Scott, B.J.; Daugherty, S.A.; Koh, Y.O. A new predictive equation for resting energy expenditure in healthy individuals. *Am. J. Clin. Nutr.* **1990**, *51*, 241–247. [CrossRef]

26. Hoddy, K.K.; Bhutani, S.; Phillips, S.A.; Varady, K.A. Effects of different degrees of insulin resistance on endothelial function in obese adults undergoing alternate day fasting. *Nutr. Healthy Aging* **2016**, *4*, 63–71. [CrossRef]

27. Goslawski, M.; Piano, M.R.; Bian, J.T.; Church, E.C.; Szczurek, M.; Phillips, S.A. Binge drinking impairs vascular function in young adults. *J. Am. Coll. Cardiol.* **2013**, *62*, 201–207. [CrossRef]

28. Thijssen, D.H.; Black, M.A.; Pyke, K.E.; Padilla, J.; Atkinson, G.; Harris, R.A.; Parker, B.; Widlansky, M.E.; Tschakovsky, M.E.; Green, D.J. Assessment of flow-mediated dilation in humans: A methodological and physiological guideline. *Am. J. Physiol. Heart. Circ. Physiol.* **2011**, *300*, H2–H12. [CrossRef]

29. Hwang, C.L.; Bian, J.T.; Thur, L.A.; Peters, T.A.; Piano, M.R.; Phillips, S.A. Tetrahydrobiopterin Restores Microvascular Dysfunction in Young Adult Binge Drinkers. *Alcohol. Clin. Exp. Res.* **2020**, *44*, 407–414. [CrossRef]

30. Inaba, Y.; Chen, J.A.; Bergmann, S.R. Prediction of future cardiovascular outcomes by flow-mediated vasodilatation of brachial artery: A meta-analysis. *Int. J. Cardiovasc. Imaging* **2010**, *26*, 631–640. [CrossRef]

31. Durrer, C.; Lewis, N.; Wan, Z.; Ainslie, P.N.; Jenkins, N.T.; Little, J.P. Short-Term Low-Carbohydrate High-Fat Diet in Healthy Young Males Renders the Endothelium Susceptible to Hyperglycemia-Induced Damage, An Exploratory Analysis. *Nutrients* **2019**, *11*, 489. [CrossRef]

32. Alian, Z.; Hashemipour, M.; Dehkordi, E.H.; Hovsepian, S.; Amini, M.; Moadab, M.H.; Javanmard, S.H. The effects of folic acid on markers of endothelial function in patients with type 1 diabetes mellitus. *Med. Arh.* **2012**, *66*, 12–15. [CrossRef]

33. Verhaar, M.C.; Wever, R.M.; Kastelein, J.J.; van Dam, T.; Koomans, H.A.; Rabelink, T.J. 5-methyltetrahydrofolate, the active form of folic acid, restores endothelial function in familial hypercholesterolemia. *Circulation* **1998**, *97*, 237–241. [CrossRef]

34. Whisner, C.M.; Angadi, S.S.; Weltman, N.Y.; Weltman, A.; Rodriguez, J.; Patrie, J.T.; Gaesser, G.A. Effects of Low-Fat and High-Fat Meals, with and without Dietary Fiber, on Postprandial Endothelial Function, Triglyceridemia, and Glycemia in Adolescents. *Nutrients* **2019**, *11*, 2626. [CrossRef]

35. Robinson, A.T.; Franklin, N.C.; Norkeviciute, E.; Bian, J.T.; Babana, J.C.; Szczurek, M.R.; Phillips, S.A. Improved arterial flow-mediated dilation after exertion involves hydrogen peroxide in overweight and obese adults following aerobic exercise training. *J. Hypertens.* **2016**, *34*, 1309–1316. [CrossRef]

36. Cavka, A.; Cosic, A.; Jukic, I.; Jelakovic, B.; Lombard, J.H.; Phillips, S.A.; Seric, V.; Mihaljevic, I.; Drenjancevic, I. The role of cyclo-oxygenase-1 in high-salt diet-induced microvascular dysfunction in humans. *J. Physiol.* **2015**, *593*, 5313–5324. [CrossRef]

37. Mahmoud, A.M.; Hwang, C.L.; Szczurek, M.R.; Bian, J.T.; Ranieri, C.; Gutterman, D.D.; Phillips, S.A. Low-Fat Diet Designed for Weight Loss But Not Weight Maintenance Improves Nitric Oxide-Dependent Arteriolar Vasodilation in Obese Adults. *Nutrients* **2019**, *11*, 1339. [CrossRef]

38. Ntaios, G.; Gatselis, N.K.; Makaritsis, K.; Dalekos, G.N. Adipokines as mediators of endothelial function and atherosclerosis. *Atherosclerosis* **2013**, *227*, 216–221. [CrossRef]

39. Korda, M.; Kubant, R.; Patton, S.; Malinski, T. Leptin-induced endothelial dysfunction in obesity. *Am. J. Physiol. Heart Circ. Physiol.* **2008**, *295*, H1514–H1521. [CrossRef]

40. Chen, H.; Montagnani, M.; Funahashi, T.; Shimomura, I.; Quon, M.J. Adiponectin stimulates production of nitric oxide in vascular endothelial cells. *J. Biol. Chem.* **2003**, *278*, 45021–45026. [CrossRef]

Nutrients **2020**, *12*, 1649

41. Gardner, C.D.; Trepanowski, J.F.; Del Gobbo, L.C.; Hauser, M.E.; Rigdon, J.; Ioannidis, J.P.A.; Desai, M.; King, A.C. Effect of Low-Fat vs Low-Carbohydrate Diet on 12-Month Weight Loss in Overweight Adults and the Association With Genotype Pattern or Insulin Secretion: The DIETFITS Randomized Clinical Trial. *JAMA* **2018**, *319*, 667–679. [CrossRef]

42. Yannoutsos, A.; Levy, B.I.; Safar, M.E.; Slama, G.; Blacher, J. Pathophysiology of hypertension: Interactions between macro and microvascular alterations through endothelial dysfunction. *J. Hypertens.* **2014**, *32*, 216–224. [CrossRef] [PubMed]

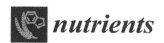

Article

Hyperhomocysteinemia and Low Folate and Vitamin B12 Are Associated with Vascular Dysfunction and Impaired Nitric Oxide Sensitivity in Morbidly Obese Patients

Mohamed Haloul [1,2], Smita Jagdish Vinjamuri [1], Dina Naquiallah [1],
Mohammed Imaduddin Mirza [1], Maryam Qureshi [1], Chandra Hassan [3], Mario Masrur [3],
Francesco M. Bianco [3], Patrice Frederick [3], Giulianotti P. Cristoforo [3], Antonio Gangemi [3],
Mohamed M. Ali [4,5], Shane A. Phillips [1,4,5] and Abeer M. Mahmoud [1,*]

[1] Division of Endocrinology, Diabetes, and Metabolism, Department of Medicine, College of Medicine, University of Illinois at Chicago, Chicago, IL 60612, USA; haloul57@uic.edu (M.H.); svinja2@uic.edu (S.J.V.); dnaqui2@uic.edu (D.N.); mmirza24@uic.edu (M.I.M.); mshafi1@uic.edu (M.Q.); shanep@uic.edu (S.A.P.)
[2] Clinical Pathology Laboratory, Children's Cancer Hospital Egypt, Cairo 57357, Egypt
[3] Departments of Surgery, College of Medicine, University of Illinois at Chicago, Chicago, IL 60612, USA; chandrar@uic.edu (C.H.); mmasrur@uic.edu (M.M.); biancofm@uic.edu (F.M.B.); pfrede1@uic.edu (P.F.); piercg@uic.edu (G.P.C.); agangemi@uic.edu (A.G.)
[4] Department of Physical Therapy, College of Applied Health Sciences, University of Illinois at Chicago, Chicago, IL 60612, USA; mali37@uic.edu
[5] Integrative Physiology Laboratory, College of Applied Health Sciences, University of Illinois at Chicago, Chicago, IL 60612, USA
[*] Correspondence: amahmo4@uic.edu

Received: 30 May 2020; Accepted: 1 July 2020; Published: 7 July 2020

Abstract: There is a high prevalence of hyperhomocysteinemia that has been linked to high cardiovascular risk in obese individuals and could be attributed to poor nutritional status of folate and vitamin B12. We sought to examine the association between blood homocysteine (Hcy) folate, and vitamin B12 levels and vascular dysfunction in morbidly obese adults using novel ex vivo flow-induced dilation (FID) measurements of isolated adipose tissue arterioles. Brachial artery flow-mediated dilation (FMD) was also measured. Subcutaneous and visceral adipose tissue biopsies were obtained from morbidly obese individuals and non-obese controls. Resistance arterioles were isolated in which FID, acetylcholine-induced dilation (AChID), and nitric oxide (NO) production were measured in the absence or presence of the NO synthase inhibitor, L-NAME, Hcy, or the superoxide dismutase mimetic, TEMPOL. Our results demonstrated that plasma Hcy concentrations were significantly higher, while folate, vitamin B12, and NO were significantly lower in obese subjects compared to controls. Hcy concentrations correlated positively with BMI, fat %, and insulin levels but not with folate or vitamin B12. Brachial and arteriolar vasodilation were lower in obese subjects, positively correlated with folate and vitamin B12, and inversely correlated with Hcy. Arteriolar NO measurements and sensitivity to L-NAME were lower in obese subjects compared to controls. Finally, Hcy incubation reduced arteriolar FID and NO sensitivity, an effect that was abolished by TEMPOL. In conclusion, these data suggest that high concentrations of plasma Hcy and low concentrations of folate and vitamin B12 could be independent predictors of vascular dysfunction in morbidly obese individuals.

Keywords: homocysteine; folate; vitamin B12; obesity; vascular dysfunction; bariatric surgery; nitric oxide

1. Introduction

Obesity is a major public health concern that affects more than one-third of the population and increases the risk of other health problems, including metabolic and cardiovascular diseases [1]. Several factors contribute to the increasing trend in obesity, including genetic predisposition and lack of physical activity, yet the most predominant factor is excess caloric intake. Despite overeating, obese individuals have a relatively high incidence of micronutrient deficiencies [2]. Some of these micronutrients act as cofactors in critical biological pathways in the body, such as energy metabolism and immune function. One of these vital biological processes that are regulated by the bioavailability of micronutrients, namely folate and other B vitamins, is One-Carbon metabolism [3].

In the "One-Carbon metabolism", dietary folate is converted to dihydrofolate (DHF) then to tetrahydrofolate (THF) that, in turn, is converted to 5-methyl THF via a series of enzymatic reactions cofactored by vitamins B6 and B12, and betaine. The final product, 5-methyl THF, donates its methyl group to homocysteine (Hcy) to produce methionine, which is critical for the formation of the ultimate methyl donor, S-Adenosylmethionine (SAM). The latter is metabolized to S-adenosylhomocysteine (SAH), which could be reversibly converted to Hcy via the enzyme SAH hydrolase. The fate of Hcy is through re-methylation to methionine via the folate-dependent pathway or transsulfuration to cystathionine, via cystathionine β-synthase [3].

Hyperhomocysteinemia refers to increased plasma levels of Hcy and has been classified into three categories: mild (15–30 μmol/L), moderate (30–100 μmol/L), and severe (100 μmol/L) [4]. Several pathological conditions could cause hyperhomocysteinemia, including dysfunction of the enzymes that are associated with homocysteine biosynthesis and metabolism such as methyl-THF reductase and cystathionine β-synthase or deficiency in cofactors such as folate and vitamins B2, B6, and B12 [5]. Hyperhomocysteinemia is considered an established, independent risk factor for cardiovascular disease (CVD), including atherosclerosis and coronary artery disease [6,7]. Despite this growing evidence of the role of hyperhomocysteinemia in vascular dysfunction, its effect and the mechanistic drive of this effect on human microvasculature are largely unexplored. In the current study, we aimed to investigate the hypothesis that hyperhomocysteinemia is associated with microvascular dysfunction in morbidly obese adults. Using the proposed ex vivo system in this study, we were able to explore the differential responses to vasoactive mediators in arterioles preconditioned with hyperhomocysteinemia compared to those isolated from subjects with normal Hcy levels. Moreover, we measured other variables that were previously proposed to contribute to hyperhomocysteinemia such as folate, vitamin B12, and insulin levels, as well as alcohol intake [5].

2. Methods

2.1. Human Participants

Subjects were 40 obese adults and 40 non-obese controls who underwent bariatric surgeries and elective surgeries (non-inflamed hernias and cholecystectomies), respectively, at the University of Illinois Medical Center. Inclusion criteria included age from 21 to 49 years old, a BMI higher than 35 kg/m^2 for the obese group and less than 30 kg/m^2 for the controls, and the absence of significant chronic or inflammatory disease that may modify vascular outcomes. Excluded subjects included those above 50 years old, postmenopausal, and pregnant women, smokers, subjects with a history of previous bariatric surgery, and individuals with current cardiac, hepatic, or renal disease, malignancy, or acute or chronic inflammatory conditions. Evaluating subjects for eligibility criteria took place before the first data collection clinical visit. The study team informed the eligible subjects about the study specifics and provided them with a written informed consent. All protocols and methods that were used in this study followed the regulations established by the most recent revision of the Declaration of Helsinki and were approved by the University of Illinois Institutional Review Board. During subject's clinical visit, blood samples and anthropometric/body composition measurements were collected, as well as brachial artery ultrasound imaging. In addition, information about alcohol administration and the intake of supplements that contain folate or vitamin B12 were obtained via questionnaires. For alcohol consumption, subjects were classified into (1) light drinkers, those who consume alcohol less than one time/month with less than 5 drinks/time, 1–3 times/month with less than 3 drinks/time or 1–2 times/week with less than 2 drinks/time; (2) moderate drinkers, those who consume alcohol 1–3 times/month with 3–4 drinks/time, 1–2 times/week with 2–4 drinks/time, or 3–6 times/week with less than 2 drinks/time; and (3) heavy drinkers, those who consume alcohol at any quantity and/or frequency that is more than moderate drinkers. On the day of bariatric surgery, adipose tissue samples, both visceral (VAT) and subcutaneous (SAT) were provided to us by the surgeon and put in ice-cold HEPES buffer for transfer to the laboratory for dissection and isolation of microvessels.

2.2. Physical Measurements and Body Composition

Physical characteristics including body mass, body mass index (BMI), and waist circumference were assessed. Dual X-ray absorptiometry (DXA; iDXA, General Electric Inc., Boston, MA, USA) was used to quantify lean, total fat, and visceral fat mass. All subjects had a single scan performed on Lunar iDXA. Subjects were positioned on the scanner following the operator's manual, and all women had confirmed negative pregnancy tests before scanning.

2.3. Cardiometabolic Measurements

Biochemical measurements of lipid profile and glucose metabolism were performed in fasting blood samples. Plasma glucose concentration was measured using a standard glucometer (LifeScan). Insulin was measured via a highly sensitive Insulin ELISA kit, ENZ-KIT141-0001 (Enzo Life Sciences, Inc., Farmingdale, NY, USA) following the producer's protocol. To assess insulin resistance, we used the homeostasis model assessment formula, HOMA-IR which is calculated by dividing the product of fasting insulin (μU/L) and fasting glucose (nmol/L) by 22.5, as previously described [8]. Triglycerides, total cholesterol, high-density lipoproteins (HDL), and direct low-density lipoproteins (LDL) were measured on a Hitachi 911 analyzer using enzymatic assays from Roche Diagnostics (Indianapolis, IN, USA) and following to the manufacturer's specification.

2.4. Plasma Hcy, Folate, and Vitamin B12

Total plasma Hcy levels were measured using a Hcy ELISA Kit (Cell Biolabs Inc., San Diego, CA, USA), following the manufacturer's guidelines. Briefly, plasma samples were diluted 2X and incubated in the Hcy conjugate coated plate for 10 min at room temperature. Then, the primary anti-Hcy antibody was added and incubated for one hour, followed by washing steps and the addition of the secondary antibody. Finally, the provided substrate was incubated for 30 min after which the reaction was stopped using the provided stop solution. Absorbance was measured via iMark Microplate Reader (BioRad, Hercules, CA, USA) using 450 nm as the primary wavelength. Plasma levels of folate and vitamin B12 were assessed via Elecsys Folate III (Roche Diagnostics; Indianapolis, IN, USA) approach that utilizes a competitive assay principle via natural, specific folate binding protein and specific intrinsic factor for vitamin B12, respectively.

2.5. Serum NO Measurements

Serum concentrations of nitrate and nitrite, stable NO metabolites, were measured using the Griess reaction (Cayman Chemicals, Ann Arbor, MI) as we previously described [9]. Briefly, serum samples were ultra-filtered through 10 KDa molecular weight cut-off filters from Millipore (Burlington, MA, USA). In filtered samples, nitrate reductase converted nitrates into nitrites, which in turn is converted into a dark purple azo compound when Griess reagents were supplied. Absorbance was measured at 540 nm using iMark Microplate Reader. A nitrate standard curve was included in the experiment and used to calculate nitrate concentrations in samples.

2.6. Brachial Artery Flow-Mediated Dilation (FMD)

Brachial imaging was performed on Hitachi Prosound Alpha 7 (Hitachi Aloka Medical America, Wallingford, CT, USA) using a linear probe placed about 5 cm above the antecubital fossa of the left arm, abducted at about 90 degrees relative to the body torso. After a 1-min baseline imaging (BSL), an inflatable blood pressure cuff was wrapped around the right mid-forearm and inflated up to 200 to 220 mmHg for 5 min. After cuff deflation, a 300-s long video sequence at three frames/second was recorded using a video grabber for offline measurement. The imaging protocol involved acquiring at least 60 s of BSL diameter before inflating the cuff and 300 s for the reactive hyperemia (RH) event induced by the cuff deflation. Blood flow velocity was acquired simultaneously using pulsed wave Doppler. Brachial Analyzer software (Medical Imaging Applications LLC, Coralville, IA, USA) was used to analyze the brachial artery diameter (Figure 1). Percent changes in FMD were calculated as follows [%FMD = (RH diameter in mm – BSL diameter in mm/BSL diameter in mm) × 100].

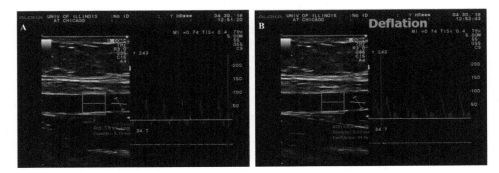

Figure 1. Duplex B-mode/pulsed wave Doppler (PWD) ultrasound of brachial artery flow-mediated dilation (FMD). This figure shows a long axis scan of brachial artery with simultaneous blood velocity profile by pulsed wave Doppler before (**A**) and after cuff deflation (**B**). For offline image analyses, a representative section of brachial artery is selected for an automated measurement of diameter. Baseline diameter (BSL) was averaged from a serial of recorded frames before cuff deflation and the maximum diameter was measured after cuff deflation during reactive hyperemia (RH).

2.7. Microvascular Preparations

Adipose tissues were cleaned of excess connective tissue and carefully dissected to isolate visceral and subcutaneous resistance arterioles. Isolated arterioles were used to measure microvascular reactivity as we previously described [9–11]. Briefly, both SAT and VAT arterioles were cannulated and mounted in an organ perfusion chamber where arteriolar ends were secured using 10-0 nylon Ethilon monofilament suture. The whole setup was then placed on the stage of an inverted microscope to which a video camera is attached. Images were displayed on a video monitor and the internal arteriolar diameter was measured via a video measuring device (model VIA-100; Boeckeler, Madison, WI, USA). To maintain arterioles under physiological conditions, warm physiological salt solution (Krebs buffer) was continuously perfused inside the organ chamber. Krebs buffer consisted of the following ingredients in mmol/L: 123 NaCl, 4.4 KCL, 20 $NaHCO_3$, 2.5 $CaCl_2$, 1.2 KH_2PO_4, 1.2 $MgSO_4$, and 11 glucose. The temperature of the buffer was maintained at 37 °C, and the pH was adjusted to 7.4. The buffer was also provided with a mixture of air that contains 21% O_2, 5% CO_2, and 74% N_2. The arteriolar ends were connected to physiological buffer-containing reservoirs that were used to adjust the intraluminal pressure gradient (10–100 cmH_2O) [12].

2.8. Flow-Induced Dilation (FID) Measurements

Endothelin-1 (Peninsula, San Carlos, CA, USA) was used to pre-constrict cannulated arterioles and those that demonstrated less than 30% constriction compared to baseline were excluded from the study since they are mostly damaged during processing [9–11,13–15]. Internal diameters of cannulated arterioles were measured at baseline conditions and during continuing increases of the intraluminal pressure gradient (10–100 cmH$_2$O), acetylcholine concentration (ACh; 10^{-9}–10^{-4} M) [10], or the NO donor, sodium nitroprusside (SNP; 10^{-9}–10^{-4} M). Measurements were repeated after incubations with the endothelial nitric oxide synthase inhibitor L-NAME (10^{-4} M). All treatments were applied for 30 min followed by measuring FID and acetylcholine-induced dilation (AchID). In a subset of subjects (ten obese and ten controls), arterioles were incubated with 100 µM of Hcy for 180 min [16] with and without L-NAME or the superoxide dismutase mimetic, 4-Hydroxy-TEMPO (TEMPOL, 10^{-5} M). Maximum dilation of arterioles was assessed at the end of each experiment using the antispasmodic, Papaverine at a concentration of 10^{-4} M. Arteriolar vasodilation was calculated as the percentage change in arteriolar diameter following different treatments relative to the diameter after ET-1-induced constriction. All the above-mentioned chemicals except endothelin-1 were acquired from Sigma Aldrich (St. Louis, MO, USA).

2.9. Measurements of Arteriolar NO and Reactive Oxygen Species (ROS)

Nitric oxide and ROS generation in the adipose tissue-isolated arterioles were measured as we previously described [17] using NO Detection Kit (Enzo Life Sciences, Inc., Farmingdale, NY, USA) and ROS green fluorescent detection reagent, 2′,7′-dichlorodihydrofluorescein diacetate (H$_2$DCFDA) (Thermo Fisher Scientific). Flow-induced generation of nitric oxide and ROS were detected in cannulated arterioles that were kept at 37 °C in Krebs solution that was supplied by a 20% O$_2$/5% CO$_2$ gas mixture. Vessels were maintained at an equilibration pressure of 60 cm H$_2$O for one hour. Vessels incubated in 10^{-5} mol/L ACh or 10^{-3} mol/L BSO served as positive controls for NO and superoxide generation, respectively. Vessels were stained, mounted on microscopic coverslips, and imaged via fluorescence microscopy (Eclipse TE 2000, Nikon, Japan) at wavelengths of 650/670 nm and 495/527 nm for NO and ROS detection, respectively. All procedures for incubation, staining, and detection were consistent among all experiments and treatment conditions. Fluorescence intensities in the developed images were measured and expressed in arbitrary units using NIH Image J software (NIH, Bethesda, MD, USA).

2.10. Statistical Analyses

All findings were reported as the mean ± standard error and a *p* value less of than 0.05 was considered statistically significant. Fluorescent intensities were analyzed using NIH Image J software (NIH, Bethesda, MD, USA) after correcting for background autofluorescence. Physical features, cardiometabolic parameters, and vascular measurements were assessed using Student's unpaired *t*-test for between group comparisons. Statistically significant linear relationship between continuous variables were tested using a bivariate Pearson Correlation. Arteriolar vasodilation was presented as a percentage increase in diameter in response to different treatment conditions relative to the pre-constricted state. Multivariate regression analysis was run to predict vasodilation (FID and AchID) from other independent variables. Analyses were conducted using SPSS statistical software (version 26.0; SPSS Inc., Chicago, IL, USA).

3. Results

3.1. Physical and Cardiometabolic Parameters

Physical characteristics, including age, gender, body weight, BMI, waist circumference, fat percentage, and cardiometabolic risk factors including blood pressure, heart rate, lipid profile, and glucose metabolism are displayed in Table 1. Body weight, waist circumference, BMI, and fat percentage were significantly higher in obese compared to non-obese subjects ($p < 10^{-10}$). Moreover, heart rate, systolic and diastolic blood pressure were higher in the obese group ($p < 0.01$). Although the average fasting blood glucose and HbAlc were not statistically different between the two groups, the average fasting plasma insulin and HOMA-IR were lower in the control group compared to obese subjects by 43% and 52%, respectively. Total cholesterol, LDL, and triglycerides did not differ between the groups; however, the average HDL level was 30% higher ($p = 0.0004$) in the non-obese compared to obese subjects. Biomarkers of inflammation namely interleukin 6 (IL6), IL8, and C-reactive protein (CRP) were 3.2-fold, 63%, and 4.4-fold higher, respectively, in the obese subject compared to the non-obese controls. These inflammatory biomarkers correlated negatively with vascular functions that were measured via brachial artery FMD or arteriolar FID.

Table 1. Physical characteristics Cardiometabolic risk factors of study participants.

Variable	Non-Obese Controls	Obese Bariatric Patients	*p*-Value
n	40 (18 ♂)	40 (12 ♂)	
Age, y	35.4 ± 1.3	36.2 ± 1	0.339
Weight, kg	74.4 ± 1.6	142.4 ± 3.7 *	<0.001
BMI, kg/ m^2	24.9 ± 0.5	50.6 ± 1.1 *	<0.001
WC, cm	131.5 ± 4	91.5 ± 2 *	<0.001
Body fat, %	32.2 ± 2.5	52.3 ± 1.0 *	<0.001
Body lean, %	65.3 ± 2.4	46.5 ± 0.9 *	<0.001
VAT mass, kg	0.7 ± 0.1	2.0 ± 0.2 *	0.0002
HR, bpm	74 ± 2	81 ± 1 *	0.004
SBP, mmHg	118 ± 2	132 ± 2 *	<0.001
DBP, mmHg	75 ± 1	80 ± 1 *	0.013
FPG, mg/dL	92 ± 2	103 ± 5	0.112
FPI, μU/mL	8.4 ± 1.4	14.9 ± 2.8 *	<0.001
HOMA-IR	1.9 ± 0.1	4.1 ± 0.4 *	0.002
HbAlc, %	5.3 ± 0.1	5.8 ± 0.2	0.148
Total chol, mg/dL	155 ± 9	165 ± 4	0.171
HDL, mg/dL	56 ± 6	43 ± 1 *	<0.001
LDL, mg/dL	87 ± 7	99 ± 4	0.116
TG, mg/dL	92 ± 11	115 ± 8	0.136
IL6, pg/mL	5.2 ± 0.7	21.6 ± 3.6 *	0.001
IL8, pg/mL	3.0 ± 0.1	4.9 ± 0.4 *	<0.001
CRP, mg/L	0.7 ± 0.1	3.8 ± 0.2 *	<0.0001

BMI, body mass index; Chol, cholesterol; cm, centimeters; CRP, C-reactive protein; DBP, diastolic blood pressure; FPG, fasting plasma glucose; FPI, fasting plasma insulin; HDL, high density lipoprotein; HOMA-IR, Homeostatic model assessment for insulin resistance; HR, heart rate; IL6, interleukin 6; IL8, interleukin 8; kg, kilograms; LDL, low density lipoprotein; n, number; SBP. Systolic blood pressure; TG, triglycerides; VAT, visceral adipose tissue; WC, waist circumference; y, years; ♂, males; * $p < 0.05$.

3.2. Plasma Hcy, Folate, and Vitamin B12 and Serum NO Measurements

The average total plasma Hcy was found to be significantly higher in the obese group (1.5 ± 0.04 μg/mL; equivalent to 11.4 ± 0.3 μmol/L) compared to the non-obese group (1.2 ± 0.03 μg/mL; equivalent to 8.7 ± 0.2 μmol/L; $p < 0.0001$) (Figure 2A). Plasma Hcy correlated positively with body weight ($r = 0.41$, $p = 0.004$), waist circumference ($r = 0.43$, $p = 0.014$), BMI ($r = 0.45$, $p = 0.002$), and fat percentage ($r = 0.41$, $p = 0.016$), and negatively with lean percentage ($r = -0.40$, $p = 0.017$). Interestingly, plasma Hcy correlated significantly with fasting insulin levels ($r = 0.47$, $p = 0.001$) and when obese subjects were divided into hyperinsulinemic (>9 μU/mL) and normoinsulinemic (<9 μU/mL) groups, the hyperinsulinemic group had a higher level of Hcy (12.9 ± 0.2 μmol/L) compared to the normoinsulinemic one (8.9 ± 0.4 μmol/L, $p < 0.01$). The average of plasma folate was ~27% higher in the non-obese controls compared to obese subjects (18.7 ± 0.7 ng/mL vs. 14.8 ± 0.8 ng/mL; $p = 0.0004$) (Figure 2B). Plasma folate correlated negatively with body weight ($r = -0.36$, $p < 0.0001$), VAT mass ($r = -0.49$, $p = 0.008$), and fasting plasma insulin ($r = -0.21$, $p = 0.044$). Similarly, vitamin B12 levels were ~41% higher in the non-obese compared to obese subjects (561.8 ± 17.9 ng/L vs. 397.5 ± 26.3 ng/L;

$p < 0.0001$) (Figure 2C) and correlated negatively with body weight ($r = -0.39$, $p < 0.0001$), total fat mass ($r = -0.41$, $p = 0.004$), fasting plasma insulin ($r = -0.30$, $p = 0.005$), and HOMA-IR ($r = -0.23$, $p = 0.028$). Finally, serum levels of nitrates and nitrites, as a surrogate marker of NO bioavailability, were ~32% higher in the non-obese compared to obese subjects (4.9 ± 0.6 μmol/L vs. 3.7 ± 0.4 μmol/L; $p = 0.047$) (Figure 2D).

3.3. Brachial Artery FMD

Baseline arterial diameter was not statistically different between the two groups, obese (6.1 ± 0.6) and non-obese ((5.2 ± 0.2), $p = 0.619$). The %FMD, calculated as described in the methods, was 1.6-fold lower in the obese subjects compared to the non-obese controls ($p = 0.017$; Figure 2E). Percentage FMD correlated positively with lean % ($r = 0.71$, $p < 0.0001$), folate ($r = 0.32$, $p = 0.030$), and vitamin B12 ($r = 0.67$, $p < 0.0001$) and negatively with body weight ($r = -0.87$, $p < 0.0001$), BMI ($r = -0.89$, $p < 0.0001$), total fat % ($r = -0.57$, $p = 0.001$), VAT mass ($r = -0.77$, $p < 0.0001$), Hcy ($r = -0.47$, $p = 0.007$), and HOMA-IR ($r = -0.32$, $p = 0.024$).. Furthermore, there were significant direct correlations between %FMD and arteriolar FID (at Δ 60, $r = 0.43$, $p = 0.004$) and AchID (at 10^{-5} mole/L, $r = 0.51$, $p = 0.001$) among the subjects.

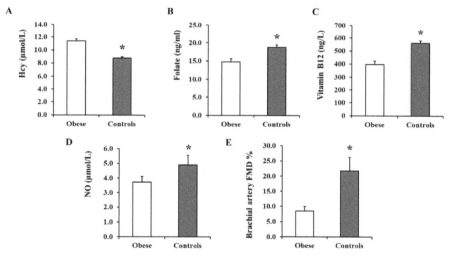

Figure 2. Plasma Hcy, folate, vitamin B12, and NO concentrations and brachial artery FMD measurements. Plasma from obese subjects ($n = 40$) and non-obese controls ($n = 40$) were analyzed for Hcy (**A**), folate (**B**), and vitamin B12 (**C**) using specific ELISA assays and for nitrates + nitrites (NO metabolites) using the Griess chemical reaction assay (**D**). Percentage of brachial artery FMD was calculated by subtracting the mean baseline diameter from the largest mean values obtained after cuff deflation in obese subjects ($n = 40$) and non-obese controls ($n = 40$) (**E**). All measurements are presented as means ± standard error (SE). * ($p < 0.05$) for comparing obese subjects with controls.

3.4. Arteriolar Vasoreactivity and NO and ROS Production

Figure 3 shows the response of isolated SAT arterioles to increasing the intraluminal pressure gradient (Δ 10–Δ 100 cmH$_2$O). Arteriolar FID was higher in the non-obese compared to obese subjects across all pressure gradients. The maximum dilation (MD) at Δ 60 cmH$_2$O, which corresponds to physiological shear stress, was 60% higher in the controls (Figure 3A). Similar results were obtained in response to Ach (Figure 3B). The reduction in FID and AchID observed in SAT arterioles in response to endothelial nitric oxide synthase (eNOS) inhibition by L-NAME (Figure 3C,D) were of a higher magnitude in the controls compared to obese subjects (1.8 fold higher at Δ 60 cmH$_2$O, $p < 0.0001$).

The observed low sensitivity of SAT arterioles to NO inhibition in obese subjects might indicate a disruption in the NO-dependent vasodilation mechanism in this group. Similar patterns of differences in the FID and AchID between obese and non-obese subjects were observed in the VAT arterioles (Figure 4A,B). The response of VAT arterioles to NO inhibition via L-NAME was less than that seen in SAT arterioles in both the obese (reduction in % vasodilation by 35 in SAT vs. 6 in VAT at Δ 60 cmH_2O) and non-obese (reduction in % vasodilation by 12 in SAT vs. 2 in VAT at Δ 60 cmH_2O) groups, indicating lower sensitivity of VAT arterioles to NO-induced vasoreactivity (Figure 4C,D). Furthermore, arteriolar FID and AchID were lower in the VAT compared to SAT arterioles in the non-obese (24% lower at Δ 60 cmH_2O, $p < 0.01$) and obese subjects (1.3 fold lower at Δ 60 cmH_2O, $p < 0.0001$); yet, the magnitude of reduction was much higher in the latter group across all pressure gradients and Ach doses. Baseline FID and AchID in SAT and VAT arterioles correlated significantly with anthropometric and cardiometabolic risk factors, as shown in Table 2 (only FID is shown). Using multivariate regression analysis, Hcy, folate, and vitamin B12 were independent predictive factors for the FID and AchID in both SAT and VAT arterioles. The magnitude of FID reductions following L-NAME incubation, which reflects NO sensitivity correlated negatively with weight, waist circumference, BMI, DEXA-estimated fat% and VAT mass, systolic blood pressure, HbA1c, fasting plasma insulin, HOMA-IR, triglycerides, and Hcy and positively with DEXA-estimated lean%, HDL, NO, folate, and vitamin B12 (Table 3). These correlations were more significant in SAT arterioles compared to VAT arterioles, indicating a higher NO sensitivity in the former.

Table 2. Pearson correlations between subcutaneous (SAT) and visceral (VAT) arteriolar FID at Δ 60 and different physical and cardiometabolic variables.

	SAT Arteriole FID at Δ 60		VAT Arteriole FID at Δ 60	
	Pearson Correlation	*p* Value	Pearson Correlation	*p* Value
Weight	−0.856	<0.0001	−0.873	<0.0001
WC	−0.761	<0.0001	−0.761	<0.0001
BMI	−0.916	<0.0001	−0.937	<0.0001
Fat%	−0.839	<0.0001	−0.843	<0.0001
Lean%	0.833	<0.0001	0.837	<0.0001
VAT Mass	−0.625	<0.0001	−0.635	<0.0001
HR	−0.185	0.045	−0.187	0.043
SBP	−0.357	<0.0001	−0.355	<0.0001
DBP	−0.181	0.048	−0.172	0.057
FPI	−0.516	<0.0001	−0.500	<0.0001
HOMA-IR	−0.293	0.006	−0.289	0.006
HDL	0.350	0.004	0.373	0.002
Hcy	−0.427	0.003	−0.420	0.004
Folate	0.344	0.002	0.341	0.002
VitB12	0.432	<0.0001	0.421	<0.0001
Alcohol	−0.212	0.035	−0.206	0.039
FMD%	0.434	0.004	0. 349	0.017

Table 3. Pearson correlations between No sensitivity in SAT and VAT isolated arterioles and different physical and cardiometabolic variables.

	% Reduction in FID at Δ 60 cmH$_2$O Following L-NAME Incubation (NO Sensitivity)			
	SAT Arteriole		VAT Arteriole	
	Pearson Correlation	p Value	Pearson Correlation	p Value
Weight	−0.844	<0.0001	−0.428	<0.0001
WC	−0.649	<0.0001	−0.079	0.317
BMI	−0.914	<0.0001	−0.264	0.007
Fat%	−0.715	<0.0001	−0.173	0.126
Lean%	0.711	<0.0001	0.172	0.126
VAT Mass	−0.529	0.002	−0.051	0.399
SBP	−0.332	0.001	−0.220	0.021
HbA1c	−0.241	0.043	−0.326	0.009
FPI	−0.506	<0.0001	−0.363	0.001
HOMA-IR	−0.248	0.017	−0.266	0.011
HDL	0.385	0.002	0.392	0.001
Triglycerides	−0.245	0.036	−0.043	0.379
Hcy	−0.437	0.003	−0.298	0.033
NO	0.273	0.047	0.100	0.273
Folate	0.496	0.001	0.210	0.100
VitB12	0.435	<0.0001	0.231	0.029

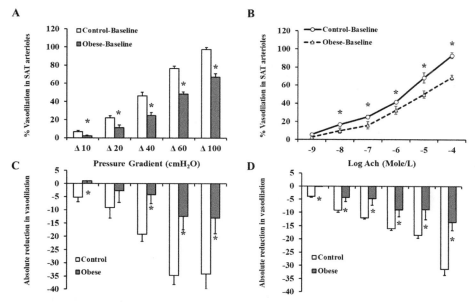

Figure 3. FID and acetylcholine-induced dilation (AchID) in SAT isolated resistance arterioles. FID measurements in SAT arterioles isolated from obese ($n = 40$) and non-obese ($n = 40$) subjects corresponding to increasing intraluminal pressure gradients of 10–100 cmH$_2$O (**A**). AchID measurements in SAT arterioles corresponding to increasing concentrations of Ach (10^{-9} to 10^{-4} M) (**B**). Absolute reduction in FID in response to eNOS inhibition via L-NAME (10^{-4} M) (**C**). Absolute reduction in AchID in response to eNOS inhibition via L-NAME (**D**). All measurements are presented as means ± standard error (SE). * ($p < 0.05$) for comparing obese subjects with controls.

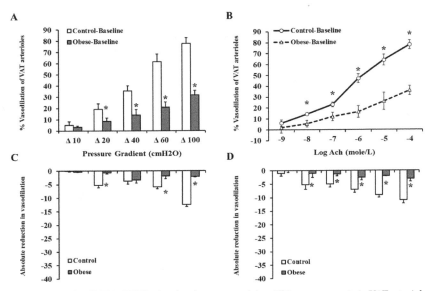

Figure 4. FID and AChID in VAT isolated resistance arterioles. FID measurements in VAT arterioles isolated from obese ($n = 40$) and non-obese ($n = 40$) subjects corresponding to increasing intraluminal pressure gradients of 10–100 cmH$_2$O (**A**). AchID measurements in VAT arterioles corresponding to increasing concentrations of Ach (10^{-9} to 10^{-4} M) (**B**). Absolute reduction in FID in response to eNOS inhibition via L-NAME (10^{-4} M) (**C**). Absolute reduction in AchID in response to eNOS inhibition via L-NAME (**D**). All measurements are presented as means ± standard error (SE). * ($p < 0.05$) for comparing obese subjects with controls.

Exogenous incubation with Hcy reduced arteriolar vasodilation in both SAT (Figure 5A) and VAT (Figure 5C) arterioles. These reductions were of a higher magnitude in the controls compared to obese subjects. At Δ 60 cm H$_2$O, the average absolute reduction in % vasodilation was 30 in control SAT arterioles and 6 in obese SAT arterioles. Similar patterns were obtained in VAT arterioles. These findings could be explained by the higher baseline FID measurements in controls compared to obese subjects. These high measurements provide a chance for a more perceptible magnitude of reduction in the control arterioles in response to Hcy. In Hcy-preconditioned arterioles, L-NAME-mediated FID reductions were of very low magnitude in obese and non-obese subjects in both SAT (Figure 5B) and VAT (Figure 5D) arterioles. The observed low sensitivity of Hcy-preconditioned arterioles to NO inhibition might indicate a disruption in the NO-dependent vasodilation mechanism in these arterioles following incubation with Hcy. Vessels that were incubated with Hcy and TEMPOL, the superoxide dismutase mimetic, had higher FID measurements compared to Hcy alone in both obese and control subjects (Figure 6 A,B). For example, When TEMPOL was combined with Hcy, FID in SAT arterioles at Δ 60 cm H$_2$O pressure increased by 55% in controls and 36% in obese subjects compared to Hcy only. Similarly, FID in VAT arterioles at Δ 60 cm H$_2$O pressure increased by 74% in controls and 77% in obese subjects. Endothelium-independent vasodilation to SNP was not different between obese and control subjects in either SAT (Figure 7A) or VAT (Figure 7B) arterioles. Moreover, SNP-induced vasodilation in Hcy-preconditioned arterioles was mostly preserved and showed little reductions compared to those in unconditioned arterioles (Figure 7C,D).

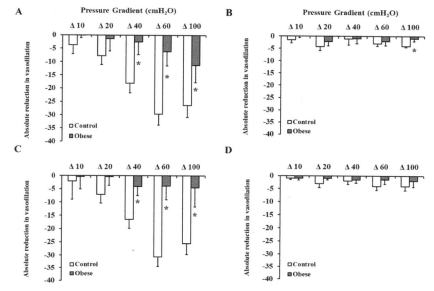

Figure 5. Effect of Hcy incubation on baseline FID and L-NAME-mediated reduction in FID. SAT (**A,B**) and VAT (**C,D**) isolated arterioles from obese subjects ($n = 10$) and non-obese controls ($n = 10$) were incubated in100 µM of Hcy for 180 min followed by measuring FID with and without eNOS inhibition via L-NAME (10^{-4} M). Charts (**A,C**) present absolute reductions in FID in Hcy preconditioned arterioles compared to corresponding unconditioned arterioles. Charts (**B,D**) present absolute reduction in FID caused by L-NAME in Hcy preconditioned arterioles compared with baseline FID after Hcy incubation. All measurements are presented as means ± standard error (SE). * ($p < 0.05$) for comparing obese subjects with controls.

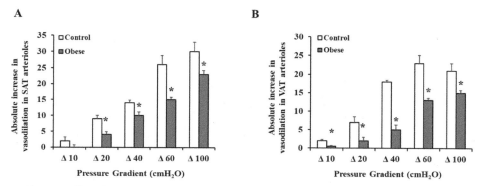

Figure 6. Effect of TEMPOL on restoring FID in Hcy preconditioned arterioles. Isolated arterioles from obese subjects ($n = 10$) and non-obese controls ($n = 10$) were incubated in100 µM of Hcy and the superoxide dismutase mimetic, TEMPOL (10^{-5} M) for 180 min followed by measuring the FID. Charts (**A**) and (**B**) present the absolute increase in FID in response to combined incubation with Hcy and TEMPOL relative to Hcy alone in SAT and VAT arterioles, respectively. All measurements are presented as means ± standard error (SE). * ($p < 0.05$) for comparing obese subjects with controls.

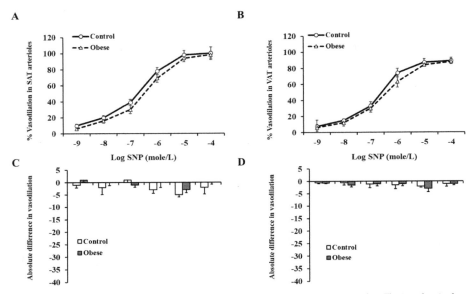

Figure 7. Endothelium-independent vasodilation in SAT and VAT isolated arterioles. The intraluminal diameter of SAT (**A**) and VAT (**B**) isolated arterioles was measured in response to increasing concentrations of SNP (10^{-9}–10^{-4} M) in obese subjects ($n = 40$) and non-obese controls ($n = 40$). The absolute difference in SNP-induced vasodilation between Hcy-preconditioned and unconditioned SAT (**C**) and VAT (**D**) arterioles in obese subjects ($n = 10$) and non-obese controls ($n = 10$). All measurements are presented as means ± standard error (SE).

Consistent with the FID data, arteriolar NO staining intensity (measured by ImageJ and expressed in arbitrary units) was lower in the obese compared to non-obese subjects in both SAT (obese: 12.6 ± 1.9, control: 30.6 ± 2.5, $p < 0.0001$) and VAT arterioles (obese: 9.9 ± 1.2, control: 24.7 ± 2.4, $p < 0.0001$) (Figure 8A,B). As opposed to NO, ROS staining was higher in obese subjects compared to controls in SAT (obese: 24.9 ± 2.6, control: 9.6 ± 2.5, $p < 0.0001$) and VAT arterioles (obese: 27.5 ± 1.0, control: 9.5 ± 3.1, $p < 0.0001$) (Figure 8A,C). Arteriolar NO was attenuated in response to L-NAME incubation in controls (% reduction in SAT = 56% and VAT = 51%, $p < 0.0001$) and obese subjects (% reduction in SAT = 18% and VAT = 9%, $p > 0.05$) (Figure 8). Similarly, Hcy incubation resulted in reductions in NO generation in controls (% reduction in SAT= 53% and VAT = 49%, $p < 0.0001$) and obese subjects (% reduction in SAT = 41% and VAT = 12%, $p < 0.05$) (Figure 9A,B). The L-NAME- and Hcy-mediated reductions in arteriolar NO were of a higher magnitude in controls compared to obese subjects and in SAT compared to VAT arterioles. This differential response could be attributed to higher baseline levels of NO in controls and SAT arterioles and accordingly, higher NO sensitivity. ROS staining increased in response to Hcy incubation in all participants (% increase in SAT = 104% and 43% and VAT = 137% and 38% in controls and obese, respectively) (Figure 9A,C). This induction in ROS was abolished in response to TEMPOL (% reduction in SAT = 45% and 56% and VAT = 39% and 50% in controls and obese, respectively). Reductions in ROS generation in response to TEMPOL was also associated with improvements in arteriolar NO staining (% increase in SAT = 1.2 and 1.6 folds and VAT = 1.4 and 17 folds in controls and obese, respectively) (Figure 9A,B).

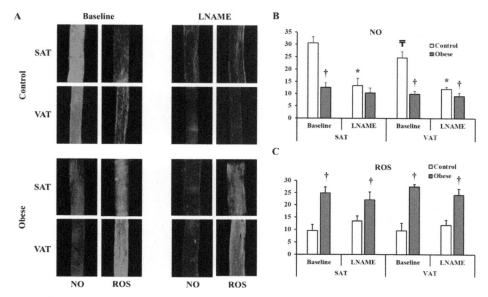

Figure 8. NO and Reactive Oxygen Species (ROS) production in isolated adipose tissue arterioles. (**A**): Representative images by fluorescence microscopy of NO (red fluorescence) and ROS (green fluorescence) generation at baseline conditions and after incubation with L-NAME in adipose tissue arterioles collected obese subjects ($n = 40$) and non-obese controls ($n = 40$). The charts present NO (**B**) and ROS (**C**) fluorescent signals that were measured and expressed in arbitrary units using NIH Image J software. All measures are represented as means± SE. * ($p < 0.05$) for comparing L-NAME to baseline in each group, † ($p < 0.05$) for comparing obese subjects with controls, and ⊤ ($p < 0.05$) for comparing SAT and VAT arterioles in each treatment condition.

Table 4 summarizes folate and vitamin B12 administration in obese and non-obese subjects. In subjects who administered supplements that contain folate or vitamin B12 before surgery, we observed no differences in arteriolar FID compared to those who were not taking supplementation. Moreover, the effect of L-NAME on inhibiting vasodilation in participants taking folate or vitamin B12 supplementation followed the same patterns observed in all participants. Data about alcohol consumption (frequency and quantity) were collected from all participants and summarized in Table 4. Using drinking level categories modified from those of Cahalan et al. [18], participants were classified as abstainers, light, moderate, and heavy drinkers. The criteria for this classification are shown under the table. Alcohol consumption was found to correlate negatively with folate levels ($r = -0.367$, $p = 0.015$), vitamin B12 concentrations ($r = -0.207$, $p = 0.047$), and SAT and VAT arteriolar FID at $\Delta 60$ cmH$_2$O ($r = -0.212$, $p = 0.035$ and $r = -0.206$, $p = 0.039$, respectively).

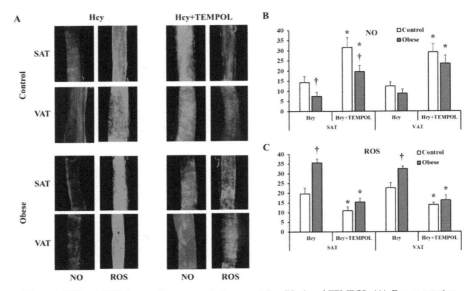

Figure 9. NO and ROS changes in response to homocysteine (Hcy) and TEMPOL. (**A**): Representative images by fluorescence microscopy of NO (red fluorescence) and ROS (green fluorescence) generation in response to Hcy and Hcy + TEMPOL treatment conditions in adipose tissue arterioles collected obese subjects ($n = 10$) and non-obese controls ($n = 10$). The charts present NO (**B**) and ROS (**C**) fluorescent signals that were measured and expressed in arbitrary units using NIH Image J software. All measures are represented as means± SE. * ($p < 0.05$) for comparing L-NAME to baseline in each group, and † ($p < 0.05$) for comparing obese subjects with controls.

Table 4. Consumption of alcohol and vitamin B12 and folate supplements.

Supplement	Non-Obese Controls ($n = 40$)	Obese Bariatric Patients ($n = 40$)
Folate (1 mg/d)	0 (0%)	3 (7.5%)
Vitamin B12 (250–5000 mcg/d)	0 (0%)	12 (30%)
Alcohol	**Non-Obese Controls ($n = 40$)**	**Obese Bariatric Patients ($n = 40$)**
Abstainers	25 (63%)	22 (55%)
Light drinkers	8 (20%)	13 (32.5%)
Moderate drinkers	7 (17%)	5 (12.5%)
Heavy drinkers	0 (0%)	0 (0%)

Light drinkers, less than one time/month with less than 5 drinks/time, 1–3 times/month with less than 3 drinks/time or 1–2 times/week with less than 2 drinks/time. Moderate drinkers, 1–3 times/month with 3–4 drinks/time, 1–2 times/week with 2–4 drinks/time, or 3–6 times/week with less than 2 drinks/time. Heavy drinkers, any quantity, and/or frequency that is more than moderate drinkers.

4. Discussion

The main findings of the current study are that (1) plasma levels of Hcy were higher while folate, vitamin B12, and NO levels were lower in obese subjects compared to non-obese controls, (2) brachial artery FMD and arteriolar FID and AchID were lower in the obese compared to the non-obese subjects and were not affected by mild or moderate alcohol consumption or administration of vitamin B12 or folic acid, (3) sensitivity to eNOS inhibition via L-NAME was higher in the non-obese controls especially in the SAT-isolated arterioles, (4) exogenous Hcy incubation reduced arteriolar FID to a greater extent in the controls compared to obese subject (5) Hcy-preconditioned arterioles lost sensitivity to eNOS inhibition via L-NAME, and (6) endothelium-independent vasodilation was not significantly different between obese and non-obese subjects, and was mostly preserved after incubation with Hcy.

Hyperhomocysteinemia has been classified as mild (15–20 μmol/L), moderate (21–100 μmol/ L), and severe (>100 μmol/L). Nevertheless, there are also expected graded increased risks for subjects with Hcy concentrations of 10–15 μmol/L. In support of this, some epidemiological studies reported a higher risk of developing peripheral arterial disease and cardiovascular events in subjects with Hcy concentrations above 10 μmol/L [19–21]. In the current study, Hcy concentrations were not severely elevated in the obese group (11.4 ± 0.3 μmol/L) and might be considered within the normal range by some classifications. Nevertheless, Hcy levels were significantly higher in obese subjects compared to non-obese controls (8.7 ± 0.2 μmol/L) and correlated significantly with higher body weight, waist circumference, BMI, and fat percentage. Comparable concentrations of Hcy have been shown by Vaya et al. [22] in morbidly obese patients (12.76 ± 5.30 μmol/L) and normal-weight subjects (10.67 ± 2.50 μmol/L). In the latter study, obese patients had significantly higher Hcy levels than controls. Moreover, waist circumference and abdominal obesity were independent predictors of higher Hcy levels. Similarly, other clinical studies have reported concentrations of Hcy that ranged between 7 and 14 μmol/L in obese subjects [23–26]. Therefore, our data and results from previous studies may indicate that obesity-related hyperhomocysteinemia lies within the mild range.

Interestingly, within obese subjects, those with insulin resistance and hyperinsulinemia were shown to have higher levels of Hcy than obese insulin-sensitive individuals. For example, a study by Martos et al. [26] reported blood Hcy of 7.81 ± 0.52 μmol/L in obese hyperinsulinemic subjects versus 6.41 ± 0.17 μmol/L in obese normoinsulinemic ($p = 0.002$). Similar results were demonstrated by Sanchez-Margalet et al. [23]; average Hcy levels were 12.4 ± 0.5 μmol/L in obese hyperinsulinemic subjects versus 7.1 ± 0.7 μmol/L in obese normoinsulinemic subjects ($p < 0.05$). Our data are consistent with these findings and support the association between hyperinsulinemia and hyperhomocysteinemia in obese individuals. In the current study, we found higher Hcy concentrations in obese subjects with insulin levels more than 10 μU/mL (12.9 ± 0.2 μmol/L) compared with obese subjects with insulin levels less than 10 μU/mL (8.9 ± 0.4 μmol/L). Nevertheless, these correlations do not provide a clear mechanistic understanding of the relationship between elevated levels of insulin and Hcy and it is still unknown whether hyperhomocysteinemia is a consequence or a cause of hyperinsulinemia. Both conditions induce oxidative stress and they also exacerbate under oxidative stress, which could create a dangerous vicious circle.

Our results showed that plasma levels of Hcy correlate negatively with endothelial-dependent macrovascular (brachial artery FMD) and microvascular (arteriolar FID) function. Plasma Hcy was an independent predictor of vascular function even after accounting for other variables such as insulin, folate, and vitamin B12. Hyperhomocysteinemia was shown to be an independent risk factor for CVD. Several observational studies have reported positive associations between blood Hcy concentrations and CVD such as hypertension, stroke, coronary artery disease, and peripheral artery disease [27–30]. In a seminal meta-analysis by Boushey et al. [19], 27 observational studies that measured the link between Hcy levels in blood and CVD risk were included, and it was concluded that 5 μmol/L increments in plasma Hcy result in 1.6 to 1.8 fold increases in CVD risk. Endothelial dysfunction is one of the earliest signs of CVD. We have previously shown that endothelial-dependent vascular function and NO sensitivity are impaired in morbidly obese bariatric patients [14]. In these studies, we observed a role of vitamin D in improving endothelial-mediated FID in this category of morbidly obese patients, which could be achieved through the antioxidative properties of vitamin D. However, the reason behind the induction of oxidative stress in adipose tissue-isolated arterioles and whether it could be attributed to Hcy abundance is not entirely understood.

In the current study, we detected higher baseline levels of ROS and lower NO production in arterioles isolated from the non-obese group compared to obese subjects. Arteriolar levels of ROS correlated positively with plasma Hcy; however, this relationship does not imply causation. Thus, in an effort to determine the contribution of ROS production to Hcy-mediated vascular dysfunction in the current study, we measured ROS generation and FID in adipose tissue-isolated arterioles exogenously incubated in Hcy alone, and Hcy combined with the superoxide dismutase mimetic,

TEMPOL. We observed significant induction in arteriolar ROS production, reduction in NO, and impairment in the FID after Hcy incubation; these changes were inhibited by the superoxide scavenger, TEMPOL. These findings may indicate a role of oxidative stress in mediating Hcy-induced endothelial dysfunction. Indeed, oxidative stress could be upstream to most of the previously suggested molecular mechanisms by which Hcy damages endothelial function. Some of these proposed mechanisms include NO inhibition, angiotensin II receptor-1 activation, prostanoid upregulation, and endothelin-1 induction [28,29,31–33]. These mechanisms were investigated in cultured endothelial cells or animal models of genetic- and diet-induced hyperhomocysteinemia. Thus, the current study provides some mechanistic understanding of Hcy-mediated microvascular dysfunction utilizing human isolated arterioles. However, further studies are required to elucidate molecular pathways involved in Hcy-induced oxidative stress such as NADPH and xanthine oxidases that could serve as therapeutic and preventive targets in Hcy-associated CVD.

In endothelial cells, oxidative stress and the resulting ROS are expected to interfere with NO bioavailability. Thus, it is anticipated that the major outcome of induced oxidative stress in endothelial cells is the interruption of NO production and, subsequently, NO-mediated vasodilation. Findings from our study supported this statement and demonstrated an abolishment of NO sensitivity in Hcy-treated vessels, as evidenced by a lack of any further impairment in the FID in response to L-NAME.

While endothelial-dependent FID was compromised in obese subjects and Hcy-preconditioned arterioles, endothelial-independent vasodilation (SNP-induced) showed little changes compared to controls and unconditioned arterioles, respectively. The response to endothelial independent vasodilators such as SNP in obese individuals has been inconsistent among different studies at both the micro- and macrovascular levels. For example, a study by Van Guilder et al. [34] reported no differences in forearm blood flow between lean and obese subjects in response to intra-arterial infusion of SNP while significant reductions in obese subjects compared to lean controls were reported by Schinzari et al. [35] using a similar approach. A similar discrepancy has been encountered for microvascular function. While in some studies, only endothelial-mediated vasodilation was different between lean and obese individuals with preservation of SNP-mediated vasodilation [36,37], other studies reported impairments in both endothelial-dependent and -independent vasodilation in obese subjects [38]. However, these microvascular studies were conducted on cutaneous microvessels, mainly capillaries, while in the current study we targeted adipose tissue-isolated arterioles. Regarding hyperhomocysteinemia, a study by Fu et al. [39] has shown that in a hyperhomocysteinemic rat model, both endothelial-dependent and -independent vasodilation of mesenteric arterioles were impaired. Nevertheless, a study by Schlaich et al. [40] reported an intact endothelial-independent forearm blood flow in subjects with elevated Hcy levels. Collectively, findings from the current study point to impaired NO-mediated vasodilation as the primary pathogenesis in vascular dysfunction that accompanies obesity and hyperhomocysteinemia. However, due to the existing inconsistency in the literature that investigates this topic, further studies are warranted.

A possible role of nutritional deficiencies of folate and vitamin B12 in the development of hyperhomocysteinemia has been suggested in previous studies. Randomized clinical trials have demonstrated that oral supplementation with a combination of folic acid and vitamins B6 and B12 lowered blood levels of homocysteine [19,41–43]. Furthermore, epidemiological studies showed that folate and vitamin B12 are major determinants of plasma homocysteine levels, and negative correlations have been reported between hyperhomocysteinemia and low levels of folate and vitamin B12 in patients with hypertension and coronary artery diseases [44–47]. In the current study, folate and vitamin B12 were found to be significantly lower in obese subjects compared to non-obese controls. Both vitamins correlated positively with each other and negatively with BMI, fat percentage, and parameters of glucose metabolism and insulin sensitivity. However, neither folate nor vitamin B12 correlated with blood levels of homocysteine in our cohort. Previous studies that investigated this association in the context of obesity have yielded inconsistent findings. While in some of these studies, an inverse correlation between Hcy concentrations and blood levels of folate and vitamin B12 have been found [46], other studies failed to prove this relationship [23,26]. This lack of evident correlations we, and some other studies, have encountered might indicate that blood concentration of Hcy reflects the collective contribution of several integrative factors and not only the folate and vitamin B12 status. These factors may include hyperinsulinemia [24], oxidative stress [48], inflammation [49], dietary habits [50], physical activity [51], alcohol consumption [52], metabolic function [53], or undiagnosed comorbidities.

Despite the lack of significant correlation with plasma levels of Hcy, folate and vitamin B12 were independent predictive factors of vascular reactivity and NO sensitivity in our participants. These findings are supported by previous clinical trials that demonstrated improvements in brachial artery FMD in response to folate or vitamin B12 supplementation in healthy people and patients with diabetes, coronary artery diseases, peripheral arterial occlusive disease, and hypercholesterolemia [54–58]. However, the current study is the first to report these associations regardless of folate or vitamin B12 intake. Moreover, it is the first study to investigate this association at the level of microvascular function using a unique ex vivo, tissue-isolated microvascular FID approach.

Previous studies suggested a role of increased alcohol consumption in inducing the risk of developing CVDs such as hypertension, stroke, coronary artery diseases, peripheral arterial diseases, and cardiomyopathy [59]. In our current study, we did not observe correlations between alcohol intake and systemic NO levels. However, we detected significant inverse associations between alcohol intake and endothelial-mediated vasodilation and NO sensitivity in adipose tissue-isolated arterioles. Moreover, alcohol inversely correlated with folate and vitamin B12 levels in plasma, which might be another mechanism by which it contributes to impaired vascular function. This assumption is supported by several studies showing that chronic alcohol exposure interferes with intestinal absorption, hepatic uptake, and renal conservation of folate [60]. It has also been reported that even moderate alcohol intake may reduce folate and vitamin B12 levels in healthy, well-nourished adults [61]. It was suggested by some studies that alcohol induces blood Hcy concentrations via its adverse effects on folate and vitamin B12 [52,62]; however, this assumption was rejected by other studies [63,64]. In our study, we did not find any correlation between alcohol intake and plasma Hcy concentrations; nevertheless, both predicted an impaired microvascular endothelial-dependent vasodilation. The relationship between alcohol consumption and plasma Hcy should be further explored in a larger number of subjects with more accurate quantification of alcohol intake and multivariate analysis of other possible factors that may modify Hcy.

There are some limitations to this study. First, we had a relatively small sample size, which carries out the risk of a type II error due to low statistical power. Second, in order to collect visceral adipose tissues, the non-obese controls had to be candidates for electives surgeries such as hernia and abdominal wall construction. These conditions may affect the general health of controls, and accordingly, the controls, despite being non-obese and devoid of any chronic disease, they are not considered healthy. Third, the obese group consisted of morbidly obese subjects who were considered for weight loss surgery, so these findings cannot be extrapolated to individuals who are mildly or moderately obese. Finally, one of the major limitations in our study is the unbalanced female to male ratio (1.1:1 in controls vs. 2.3:1 in the obese group) since fewer male patients are scheduled for bariatric surgery at our center (12.5%). Furthermore, most of the male candidates were excluded due to chronic comorbidities that may modify vascular outcomes. Although this study was not designed to determine gender-specific differences in the vascular response to different levels of Hcy, folate, vitamin B12, and alcohol, future studies are required to determine the influence of gender on vascular function.

Author Contributions: M.H.: Data acquisition, editing and reviewing final draft, S.J.V.: Data acquisition, editing and reviewing final draft, D.N.: Patient recruitment, data acquisition, editing and reviewing final draft, M.I.M.: Data acquisition, editing and reviewing final draft, M.Q.: Data acquisition, editing and reviewing final draft, C.H.: Patient recruitment, sample collection, editing and reviewing final draft, M.M.: Patient recruitment, sample collection, editing and reviewing final draft, F.M.B.: Patient recruitment, sample collection, editing and reviewing final draft, P.F.: Patient recruitment, sample collection, editing and reviewing final draft, G.P.C.: Patient recruitment, sample collection, editing and reviewing final draft, A.G.: Patient recruitment, sample collection, editing and reviewing final draft, M.M.A.: Data acquisition, editing and reviewing final draft S.A.P.: Conceptualization, editing and reviewing final draft, A.M.M.: Conceptualization, supervision, data acquisition, editing and reviewing final draft. All authors have read and agreed to the published version of the manuscript.

Funding: This research was funded by the National Heart, Lung, and Blood Institute (NHLBI) K99HL140049 and 4 R00 HL140049-03 (AMM). SAP was funded by grants HL095701and HL130513.

Acknowledgments: We would like to thank the nurses and the staff at the General and Bariatric Surgery Clinic and the CCTS (Clinical Center for Translational Sciences) for their support with the study. The content is solely the responsibility of the authors and does not necessarily represent the official views of the National Institutes of Health.

Conflicts of Interest: The authors declare no conflict of interest.

References

1. Mitchell, N.; Catenacci, V.A.; Wyatt, H.R.; Hill, J.O. Obesity: Overview of an epidemic. *Psychiatr. Clin. N. Am.* **2011**, *34*, 717–732. [CrossRef]

2. Poli, V.F.S.; Sanches, R.B.; Moraes, A.D.S.; Fidalgo, J.P.N.; Nascimento, M.A.; Bresciani, P.; Andrade-Silva, S.G.; Cipullo, M.A.T.; Clemente, J.C.; Caranti, D.A. The excessive caloric intake and micronutrient deficiencies related to obesity after a long-term interdisciplinary therapy. *Nutrition* **2017**, *38*, 113–119. [CrossRef]

3. Selhub, J. Folate, vitamin B12 and vitamin B6 and one carbon metabolism. *J. Nutr. Health Aging* **2002**, *6*, 39–42.

4. Maron, B.A.; Loscalzo, J. The treatment of hyperhomocysteinemia. *Annu. Rev. Med.* **2009**, *60*, 39–54. [CrossRef]

5. Kim, J.; Kim, H.; Roh, H.; Kwon, Y. Causes of hyperhomocysteinemia and its pathological significance. *Arch. Pharm. Res.* **2018**, *41*, 372–383. [CrossRef]

6. Wierzbicki, A.S. Homocysteine and cardiovascular disease: A review of the evidence. *Diab. Vasc. Dis. Res.* **2007**, *4*, 143–150. [CrossRef]

7. Humphrey, L.L.; Fu, R.; Rogers, K.; Freeman, M.; Helfand, M. Homocysteine level and coronary heart disease incidence: A systematic review and meta-analysis. *Mayo Clin. Proc.* **2008**, *83*, 1203–1212. [CrossRef]

8. Matthews, D.R.; Hosker, J.P.; Rudenski, A.S.; Naylor, B.A.; Treacher, D.F.; Turner, R.C. Homeostasis model assessment: Insulin resistance and beta-cell function from fasting plasma glucose and insulin concentrations in man. *Diabetologia* **1985**, *28*, 412–419. [CrossRef]

9. Mahmoud, A.M.; Szczurek, M.R.; Blackburn, B.K.; Mey, J.T.; Chen, Z.; Robinson, A.T.; Bian, J.-T.; Unterman, T.G.; Minshall, R.D.; Brown, M.D.; et al. Hyperinsulinemia augments endothelin-1 protein expression and impairs vasodilation of human skeletal muscle arterioles. *Physiol. Rep.* **2016**, *4*, e12895. [CrossRef]

10. Phillips, S.A.; Hatoum, O.A.; Gutterman, D.D. The mechanism of flow-induced dilation in human adipose arterioles involves hydrogen peroxide during CAD. *Am. J. Physiol. Heart Circ. Physiol.* **2007**, *292*, H93–H100. [CrossRef]

11. Mahmoud, A.M.; Hwang, C.-L.; Szczurek, M.R.; Bian, J.-T.; Ranieri, C.; Gutterman, D.D.; Phillips, S.A. Low-Fat Diet Designed for Weight Loss But Not Weight Maintenance Improves Nitric Oxide-Dependent Arteriolar Vasodilation in Obese Adults. *Nutrients* **2019**, *11*, 1339. [CrossRef] [PubMed]

12. Miura, H.; Wachtel, E.R.; Liu, Y.; Loberiza, F.R.; Saito, T.; Miura, M.; Gutterman, D.D. Flow-induced dilation of human coronary arterioles: Important role of Ca(2+)-activated K(+) channels. *Circulation* **2001**, *103*, 1992–1998. [CrossRef] [PubMed]

13. Hwang, C.-L.; Ranieri, C.; Szczurek, M.R.; Ellythy, A.M.; Elokda, A.; Mahmoud, A.M.; Phillips, S.A. The Effect of Low-Carbohydrate Diet on Macrovascular and Microvascular Endothelial Function is Not Affected by the Provision of Caloric Restriction in Women with Obesity: A Randomized Study. *Nutrients* **2020**, *12*, 1649. [CrossRef]

14. Mahmoud, A.M.; Szczurek, M.R.; Hassan, C.; Masrur, M.; Gangemi, A.; Phillips, S.A. Vitamin D Improves Nitric Oxide-Dependent Vasodilation in Adipose Tissue Arterioles from Bariatric Surgery Patients. *Nutrients* **2019**, *11*, 2521. [CrossRef]

15. Bian, J.-T.; Piano, M.; Kotlo, K.U.; Mahmoud, A.M.; Phillips, S.A. MicroRNA-21 Contributes to Reduced Microvascular Function in Binge Drinking Young Adults. *Alcohol Clin. Exp. Res.* **2018**, *42*, 278–285. [CrossRef]

16. Lang, D.; Kredan, M.B.; Moat, S.J.; Hussain, S.A.; Powell, C.A.; Bellamy, M.F.; Powers, H.J.; Lewis, M.J. Homocysteine-induced inhibition of endothelium-dependent relaxation in rabbit aorta: Role for superoxide anions. *Arterioscler. Thromb. Vasc. Biol.* **2000**, *20*, 422–427. [CrossRef]

17. Robinson, A.T.; Franklin, N.; Norkeviciute, E.; Bian, J.T.; Babana, J.C.; Szczurek, M.R.; Phillips, S.A. Improved arterial flow-mediated dilation after exertion involves hydrogen peroxide in overweight and obese adults following aerobic exercise training. *J. Hypertens.* **2016**, *34*, 1309–1316. [CrossRef]

18. Clark, W.B.; Hilton, M.E. *Alcohol in America: Drinking Practices and Problems*; State University of New York Press: Albany, NY, USA, 1991.

19. Boushey, C.J.; Beresford, S.A.; Omenn, G.S.; Motulsky, A.G. A quantitative assessment of plasma homocysteine as a risk factor for vascular disease. Probable benefits of increasing folic acid intakes. *JAMA* **1995**, *274*, 1049–1057. [CrossRef]

20. Van den Bosch, M.A.; Bloemenkamp, D.G.; Willem, P.T.M.; Kemmeren, J.M.; Tanis, B.C.; Algra, A.; Rosendaal, F.R.; van der Graaf, Y. Hyperhomocysteinemia and risk for peripheral arterial occlusive disease in young women. *J. Vasc. Surg.* **2003**, *38*, 772–778. [CrossRef]

21. Taylor, B.V.; Oudit, G.Y.; Evans, M. Homocysteine, vitamins, and coronary artery disease. Comprehensive review of the literature. *Can. Fam. Physician* **2000**, *46*, 2236–2245.

22. Vayá, A.; Rivera, L.; Mijares, A.H.; De La Fuente, M.; Solá, E.; Romagnoli, M.; Alis, R.; Laiz, B. Homocysteine levels in morbidly obese patients: Its association with waist circumference and insulin resistance. *Clin. Hemorheol. Microcirc.* **2012**, *52*, 49–56. [CrossRef] [PubMed]

23. Sánchez-Margalet, V.; Valle, M.; Ruz, F.J.; Gascón, F.; Mateo, J.; Goberna, R. Elevated plasma total homocysteine levels in hyperinsulinemic obese subjects. *J. Nutr. Biochem.* **2002**, *13*, 75–79. [CrossRef]

24. Meigs, J.B.; Jacques, P.F.; Selhub, J.; Singer, D.E.; Nathan, D.M.; Rifai, N.; D'Agostino, R.B.; Wilson, P.W. Fasting plasma homocysteine levels in the insulin resistance syndrome: The Framingham offspring study. *Diabetes Care* **2001**, *24*, 1403–1410. [CrossRef] [PubMed]

25. Koehler, K.M.; Baumgartner, R.N.; Garry, P.J.; Allen, R.H.; Stabler, S.P.; Rimm, E.B. Association of folate intake and serum homocysteine in elderly persons according to vitamin supplementation and alcohol use. *Am. J. Clin. Nutr.* **2001**, *73*, 628–637. [CrossRef]

26. Martos, R.; Valle, M.; Morales, R.; Cañete, R.; Gavilan, M.I.; Sánchez-Margalet, V. Hyperhomocysteinemia correlates with insulin resistance and low-grade systemic inflammation in obese prepubertal children. *Metabolism* **2006**, *55*, 72–77. [CrossRef]

27. Cheng, Z.; Yang, X.; Wang, H. Hyperhomocysteinemia and Endothelial Dysfunction. *Curr. Hypertens. Rev.* **2009**, *5*, 158–165. [CrossRef]

28. Austin, R.C.; Lentz, S.R.; Werstuck, G.H. Role of hyperhomocysteinemia in endothelial dysfunction and atherothrombotic disease. *Cell Death Differ.* **2004**, *11*, S56–S64. [CrossRef]

29. Lai, W.K.; Kan, M.Y. Homocysteine-Induced Endothelial Dysfunction. *Ann. Nutr. Metab.* **2015**, *67*, 1–12. [CrossRef]

30. Faraci, F.M.; Lentz, S.R. Hyperhomocysteinemia, oxidative stress, and cerebral vascular dysfunction. *Stroke* **2004**, *35*, 345–347. [CrossRef]

31. Chambers, J.C.; McGregor, A.; Jean-Marie, J.; Obeid, A.O.; Kooner, J.S. Demonstration of rapid onset vascular endothelial dysfunction after hyperhomocysteinemia: An effect reversible with vitamin C therapy. *Circulation* **1999**, *99*, 1156–1160. [CrossRef]

32. Lentz, S.R.; Rodionov, R.N.; Dayal, S. Hyperhomocysteinemia, endothelial dysfunction, and cardiovascular risk: The potential role of ADMA. *Atheroscler. Suppl.* **2003**, *4*, 61–65. [CrossRef]

33. McDowell, I.F.; Lang, D. Homocysteine and endothelial dysfunction: A link with cardiovascular disease. *J. Nutr.* **2000**, *130*, 369S–372S. [CrossRef] [PubMed]

34. Van Guldener, C. Why is homocysteine elevated in renal failure and what can be expected from homocysteine-lowering? *Nephrol. Dial. Transplant.* **2006**, *21*, 1161–1166. [CrossRef] [PubMed]

35. Schinzari, F.; Iantorno, M.; Campia, U.; Mores, N.; Rovella, V.; Tesauro, M.; Di Daniele, N.; Cardillo, C. Vasodilator responses and endothelin-dependent vasoconstriction in metabolically healthy obesity and the metabolic syndrome. *Am. J. Physiol. Endocrinol. Metab.* **2015**, *309*, E787–E792. [CrossRef] [PubMed]

36. De Jongh, R.T.; Serné, E.H.; Ijzerman, R.G.; De Vries, G.; Stehouwer, C.D. Impaired microvascular function in obesity: Implications for obesity-associated microangiopathy, hypertension, and insulin resistance. *Circulation* **2004**, *109*, 2529–2535. [CrossRef] [PubMed]

37.	Baldeweg, S.; Pink, A.; Yudkin, J.; Coppack, S. The relationship between obesity, vascular reactivity and endothelial dysfunction in subjects with non-insulin dependent diabetes mellitus. *Int. J. Obes. Relat. Metab. Disord.* **2000**, *24*, S134–S135. [CrossRef] [PubMed]

38.	Patik, J.C.; Christmas, K.M.; Hurr, C.; Brothers, R.M. Impaired endothelium independent vasodilation in the cutaneous microvasculature of young obese adults. *Microvasc. Res.* **2016**, *104*, 63–68. [CrossRef] [PubMed]

39.	Fu, W.Y.; Dudman, N.P.; Perry, M.A.; Wang, X. Homocysteine attenuates hemodynamic responses to nitric oxide in vivo. *Atherosclerosis* **2002**, *161*, 169–176. [CrossRef]

40.	Schlaich, M.P.; John, S.; Jacobi, J.; Lackner, K.J.; Schmieder, R.E. Mildly elevated homocysteine concentrations impair endothelium dependent vasodilation in hypercholesterolemic patients. *Atherosclerosis* **2000**, *153*, 383–389. [CrossRef]

41.	Refsum, H.; Ueland, P.M.; Nygård, O.; Vollset, S.E. Homocysteine and cardiovascular disease. *Annu. Rev. Med.* **1998**, *49*, 31–62. [CrossRef]

42.	Wald, D.S.; Law, M.; Morris, J.K. Homocysteine and cardiovascular disease: Evidence on causality from a meta-analysis. *BMJ* **2002**, *325*, 1202. [CrossRef] [PubMed]

43.	Wang, T.J.; Gona, P.; Larson, M.G.; Tofler, G.H.; Levy, D.; Newton-Cheh, C.; Jacques, P.F.; Rifai, N.; Selhub, J.; Robins, S.J.; et al. Multiple biomarkers for the prediction of first major cardiovascular events and death. *N. Engl. J. Med.* **2006**, *355*, 2631–2639. [CrossRef] [PubMed]

44.	Ma, Y.; Peng, D.; Liu, C.; Huang, C.; Luo, J. Serum high concentrations of homocysteine and low levels of folic acid and vitamin B12 are significantly correlated with the categories of coronary artery diseases. *BMC Cardiovasc. Disord.* **2017**, *17*, 37. [CrossRef] [PubMed]

45.	Scazzone, C.; Bono, A.; Tornese, F.; Arsena, R.; Schillaci, R.; Butera, D.; Cottone, S. Correlation between low folate levels and hyperhomocysteinemia, but not with vitamin B12 in hypertensive patients. *Ann. Clin. Lab. Sci.* **2014**, *44*, 286–290.

46.	Karatela, R.A.; Sainani, G.S. Plasma homocysteine in obese, overweight and normal weight hypertensives and normotensives. *Indian Heart J.* **2009**, *61*, 156–159.

47.	Han, L.; Liu, Y.; Wang, C.; Tang, L.; Feng, X.; Astell-Burt, T.; Wen, Q.; Duan, D.; Lu, N.; Xu, G.; et al. Determinants of hyperhomocysteinemia in healthy and hypertensive subjects: A population-based study and systematic review. *Clin. Nutr.* **2017**, *36*, 1215–1230. [CrossRef]

48.	Jacobsen, D.W. Hyperhomocysteinemia and oxidative stress: Time for a reality check? *Arterioscler. Thromb. Vasc. Biol.* **2000**, *20*, 1182–1184. [CrossRef]

49.	Li, T.; Chen, Y.; Li, J.; Yang, X.; Zhang, H.; Qin, X.; Hu, Y.; Mo, Z. Serum Homocysteine Concentration Is Significantly Associated with Inflammatory/Immune Factors. *PLoS ONE* **2015**, *10*, e0138099. [CrossRef]

50.	Yakub, M.; Iqbal, M.P.; Iqbal, R. Dietary patterns are associated with hyperhomocysteinemia in an urban Pakistani population. *J. Nutr.* **2010**, *140*, 1261–1266. [CrossRef]

51.	Deminice, R.; Ribeiro, D.F.; Frajacomo, F.T. The Effects of Acute Exercise and Exercise Training on Plasma Homocysteine: A Meta-Analysis. *PLoS ONE* **2016**, *11*, e0151653. [CrossRef]

52.	Gibson, A.; Woodside, J.V.; Young, I.S.; Sharpe, P.; Mercer, C.; Patterson, C.; McKinley, M.; Kluijtmans, L.; Whitehead, A.; Evans, A. Alcohol increases homocysteine and reduces B vitamin concentration in healthy male volunteers—A randomized, crossover intervention study. *QJM* **2008**, *101*, 881–887. [CrossRef] [PubMed]

53.	Schaffer, A.; Verdoia, M.; Barbieri, L.; Cassetti, E.; Suryapranata, H.; De Luca, G. Impact of Diabetes on Homocysteine Levels and Its Relationship with Coronary Artery Disease: A Single-Centre Cohort Study. *Ann. Nutr. Metab.* **2016**, *68*, 180–188. [CrossRef] [PubMed]

54.	De Bree, A.; van Mierlo, L.A.; Draijer, R. Folic acid improves vascular reactivity in humans: A meta-analysis of randomized controlled trials. *Am. J. Clin. Nutr.* **2007**, *86*, 610–617. [CrossRef] [PubMed]

55.	Olthof, M.R.; Bots, M.L.; Katan, M.B.; Verhoef, P. Acute effect of folic acid, betaine, and serine supplements on flow-mediated dilation after methionine loading: A randomized trial. *PLoS Clin. Trials.* **2006**, *1*, e4. [CrossRef] [PubMed]

56.	Vijayakumar, A.; Kim, E.-K.; Kim, H.; Choi, Y.J.; Huh, K.B.; Chang, N. Effects of folic acid supplementation on serum homocysteine levels, lipid profiles, and vascular parameters in post-menopausal Korean women with type 2 diabetes mellitus. *Nutr. Res. Pract.* **2017**, *11*, 327–333. [CrossRef] [PubMed]

57.	Yi, X.; Zhou, Y.; Jiang, D.; Li, X.; Guo, Y.; Jiang, X. Efficacy of folic acid supplementation on endothelial function and plasma homocysteine concentration in coronary artery disease: A meta-analysis of randomized controlled trials. *Exp. Ther. Med.* **2014**, *7*, 1100–1110. [CrossRef] [PubMed]

58. Hoch, A.Z.; Pajewski, N.M.; Hoffmann, R.G.; Schimke, J.E.; Gutterman, D.D. Possible relationship of folic Acid supplementation and improved flow-mediated dilation in premenopausal, eumenorrheic athletic women. *J. Sports Sci. Med.* **2009**, *8*, 123–129.

59. Piano, M.R. Alcohol's Effects on the Cardiovascular System. *Alcohol Res.* **2017**, *38*, 219–241.

60. Halsted, C.H.; Villanueva, J.A.; Devlin, A.M.; Chandler, C.J. Metabolic interactions of alcohol and folate. *J. Nutr.* **2002**, *132*, 2367S–2372S. [CrossRef]

61. Laufer, E.M.; Hartman, T.J.; Baer, D.J.; Gunter, E.W.; Dorgan, J.F.; Campbell, W.S.; Clevidence, A.B.; Brown, E.D.; Albanes, D.; Judd, J.T.; et al. Effects of moderate alcohol consumption on folate and vitamin B(12) status in postmenopausal women. *Eur. J. Clin. Nutr.* **2004**, *58*, 1518–1524. [CrossRef]

62. Bleich, S.; Bleich, K.; Kropp, S.; Bittermann, H.-J.; Degner, D.; Sperling, W.; Rüther, E.; Kornhuber, J. Moderate alcohol consumption in social drinkers raises plasma homocysteine levels: A contradiction to the 'French Paradox'? *Alcohol Alcohol.* **2001**, *36*, 189–192. [CrossRef] [PubMed]

63. Rimm, E.B.; Willett, W.C.; Hu, F.B.; Sampson, L.; Colditz, G.A.; Manson, J.E.; Hennekens, C.; Stampfer, M.J. Folate and vitamin B6 from diet and supplements in relation to risk of coronary heart disease among women. *JAMA* **1998**, *279*, 359–364. [CrossRef] [PubMed]

64. Halsted, C.H. Lifestyle effects on homocysteine and an alcohol paradox. *Am. J. Clin. Nutr.* **2001**, *73*, 501–502. [CrossRef]

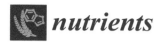 *nutrients*

Article

Compound 18 Improves Glucose Tolerance in a Hepatocyte TGR5-dependent Manner in Mice

Marlena M. Holter [1], Margot K. Chirikjian [1], Daniel A. Briere [2], Adriano Maida [3,4],
Kyle W. Sloop [2], Kristina Schoonjans [3] and Bethany P. Cummings [1,*]

[1] Department of Biomedical Sciences, College of Veterinary Medicine, Cornell University,
    Ithaca, NY 14850, USA; mmh277@cornell.edu (M.M.H.); mkc224@cornell.edu (M.K.C.)
[2] Diabetes and Complications, Lilly Research Laboratories, Eli Lilly and Company,
    Indianapolis, IN 46225, USA; briere_daniel_a@lilly.com (D.A.B); sloop_kyle_w@lilly.com (K.W.S.)
[3] Institute for Diabetes and Cancer, Helmholtz Zentrum München, 85764 Neuherberg, Germany;
    adriano.maida@helmholtz-muenchen.de (A.M.); krisitina.schoonjans@epfl.ch (K.S.)
[4] Institute of Bioengineering, École Polytechnique Fédérale de Lausanne, 1015 Lausanne, Switzerland
[*] Correspondence: bpc68@cornell.edu; Tel.: +1-607-253-3552

Received: 23 June 2020; Accepted: 15 July 2020; Published: 17 July 2020

Abstract: The bile acid receptor, TGR5, is a key regulator of glucose homeostasis, but the mechanisms by which TGR5 signaling improves glucose regulation are incompletely defined. In particular, TGR5 has an increasingly appreciated role in liver physiology and pathobiology; however, whether TGR5 signaling within the liver contributes to its glucoregulatory effects is unknown. Therefore, we investigated the role of hepatocyte TGR5 signaling on glucose regulation using a hepatocyte-specific TGR5 knockout mouse model. Hepatocyte-specific $Tgr5^{Hep+/+}$ and $Tgr5^{Hep-/-}$ mice were fed a high fat diet (HFD) for 7 weeks and then orally gavaged with three doses of a highly potent, TGR5-specific agonist, Compound 18 (10 mg/kg), or vehicle, over 72 h and underwent an oral glucose tolerance test (OGTT) after the last dose. Herein, we report that TGR5 mRNA and protein is present in mouse hepatocytes. Cumulative food intake, body weight, and adiposity do not differ between $Tgr5^{Hep+/+}$ and $Tgr5^{Hep-/-}$ mice with or without treatment with Compound 18. However, administration of Compound 18 improves glucose tolerance in $Tgr5^{HEP+/+}$ mice, but not in $Tgr5^{Hep-/-}$ mice. Further, this effect occurred independent of body weight and GLP-1 secretion. Together, these data demonstrate that TGR5 is expressed in hepatocytes, where it functions as a key regulator of whole-body glucose homeostasis.

Keywords: hepatocyte; TGR5; glucose regulation

1. Introduction

Bile acids are amphipathic steroid molecules that activate the nuclear receptor, farnesoid X receptor (FXR), and the transmembrane G-protein coupled receptor, TGR5, to integrate lipid, glucose, and energy metabolism and maintain metabolic homeostasis [1–3]. Dysregulated bile acid signaling is associated with the pathogenesis of various diseases including cholestatic liver diseases, dyslipidemia, fatty liver diseases, and type 2 diabetes [4–7]. As such, TGR5 is a key regulator of metabolic homeostasis; however, the mechanisms remain incompletely defined.

TGR5 is expressed in many tissues including endocrine glands, adipocytes, muscle, liver, brain, and the gastrointestinal tract [8–12]. TGR5 signaling in many of these tissue types has been shown to contribute to glucose regulation [3,13]. For example, in gastrointestinal enteroendocrine L cells, TGR5 signaling promotes glucagon-like peptide-1 (GLP-1) secretion [3,14,15]. Furthermore, in mice fed a high fat diet (HFD), TGR5 agonists have been shown to increase in GLP-1 secretion from L cells, which was associated with an improvement in insulin sensitivity and measures of hepatic steatosis [16].

TGR5 is also found on pancreatic beta-cells where its activation increases glucose-stimulated insulin secretion [17]. It has also been demonstrated that TGR5 signaling increases energy expenditure by increasing the activity of the cyclic-AMP-dependent thyroid hormone activating enzyme type 2 iodothyronine deiodinase, mitochondrial thermogenesis, and fat mass oxidation to enhance basal metabolic rate [13,18,19]. TGR5 signaling in adipocytes promotes beiging of white adipose tissue in mice [19] and enhances energy expenditure to improve glucose regulation [13,20]. Finally, TGR5 signaling in immune cells decreases inflammatory cytokine secretion [11,21,22], which likely decreases systemic inflammation to improve insulin sensitivity [23].

TGR5 is also robustly expressed in the liver, but the role of hepatic TGR5 signaling in glucose regulation remains poorly understood. Various studies have identified anti-inflammatory, anti-apoptotic, choleretic, and proliferative effects of TGR5 signaling in nonparenchymal cell types of the liver. Within the liver, TGR5 is highly expressed on Kupffer cells [9], sinusoidal endothelial cells [10], and cholangiocytes [24,25]. In Kupffer cells and resident macrophages, bile acid signaling through TGR5 activates a cAMP-dependent pathway that attenuates LPS-induced cytokine expression and reduces the NF-kB-dependent inflammatory response, thereby dampening hepatic inflammation and promoting tissue remodeling [9,21]. Further, activation of TGR5 on sinusoidal endothelial cells functions to modulate liver microcirculation through increased production of nitric oxide [10,26]. This serves to both mitigate portal hypertension and enable adaptation of hepatic blood flow to nutrient uptake [26,27]. TGR5 activation of biliary epithelial cells results in CFTR-dependent chloride and bicarbonate secretion into bile, which reduces bile acid protonation to protect the liver parenchyma from bile acid toxicity [25,28–30]. Additionally, TGR5 stimulates relaxation of gallbladder smooth muscle cells to induce gallbladder filling [31,32]. TGR5 has also been shown to induce cholangiocyte proliferation [33] and promote barrier function by reinforcing cholangiocyte tight junctions [30].

Previous studies highlight a role for TGR5 in liver biology and pathobiology. For example, the genetic ablation of TGR5 or the inactivation of TGR5 signaling has been shown to make mice more susceptible of cholestatic liver injuries [30,33–35]. This is thought to be due to a role for TGR5 in maintaining a healthy bile acid profile. Specifically, mice with homozygous deficiency of TGR5 exhibit decreased total bile acid pool size [8,24,32], an excessively hydrophobic bile acid pool [32,36], as well as protection from gallstone formation when fed a lithogenic diet [24]. In addition, treatment of HFD-fed mice with a TGR5-specific agonist, INT-777, decreased liver steatosis [3,24], suggesting that TGR5 signaling in the liver attenuates triglyceride accumulation. Furthermore, HFD-fed whole body $Tgr5^{-/-}$ mice are more susceptible to liver injury than littermate controls as evidenced by an elevation of serum liver enzymes due to increased cytokine mRNA levels, more pronounced inflammatory infiltrates, and increased liver necrosis [34,37], highlighting the hepatoprotective role of TGR5 signaling. Together, these data demonstrate that TGR5 exerts important effects on various aspects of liver health. As the liver is a key organ involved in whole body glucose regulation, this suggests that liver TGR5 signaling may be a critical contributor to the overall metabolic benefits of TGR5 agonists.

Despite the growing body of literature regarding the role of TGR5 in liver health, it is unknown if TGR5 signaling within the liver contributes to TGR5's role in glucose regulation, largely due to a lack of cell-type specific in vivo studies of liver TGR5 function. As the hepatocyte is the predominant cell type in the liver, here, we tested the hypothesis that TGR5 signaling in the hepatocyte improves glucose regulation. It is thought that TGR5 is, at most, lowly expressed on hepatocytes; however, this has not been extensively studied. TGR5 expression has been identified in a human hepatocellular carcinoma cell line [38], in canine hepatocytes [39], and here, in mouse hepatocytes. In this study, we employed a highly potent and specific non-bile acid TGR5 agonist, Compound 18 [40], as well as hepatocyte-specific TGR5 knockout mice to investigate the role of hepatocyte TGR5 on glucose regulation. Our results demonstrate that Compound 18 enhances glucose regulation in a hepatocyte TGR5-dependent manner.

2. Materials and Methods

2.1. Animals and Diet

All experiments were performed in accordance with the Guide for the Care and Use of Laboratory Animals and approved by the Institutional Animal Care and Use Committee of Cornell University (approved animal protocol number: 2013-0065). Study mice were individually housed and maintained in a temperature and humidity-controlled room, with a 14:10 h light-dark cycle. Whole body TGR5 knockout mice (B6.Gpbar1 $^{tm1(KOMP)Vlcg}$) (KOMP Repository, The Knockout Mouse Project; University of California, Davis, CA, USA) were used for immunofluorescence analysis of hepatocyte TGR5 expression. Hepatocyte-specific TGR5 knockout mice were generated by crossing a TGR5 floxed mouse line (B6.Gpbar1 $^{<tm1.1Auw}$/J) [23] with hepatocyte-specific albumin-Cre mouse line (B6N.Cg-Tg (Alb-cre)^{21Mgn}/J). To validate this model, hepatocytes were isolated from $Tgr5^{HEP+/+}$ and $Tgr5^{HEP-/-}$ mice and analyzed by RT-PCR to confirm the presence of $Tgr5$ mRNA in $Tgr5^{HEP+/+}$ mice and loss of $Tgr5$ mRNA in the hepatocytes of $Tgr5^{HEP-/-}$ mice (Figure S1). Starting at 8 weeks of age, male and female $Tgr5^{HEP+/+}$ and $Tgr5^{HEP-/-}$ littermates were fed a HFD consisting of ground chow (5012 LabDiets; St. Louis, MO, USA) supplemented with 3.4% butter fat, 8.5% tallow, 13.1% soybean oil, 3.5% mineral mix, and 1% vitamin mix (Dyets; Bethlehem, PA, USA) by weight for 7 weeks to produce an obese, insulin resistant phenotype. Mice were matched for baseline body weight at the start of the HFD. Food intake and body weight were measured once per week ($Tgr5^{HEP+/+}$ $n = 16$, 8 males, 8 females; $Tgr5^{HEP-/-}$; $n = 12$; 7 males, 5 females). In a separate cohort of mice, following 7 weeks of the HFD, mice received 3 consecutive, daily doses of either vehicle (20% Captisol w/v with water, CyDex Pharmaceuticals) or Compound 18 (10 mg/kg/day, Eli Lilly & Company-molecular weight = 508.62) by oral gavage. Compound 18 was formulated in 20% Captisol w/v with water, as previously described [40]. An oral glucose tolerance test (OGTT, 2 g/kg body weight oral gavage with dextrose), following an overnight (12 h) fast, was performed as previously described [41]. To minimize the contribution of TGR5-stimulated GLP-1 release, the OGTT was performed 1 h after the last dose of Compound 18 [40]. Blood glucose measurements were made using a glucometer (One-Touch Ultra, Lifescan; Milpitas, CA, USA). Serum insulin concentrations were measured by ELISA (Millipore; Burlington, MA, USA) and serum total GLP-1 concentrations were measured by sandwich electrochemiluminescence immunoassay (Meso Scale Discovery; Gaithersburg, MD, USA). Immediately following the OGTT, mice were euthanized by an overdose of pentobarbital (200 mg/kg i.p.) and tissues were weighed and collected. The following groups were studied: Vehicle $Tgr5^{HEP+/+}$ (VEH $Tgr5^{HEP+/+}$; $n = 9$; 4 males, 5 females), Compound 18 $Tgr5^{HEP+/+}$ (C18 $Tgr5^{HEP+/+}$; $n = 8$; 4 males, 4 females), Vehicle $Tgr5^{HEP-/-}$ (VEH $Tgr5^{HEP-/-}$; $n = 9$; 4 males, 5 females), and Compound 18 $Tgr5^{HEP-/-}$ (C18 $Tgr5^{HEP-/-}$; $n = 9$; 4 males, 5 females).

2.2. HOMA-IR Calculation

The HOMA-IR (homeostasis model assessment of insulin resistance) index was calculated as (fasting serum glucose × fasting serum insulin/22.5) to assess insulin resistance [42]. Log (HOMA-IR) was used as a surrogate index of insulin resistance, which has been validated for use in rodents, as previously described [43].

2.3. Immunofluorescence

Liver samples from whole body TGR5 wildtype ($Tgr5^{+/+}$) and knockout ($Tgr5^{-/-}$) mice were used for immunofluorescence analysis, as previously described [41]. Briefly, samples were collected, fixed in 4% paraformaldehyde, and paraffin embedded. Sections were deparafinized in a xylene ethanol series, placed in Tris-EDTA buffer for antigen retrieval (10 mM Tris, 1 mM EDTA, 0.05% Tween, pH = 9.0), and then blocked in 5% bovine serum albumin. Sections were immunostained for TGR5 using a polyclonal anti-rabbit antibody (LSBio; Seattle, WA, USA; 1:500) and for albumin using a monoclonal anti-mouse antibody (Santa Cruz Biotechnology; Dallas, TX, USA; 1:500). The antibody against TGR5 was validated on adipose samples from whole-body TGR5 wildtype ($Tgr5^{+/+}$) and knockout ($Tgr5^{-/-}$) (Figure 1). Detection of the primary antibodies was performed using Alexa Flour 488 anti-rabbit and Alexa Fluor 633 anti-mouse secondary antibodies (1:500) (Invitrogen; Foster City, CA, USA). Nuclei were detected using 4′,6′-diamino-2-phenyl inodole (DAPI), which was included in the mounting solution (Invitrogen; Foster City, CA, USA). Images were captured using Nikon Eclipse E400 fluorescent microscope with Olympus DP73 color camera (final magnification 20× for adipose and 100× for liver).

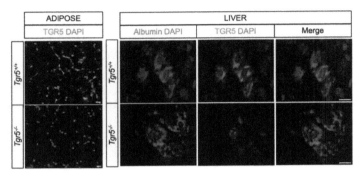

Figure 1. TGR5 is expressed in hepatocytes. Representative images of whole body TGR5 wild-type ($Tgr5^{+/+}$) and knockout ($Tgr5^{-/-}$) mouse adipose and liver sections immunostained for TGR5 (green), albumin (red), and DAPI. Scale bar = 20 um.

2.4. Statistics and Data Analysis

Data are presented as mean ± SEM. The main effect of sex was not significant so the data for males and females were combined. All statistical analyses were performed using GraphPad Prism 8.00 for Mac (GraphPad Software, San Diego, CA, USA). Data were analyzed by two-factor ANOVA with Bonferroni's post-test or Student's *t*-test, as indicated. Differences were considered significant at $p < 0.05$.

3. Results

3.1. TGR5 Is Expressed in Hepatocytes

TGR5 is highly expressed in the liver [9,10,24,25]; however, whether TGR5 is expressed in mouse hepatocytes has not been previously reported. Therefore, we assessed TGR5 expression in mouse liver sections. Adipose tissue sections from a whole body TGR5 knockout mouse model were used for antibody validation (Figure 1). As previously reported [11,44], TGR5 was highly expressed in adipocytes. TGR5 was not detected in adipocytes from $Tgr5^{-/-}$ mice, confirming antibody specificity. TGR5 expression was also detected in some, but not all, hepatocytes in $Tgr5^{+/+}$, but not $Tgr5^{-/-}$ mice (Figure 1). These data are the first to demonstrate that while lowly expressed, TGR5 is present in mouse hepatocytes. Given that hepatocytes comprise the majority of the liver parenchyma and are a key determinant of whole body glucose homeostasis, we used a hepatocyte-specific TGR5 knockout mouse model to determine the role of hepatocyte TGR5 signaling in metabolic health.

3.2. Hepatocyte TGR5 Does Not Contribute to Regulation of Food Intake, Body Weight, or Adiposity

To assess the role of hepatocyte TGR5 on the regulation of body weight, we measured body weight and food intake in $Tgr5^{HEP+/+}$ and $Tgr5^{HEP-/-}$ mice over the course of 7 weeks of HFD (Figure 2A). Similar to previous work in whole body TGR5 knockout mouse models [24,41,45], cumulative food intake and body weight did not differ between $Tgr5^{HEP+/+}$ and $Tgr5^{HEP-/-}$ mice (Figure 2B,C), which allowed us to assess the body weight-independent effects of hepatocyte TGR5 signaling on glucose regulation. In addition, final body weight and adiposity, measured after 3 consecutive daily doses of

Compound 18 or vehicle, did not differ between genotype or treatment (Figure 2D–H). These data demonstrate that hepatocyte TGR5 does not regulate food intake, body weight, or adiposity under basal conditions or following stimulation by Compound 18.

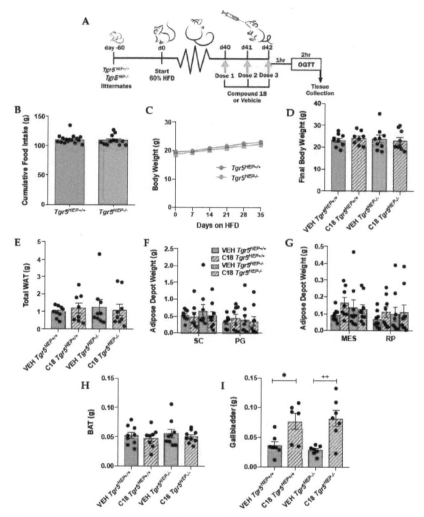

Figure 2. Hepatocyte TGR5 does not contribute to regulation of food intake, body weight, or adiposity. (**A**) Study design. (**B**) Cumulative food intake and (**C**) body weight over 7 weeks of high fat diet (HFD) feeding in $Tgr5^{HEP+/+}$ and $Tgr5^{HEP-/-}$ mice. n = 12–16. (**D**) Body weight at the time of euthanasia; (**E**) total white adipose tissue (WAT) weight; (**F**) subcutaneous (SC) and perigonadal (PG); (**G**) mesenteric (MES) and retroperitoneal (RP) adipose tissue weights; (**H**) brown adipose tissue (BAT) weights; and (**I**) gallbladder weight in $Tgr5^{HEP+/+}$ and $Tgr5^{HEP-/-}$ mice treated with Compound 18 (C18) or vehicle (VEH). n = 6–9. * $p < 0.05$ compared with VEH $Tgr5^{HEP+/+}$; ++ $p < 0.01$ compared with VEH $Tgr5^{HEP-/-}$ by two-factor ANOVA.

TGR5 is highly enriched in the biliary tract [24,25] and its absence has been shown to slow bile flow and reduce gallbladder volume [31,32]. Consistent with this, Compound 18 and other synthetic

TGR5 agonists have been reported to increase gallbladder filling [40,46,47]. Therefore, we assessed gallbladder weight at the time of euthanasia in a sub-set of mice to determine the impact of Compound 18 treatment on this negative side-effect. Treatment with Compound 18 increased gallbladder weight in both $Tgr5^{HEP+/+}$ and $Tgr5^{HEP-/-}$ mice (Figure 2I, $p < 0.05$). These data demonstrate that Compound 18 promotes gallbladder filling independently of hepatocyte TGR5 signaling.

3.3. Compound 18 Improves Glucose Regulation in a Hepatocyte TGR5-dependent Manner

To assess the role of hepatocyte TGR5 on glucose regulation, we performed an OGTT in HFD-fed $Tgr5^{HEP+/+}$ and $Tgr5^{HEP-/-}$ mice with and without Compound 18 treatment. Compound 18 improved glucose tolerance compared with vehicle-treated controls in $Tgr5^{HEP+/+}$ mice, but not $Tgr5^{HEP-/-}$ mice (Figure 3A, $p < 0.05$). Furthermore, Compound 18-treated $Tgr5^{HEP+/+}$ mice exhibited lower blood glucose excursions compared with Compound 18-treated $Tgr5^{HEP-/-}$ mice (Figure 3A, $p < 0.05$).

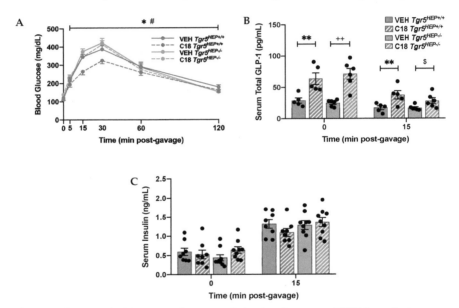

Figure 3. Compound 18 improves glucose regulation in a hepatocyte TGR5-dependent manner. (**A**) Blood glucose, (**B**) serum total GLP-1, and (**C**) serum insulin concentrations during an OGTT in $Tgr5^{HEP+/+}$ and $Tgr5^{HEP-/-}$ mice after 3 doses of Compound 18 (C18) or vehicle (VEH). $n = 5$–9. * $p < 0.05$, ** $p < 0.01$ C18 $Tgr5^{HEP+/+}$ vs. VEH $Tgr5^{HEP+/+}$; ++ $p < 0.01$ C18 $Tgr5^{HEP-/-}$ vs. VEH $Tgr5^{HEP-/-}$; # $p < 0.05$ C18 $Tgr5^{HEP-/-}$ vs. C18 $Tgr5^{HEP+/+}$ by two-factor ANOVA; \$ $p < 0.05$ compared with VEH $Tgr5^{HEP-/-}$ by Student's *t*-test.

A key mechanism by which TGR5 agonists improve glucose tolerance is through induction of GLP-1 secretion and subsequent enhancement of glucose-stimulated insulin secretion [3]. Previous work finds that while Compound 18 potently promotes GLP-1 secretion, GLP-1 levels return to baseline within approximately 1 h of Compound 18 administration in mice [40]. Therefore, to control for the effect of GLP-1, we performed the OGTT 1 h following the last dose of Compound 18 or vehicle. As baseline fasting blood samples were collected approximately 45 min after the last Compound 18 dose, fasting total serum GLP-1 levels were still elevated in Compound 18-treated $Tgr5^{HEP+/+}$ and $Tgr5^{HEP-/-}$ mice compared to vehicle controls (Figure 3B, $p < 0.05$). While this Compound 18-induced increase in serum GLP-1 levels was diminished by 15 min post-glucose gavage, there remained an elevation of serum GLP-1 levels in Compound 18-treated mice compared with control ($p < 0.05$ by 2-factor

ANOVA in the $Tgr5^{HEP+/+}$ mice and $p < 0.05$ by Student's *t*-test in the $Tgr5^{HEP-/-}$ mice). Nevertheless, fasting serum insulin concentrations and serum insulin concentrations at 15 min after the glucose gavage did not differ between the genotype or treatment condition (Figure 3C). As expected, serum insulin levels at 15 min post-glucose gavage were elevated compared with fasting serum insulin concentrations in all groups. Of note, the lack of a difference in fasting serum insulin concentrations despite marked elevations in fasting serum GLP-1 concentrations points to the glucose-dependent actions of GLP-1 to promote insulin secretion. Together, these data demonstrate that hepatocyte TGR5 signaling contributes to the effect of Compound 18 to improve glucose tolerance, independently of insulin and GLP-1 secretion.

3.4. An Index of Insulin Sensitivity Is Impaired in Compound 18-treated Mice Lacking Hepatocyte TGR5

As expected, we did not observe alterations in insulin secretion during the OGTT between genotype or between treatment. It has been previously shown that enhanced TGR5 signaling improves insulin resistance in various tissues by decreasing inflammation [23] and lipotoxicity [16] and increasing energy expenditure [13,20], but the hepatocyte-specific effect of TGR5 signaling on insulin resistance has not been investigated. Therefore, we evaluated an index of insulin resistance in $Tgr5^{HEP+/+}$ and $Tgr5^{HEP-/-}$ mice with and without Compound 18 treatment. We chose the log(HOMA-IR) as a surrogate index of insulin sensitivity as it has been shown to have improved predictive accuracy compared with other indices [43].

There was no significant difference in fasting blood glucose (Figure 4A) or fasting serum insulin concentrations (Figure 4B) between genotype or treatment. However, Compound 18-treated $Tgr5^{HEP+/+}$ mice exhibited a lower log(HOMA-IR) compared to Compound 18-treated $Tgr5^{HEP-/-}$ mice (Figure 4C, $p < 0.05$ by Student's *t*-test). Together, with a lack of a difference in glucose-stimulated insulin secretion, these data suggest that hepatocyte TGR5 signaling may improve glucose homeostasis, in part, through an improvement in insulin sensitivity. Nevertheless, further work is needed to define the impact of hepatocyte TGR5 signaling on insulin sensitivity.

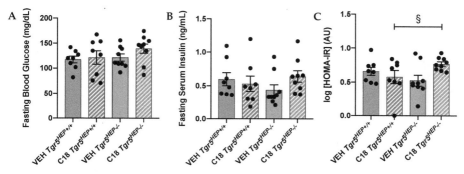

Figure 4. Compound 18 improves insulin sensitivity in a hepatocyte TGR5-dependent manner. (**A**) Fasting blood glucose, (**B**) fasting serum insulin concentrations, and (**C**) log(HOMA-IR) in $Tgr5^{HEP+/+}$ and $Tgr5^{HEP-/-}$ mice after 3 doses of Compound 18 (C18) or vehicle (VEH). $n = 8–9$. § $p < 0.05$ compared with Compound 18 $Tgr5^{HEP+/+}$ by one-tailed Student's *t*-test.

4. Discussion

The TGR5 receptor is ubiquitously expressed throughout the body and has a well-defined role in many regulatory functions that affect hepatic metabolism and extrahepatic glucose homeostasis [3,9,13,21]; however, the expression of TGR5 and its functional significance in hepatocytes remained unknown to date. In this study, we performed the first targeted assessment of TGR5 expression in mouse hepatocytes. TGR5 was detected in hepatocytes of paraffin embedded liver sections by immunofluorescence staining. Our understanding of the liver-specific effects of TGR5 on glucose regulation remain limited due to a lack of cell-type specific in vivo studies of liver TGR5 function. To this end, we employed a hepatocyte-specific TGR5 knockout mouse model in order to dissect the functional significance of hepatocyte TGR5 signaling. Herein, we provide compelling data that TGR5 is expressed in hepatocytes, where it functions as a regulator of whole body glucose homeostasis.

TGR5 has been implicated in body weight regulation through its role in energy metabolism. Specifically, TGR5 regulates energy expenditure by inducing mitochondrial biogenesis and thereby increasing basal metabolism in thermogenically competent tissues, such as brown adipose tissue and skeletal muscle and through the beiging of white adipose tissue [13,18,19,48]. In this study, there was no difference in body weight or adiposity between $Tgr5^{HEP+/+}$ and $Tgr5^{HEP-/-}$ mice with or without treatment with Compound 18, demonstrating that hepatocyte TGR5 signaling does not regulate body weight, food intake, or adiposity. While Briere et al. reported that 14 days of Compound 18 administration at 60 mg/kg reduced body weight and fat mass gain in HFD-fed mice [40], it is likely that our 3-day dosing paradigm at 10 mg/kg was not long enough or robust enough to induce Compound 18-dependent reductions in adiposity. Nevertheless, the absence of genotype-dependent and Compound 18-dependent effects on adiposity and body weight in this study enabled us to assess the body weight-independent effects of hepatocyte TGR5 signaling on glucose homeostasis.

While our data are consistent with previous work demonstrating that TGR5 ablation contributes to metabolic dysregulation in mouse models [3,19,34,37,49], our data are the first to demonstrate that TGR5 signaling specifically within the hepatocyte plays a significant role in whole body glucose regulation. Until now, the role of TGR5 in the maintenance of glucose homeostasis and insulin sensitivity has been attributed to its effects on mitochondrial function in muscle and BAT and/or insulin release from the pancreas, enhanced by enteroendocrine L cell GLP-1 secretion [3,13–15,17,20]. For example, various TGR5 agonists have been shown to ameliorate glucose intolerance in obese and diabetic mice [3,13,50,51]. While in some studies, this improvement in glucose tolerance was associated with increased energy expenditure and subsequent weight loss [3,50], other studies attributed body weight-independent improvements in hyperglycemia to enhanced GLP-1 secretion [40,52]. In contrast, our data show that Compound 18 improves glucose tolerance in a hepatocyte TGR5-dependent manner. Further, in contrast to the aforementioned studies, this effect can occur independently of body weight, GLP-1 secretion, and glucose-stimulated insulin secretion. Thus, we provide evidence that TGR5 agonists improve glucose homeostasis through an additional novel mechanism specific to hepatocyte TGR5 signaling.

The hepatocyte TGR5-dependent improvement in glucose tolerance occurred in the absence of a difference in insulin secretion, suggesting that hepatocyte TGR5 signaling regulates hepatic glucose metabolism and/or insulin sensitivity. Hepatic glucose metabolism is dictated predominantly by hepatic glucose output and insulin sensitivity [53]. Using an index of insulin resistance, our data suggest that hepatocyte TGR5 signaling may regulate insulin sensitivity. Recent studies have proposed that HOMA-IR measurements of insulin resistance refer mostly to the liver, rather than describing peripheral insulin sensitivity [54,55]. This is of particular interest in our model as we sought to understand how liver TGR5 regulates glucose homeostasis. Consistent with our findings, previous work has shown that administration of INT-777 reduced insulin resistance in liver and muscle in obese mice, as assessed by a hyperinsulinemic euglycemic clamp and ^{14}C-2-deoxy-glucose tracers [3]. It is also possible that the improved hepatic insulin resistance in $Tgr5^{HEP+/+}$ mice, as compared to $Tgr5^{HEP-/-}$ mice, following treatment with Compound 18 is mediated by reduced inflammation and decreased ectopic triglyceride deposition, characteristic of enhanced liver TGR5 signaling [3,24]. Nevertheless, further work is needed to determine the mechanisms by which hepatocyte TGR5 signaling improves glucose tolerance.

A growing body of literature has highlighted the potential value of TGR5 agonists in the treatment of various metabolic and liver diseases [3,13,20,23,40,41,52]. However, the clinical development of TGR5 agonists is complicated by the wide range of effects associated with systemic TGR5 activation. TGR5 expression in mouse and human gallbladder is estimated to be 10-fold higher than any other tissue [24,25,40]. Studies in whole body *Tgr5*$^{-/-}$ mice have documented decreased bile flow from the liver [32] and reduced gallbladder volume [31,32], which is explained by reduced TGR5-dependent biliary secretion and impaired smooth muscle relaxation of the gallbladder, respectively. In contrast, the oral administration of TGR5 agonists, including INT-777, oleanolic acid, Compound 23g, and RO552739, has been shown to induce hepatic bile flow [32,52] and increase gallbladder filling in wild type mice [32,46,47,50]. Similarly, Compound 18 has been shown to have a dose-dependent effect on gallbladder filling, an effect that is lost in whole body *Tgr5*$^{-/-}$ mice [40]. To this end, a major side effect of TGR5 agonists is the inhibition of gallbladder emptying, ultimately leading to cholestatic liver injury [24,32,40]. As expected, in this present study, we found no difference in gallbladder weight between *Tgr5*$^{HEP+/+}$ and *Tgr5*$^{HEP-/-}$ mice in the absence of Compound 18. However, in response to Compound 18 administration, our data demonstrate a significant increase in gallbladder weight in both *Tgr5*$^{HEP+/+}$ and *Tgr5*$^{HEP-/-}$ mice. Together, these results suggest that hepatocyte TGR5 does not contribute to the role of TGR5 in gallbladder filling under basal conditions or in the presence of a TGR5 agonist. Further, our results highlight the need to identify cell-type specific effects and downstream signaling targets of TGR5 signaling in order to develop better bile acid-based therapeutics to treat diabetes and metabolic disease.

5. Conclusions

In conclusion, TGR5 is a promising therapeutic target, but its breadth of actions, particularly in the gallbladder, complicates this task. As such, there is a growing need to identify cell-type specific effects of TGR5 signaling in order to begin to identify and target the downstream effectors of TGR5 signaling. Our findings provide additional insight into the underlying mechanisms by which TGR5 agonists improve whole body glucose homeostasis. Importantly, our data demonstrate that hepatocyte TGR5 signaling regulates whole body glucose homeostasis.

Supplementary Materials: The following are available online at http://www.mdpi.com/2072-6643/12/7/2124/s1, Figure S1: Validation of hepatocyte-specific TGR5 knockout mouse model.

Author Contributions: Investigation: M.M.H., M.K.C., A.M., and B.P.C.; Conceptualization, Resources: D.A.B., K.W.S., K.S., and B.P.C.; Methodology: M.M.H., M.K.C., A.M., D.A.B., K.W.S., K.S., and B.P.C.; Formal Analysis, Validation: M.M.H. and B.P.C.; Writing—Original Draft Preparation: M.M.H.; Writing—Review & Editing: M.K.C., A.M., D.A.B., K.W.S., K.S., and B.P.C.; Supervision, Funding Acquisition: B.P.C.; All authors have read and agreed to the published version of the manuscript.

Funding: This research was funded by Nutracia 2018-55 and NIH/NCI 5R21CA195002.

Acknowledgments: We thank Eli Lilly & Company for supplying Compound 18. We thank the Animal Health and Diagnostic Center Histopathology Core for preparation of samples for histological analysis. We would like to thank Jackie Belliveau for assistance with animal care.

Conflicts of Interest: The authors have no conflicts of interest to disclose, except KWS and DAB are employees of Eli Lilly & Company. The funders had no role in the design of the study; in the collection, analyses, or interpretation of data; in the writing of the manuscript, or in the decision to publish the results.

References

1. Pathak, P.; Liu, H.; Boehme, S.; Xie, C.; Krausz, K.W.; Gonzalez, F.; Chiang, J.Y.L. Farnesoid X receptor induces Takeda G-protein receptor 5 cross-talk to regulate bile acid synthesis and hepatic metabolism. *J. Biol. Chem.* **2017**, *292*, 11055–11069. [CrossRef]
2. Cariou, B.; van Harmelen, K.; Duran-Sandoval, D.; van Dijk, T.H.; Grefhorst, A.; Abdelkarim, M.; Caron, S.; Torpier, G.; Fruchart, J.C.; Gonzalez, F.J.; et al. The farnesoid X receptor modulates adiposity and peripheral insulin sensitivity in mice. *J. Biol. Chem.* **2006**, *281*, 11039–11049. [CrossRef] [PubMed]
3. Thomas, C.; Gioiello, A.; Noriega, L.; Strehle, A.; Oury, J.; Rizzo, G.; Macchiarulo, A.; Yamamoto, H.; Mataki, C.; Pruzanski, M.; et al. TGR5-mediated bile acid sensing controls glucose homeostasis. *Cell Metab.* **2009**, *10*, 167–177. [CrossRef]
4. Li, T.; Chiang, J.Y. Bile acid signaling in metabolic disease and drug therapy. *Pharmacol. Rev.* **2014**, *66*, 948–983. [CrossRef] [PubMed]

5. Erickson, S.K.; Lear, S.R.; Deane, S.; Dubrac, S.; Huling, S.L.; Nguyen, L.; Bollineni, J.S.; Shefer, S.; Hyogo, H.; Cohen, D.E.; et al. Hypercholesterolemia and changes in lipid and bile acid metabolism in male and female cyp7A1-deficient mice. *J. Lipid Res.* **2003**, *44*, 1001–1009. [CrossRef]

6. Ferslew, B.C.; Xie, G.; Johnston, C.K.; Su, M.; Stewart, P.W.; Jia, W.; Brouwer, K.L.; Barritt, A.S.T. Altered Bile Acid Metabolome in Patients with Nonalcoholic Steatohepatitis. *Dig. Dis. Sci.* **2015**, *60*, 3318–3328. [CrossRef] [PubMed]

7. Brufau, G.; Stellaard, F.; Prado, K.; Bloks, V.W.; Jonkers, E.; Boverhof, R.; Kuipers, F.; Murphy, E.J. Improved glycemic control with colesevelam treatment in patients with type 2 diabetes is not directly associated with changes in bile acid metabolism. *Hepatology* **2010**, *52*, 1455–1464. [CrossRef] [PubMed]

8. Maruyama, T.; Miyamoto, Y.; Nakamura, T.; Tamai, Y.; Okada, H.; Sugiyama, E.; Nakamura, T.; Itadani, H.; Tanaka, K. Identification of membrane-type receptor for bile acids (M-BAR). *Biochem. Biophys. Res. Commun.* **2002**, *298*, 714–719. [CrossRef]

9. Keitel, V.; Donner, M.; Winandy, S.; Kubitz, R.; Haussinger, D. Expression and function of the bile acid receptor TGR5 in Kupffer cells. *Biochem. Biophys. Res. Commun.* **2008**, *372*, 78–84. [CrossRef]

10. Keitel, V.; Reinehr, R.; Gatsios, P.; Rupprecht, C.; Gorg, B.; Selbach, O.; Haussinger, D.; Kubitz, R. The G-protein coupled bile salt receptor TGR5 is expressed in liver sinusoidal endothelial cells. *Hepatology* **2007**, *45*, 695–704. [CrossRef]

11. Kawamata, Y.; Fujii, R.; Hosoya, M.; Harada, M.; Yoshida, H.; Miwa, M.; Fukusumi, S.; Habata, Y.; Itoh, T.; Shintani, Y.; et al. A G protein-coupled receptor responsive to bile acids. *J. Biol. Chem.* **2003**, *278*, 9435–9440. [CrossRef] [PubMed]

12. Poole, D.P.; Godfrey, C.; Cattaruzza, F.; Cottrell, G.S.; Kirkland, J.G.; Pelayo, J.C.; Bunnett, N.W.; Corvera, C.U. Expression and function of the bile acid receptor GpBAR1 (TGR5) in the murine enteric nervous system. *Neurogastroenterol. Motil.* **2010**, *22*, 814-e228. [CrossRef] [PubMed]

13. Watanabe, M.; Houten, S.M.; Mataki, C.; Christoffolete, M.A.; Kim, B.W.; Sato, H.; Messaddeq, N.; Harney, J.W.; Ezaki, O.; Kodama, T.; et al. Bile acids induce energy expenditure by promoting intracellular thyroid hormone activation. *Nature* **2006**, *439*, 484–489. [CrossRef] [PubMed]

14. Katsuma, S.; Hirasawa, A.; Tsujimoto, G. Bile acids promote glucagon-like peptide-1 secretion through TGR5 in a murine enteroendocrine cell line STC-1. *Biochem. Biophys. Res. Commun.* **2005**, *329*, 386–390. [CrossRef]

15. Li, Y.; Cheng, K.C.; Niu, C.-S.; Lo, S.-H.; Cheng, J.-T.; Niu, H.-S. Investigation of triamterene as an inhibitor of the TGR5 receptor: Identification in cells and animals. *Drug Des. Dev. Ther.* **2017**, *11*, 1127–1134. [CrossRef] [PubMed]

16. Finn, P.D.; Rodriguez, D.; Kohler, J.; Jiang, Z.; Wan, S.; Blanco, E.; King, A.J.; Chen, T.; Bell, N.; Dragoli, D.; et al. Intestinal TGR5 agonism improves hepatic steatosis and insulin sensitivity in Western diet-fed mice. *Am. J. Physiol. Gastrointest. Liver Physiol.* **2019**, *316*, G412–G424. [CrossRef]

17. Kumar, D.P.; Rajagopal, S.; Mahavadi, S.; Mirshahi, F.; Grider, J.R.; Murthy, K.S.; Sanyal, A.J. Activation of transmembrane bile acid receptor TGR5 stimulates insulin secretion in pancreatic beta cells. *Biochem. Biophys. Res. Commun.* **2012**, *427*, 600–605. [CrossRef]

18. Broeders, E.P.; Nascimento, E.B.; Havekes, B.; Brans, B.; Roumans, K.H.; Tailleux, A.; Schaart, G.; Kouach, M.; Charton, J.; Deprez, B. The bile acid chenodeoxycholic acid increases human brown adipose tissue activity. *Cell Metab.* **2015**, *22*, 418–426. [CrossRef]

19. Velazquez-Villegas, L.A.; Perino, A.; Lemos, V.; Zietak, M.; Nomura, M.; Pols, T.W.H.; Schoonjans, K. TGR5 signalling promotes mitochondrial fission and beige remodelling of white adipose tissue. *Nat. Commun.* **2018**, *9*, 1–13. [CrossRef]

20. Huang, S.; Ma, S.; Ning, M.; Yang, W.; Ye, Y.; Zhang, L.; Shen, J.; Leng, Y. TGR5 agonist ameliorates insulin resistance in the skeletal muscles and improves glucose homeostasis in diabetic mice. *Metabolism* **2019**, *99*, 45–56. [CrossRef]

21. Wang, Y.D.; Chen, W.D.; Yu, D.; Forman, B.M.; Huang, W. The G-protein-coupled bile acid receptor, Gpbar1 (TGR5), negatively regulates hepatic inflammatory response through antagonizing nuclear factor kappa light-chain enhancer of activated B cells (NF-kappaB) in mice. *Hepatology* **2011**, *54*, 1421–1432. [CrossRef] [PubMed]

22. Guo, C.; Qi, H.; Yu, Y.; Zhang, Q.; Su, J.; Yu, D.; Huang, W.; Chen, W.D.; Wang, Y.D. The G-Protein-Coupled Bile Acid Receptor Gpbar1 (TGR5) Inhibits Gastric Inflammation Through Antagonizing NF-kappaB Signaling Pathway. *Front. Pharmacol.* **2015**, *6*, 287. [CrossRef] [PubMed]

23. Perino, A.; Pols, T.W.; Nomura, M.; Stein, S.; Pellicciari, R.; Schoonjans, K. TGR5 reduces macrophage migration through mTOR-induced C/EBPbeta differential translation. *J. Clin. Investig.* **2014**, *124*, 5424–5436. [CrossRef]

24. Vassileva, G.; Golovko, A.; Markowitz, L.; Abbondanzo, S.J.; Zeng, M.; Yang, S.; Hoos, L.; Tetzloff, G.; Levitan, D.; Murgolo, N.J.; et al. Targeted deletion of Gpbar1 protects mice from cholesterol gallstone formation. *Biochem. J.* **2006**, *398*, 423–430. [CrossRef] [PubMed]

25. Keitel, V.; Cupisti, K.; Ullmer, C.; Knoefel, W.T.; Kubitz, R.; Haussinger, D. The membrane-bound bile acid receptor TGR5 is localized in the epithelium of human gallbladders. *Hepatology* **2009**, *50*, 861–870. [CrossRef] [PubMed]

26. Renga, B.; Cipriani, S.; Carino, A.; Simonetti, M.; Zampella, A.; Fiorucci, S. Reversal of Endothelial Dysfunction by GPBAR1 Agonism in Portal Hypertension Involves a AKT/FOXOA1 Dependent Regulation of H2S Generation and Endothelin-1. *PLoS ONE* **2015**, *10*, e0141082. [CrossRef]

27. Klindt, C.; Reich, M.; Hellwig, B.; Stindt, J.; Rahnenführer, J.; Hengstler, J.G.; Köhrer, K.; Schoonjans, K.; Häussinger, D.; Keitel, V. The G Protein-Coupled Bile Acid Receptor TGR5 (Gpbar1) Modulates Endothelin-1 Signaling in Liver. *Cells* **2019**, *8*, 1467. [CrossRef]

28. Baghdasaryan, A.; Claudel, T.; Gumhold, J.; Silbert, D.; Adorini, L.; Roda, A.; Vecchiotti, S.; Gonzalez, F.J.; Schoonjans, K.; Strazzabosco, M.; et al. Dual farnesoid X receptor/TGR5 agonist INT-767 reduces liver injury in the Mdr2−/− (Abcb4−/−) mouse cholangiopathy model by promoting biliary HCO(-)(3) output. *Hepatology* **2011**, *54*, 1303–1312. [CrossRef]

29. de Buy Wenniger, L.J.M.; Hohenester, S.; Maroni, L.; van Vliet, S.J.; Elferink, R.P.O.; Beuers, U. The Cholangiocyte Glycocalyx Stabilizes the 'Biliary HCO3-Umbrella': An Integrated Line of Defense against Toxic Bile Acids. *Dig. Dis.* **2015**, *33*, 397–407. [CrossRef]

30. Merlen, G.; Kahale, N.; Ursic-Bedoya, J.; Bidault-Jourdainne, V.; Simerabet, H.; Doignon, I.; Tanfin, Z.; Garcin, I.; Pean, N.; Gautherot, J.; et al. TGR5-dependent hepatoprotection through the regulation of biliary epithelium barrier function. *Gut* **2020**, *69*, 146–157. [CrossRef]

31. Lavoie, B.; Balemba, O.B.; Godfrey, C.; Watson, C.A.; Vassileva, G.; Corvera, C.U.; Nelson, M.T.; Mawe, G.M. Hydrophobic bile salts inhibit gallbladder smooth muscle function via stimulation of GPBAR1 receptors and activation of KATP channels. *J. Physiol.* **2010**, *588*, 3295–3305. [CrossRef]

32. Li, T.; Holmstrom, S.R.; Kir, S.; Umetani, M.; Schmidt, D.R.; Kliewer, S.A.; Mangelsdorf, D.J. The G protein-coupled bile acid receptor, TGR5, stimulates gallbladder filling. *Mol. Endocrinol.* **2011**, *25*, 1066–1071. [CrossRef]

33. Reich, M.; Deutschmann, K.; Sommerfeld, A.; Klindt, C.; Kluge, S.; Kubitz, R.; Ullmer, C.; Knoefel, W.T.; Herebian, D.; Mayatepek, E.; et al. TGR5 is essential for bile acid-dependent cholangiocyte proliferation in vivo and in vitro. *Gut* **2016**, *65*, 487–501. [CrossRef]

34. Pean, N.; Doignon, I.; Garcin, I.; Besnard, A.; Julien, B.; Liu, B.; Branchereau, S.; Spraul, A.; Guettier, C.; Humbert, L.; et al. The receptor TGR5 protects the liver from bile acid overload during liver regeneration in mice. *Hepatology* **2013**, *58*, 1451–1460. [CrossRef]

35. Merlen, G.; Bidault-Jourdainne, V.; Kahale, N.; Glenisson, M.; Ursic-Bedoya, J.; Doignon, I.; Garcin, I.; Rainteau, D.; Tordjmann, T. Hepatoprotective impact of the bile acid receptor TGR5. *Liver Int.* **2020**, *40*, 1005–1015. [CrossRef] [PubMed]

36. Donepudi, A.C.; Boehme, S.; Li, F.; Chiang, J.Y.L. G-protein-coupled bile acid receptor plays a key role in bile acid metabolism and fasting-induced hepatic steatosis in mice. *Hepatology* **2017**, *65*, 813–827. [CrossRef] [PubMed]

37. Keitel, V.; Reich, M.; Sommerfeld, A.; Kluge, S.; Kubitz, R.; Häussinger, D. Role of the bile acid receptor TGR5 (Gpbar-1) in liver damage and regeneration. *Eur. J. Med. Res.* **2014**, *19*, S21. [CrossRef]

38. Yang, J.I.; Yoon, J.H.; Myung, S.J.; Gwak, G.Y.; Kim, W.; Chung, G.E.; Lee, S.H.; Lee, S.M.; Kim, C.Y.; Lee, H.S. Bile acid-induced TGR5-dependent c-Jun-N terminal kinase activation leads to enhanced caspase 8 activation in hepatocytes. *Biochem. Biophys. Res. Commun.* **2007**, *361*, 156–161. [CrossRef] [PubMed]

39. Giaretta, P.R.; Suchodolski, J.S.; Blick, A.K.; Steiner, J.M.; Lidbury, J.A.; Rech, R.R. Distribution of bile acid receptor TGR5 in the gastrointestinal tract of dogs. *Histol. Histopathol.* **2018**, *34*, 69–79. [CrossRef]

40. Briere, D.A.; Ruan, X.; Cheng, C.C.; Siesky, A.M.; Fitch, T.E.; Dominguez, C.; Sanfeliciano, S.G.; Montero, C.; Suen, C.S.; Xu, Y.; et al. Novel Small Molecule Agonist of TGR5 Possesses Anti-Diabetic Effects but Causes Gallbladder Filling in Mice. *PLoS ONE* **2015**, *10*, e0136873. [CrossRef]

41. McGavigan, A.K.; Garibay, D.; Henseler, Z.M.; Chen, J.; Bettaieb, A.; Haj, F.G.; Ley, R.E.; Chouinard, M.L.; Cummings, B.P. TGR5 contributes to glucoregulatory improvements after vertical sleeve gastrectomy in mice. *Gut* **2017**, *66*, 226–234. [CrossRef] [PubMed]

42. Matthews, D.R.; Hosker, J.P.; Rudenski, A.S.; Naylor, B.A.; Treacher, D.F.; Turner, R.C. Homeostasis model assessment: Insulin resistance and beta-cell function from fasting plasma glucose and insulin concentrations in man. *Diabetologia* **1985**, *28*, 412–419. [CrossRef] [PubMed]

43. Lee, S.; Muniyappa, R.; Yan, X.; Chen, H.; Yue, L.Q.; Hong, E.G.; Kim, J.K.; Quon, M.J. Comparison between surrogate indexes of insulin sensitivity and resistance and hyperinsulinemic euglycemic clamp estimates in mice. *Am. J. Physiol. Endocrinol. Metab.* **2008**, *294*, E261–E270. [CrossRef] [PubMed]

44. Svensson, P.-A.; Olsson, M.; Andersson-Assarsson, J.C.; Taube, M.; Pereira, M.J.; Froguel, P.; Jacobson, P. The TGR5 gene is expressed in human subcutaneous adipose tissue and is associated with obesity, weight loss and resting metabolic rate. *Biochem. Biophys. Res. Commun.* **2013**, *433*, 563–566. [CrossRef] [PubMed]

45. Hao, Z.; Leigh Townsend, R.; Mumphrey, M.B.; Gettys, T.W.; Yu, S.; Munzberg, H.; Morrison, C.D.; Berthoud, H.R. Roux-en-Y Gastric Bypass Surgery-Induced Weight Loss and Metabolic Improvements Are Similar in TGR5-Deficient and Wildtype Mice. *Obes. Surg.* **2018**, *28*, 3227–3236. [CrossRef]

46. Duan, H.; Ning, M.; Chen, X.; Zou, Q.; Zhang, L.; Feng, Y.; Zhang, L.; Leng, Y.; Shen, J. Design, synthesis, and antidiabetic activity of 4-phenoxynicotinamide and 4-phenoxypyrimidine-5-carboxamide derivatives as potent and orally efficacious TGR5 agonists. *J. Med. Chem.* **2012**, *55*, 10475–10489. [CrossRef]

47. Ullmer, C.; Alvarez Sanchez, R.; Sprecher, U.; Raab, S.; Mattei, P.; Dehmlow, H.; Sewing, S.; Iglesias, A.; Beauchamp, J.; Conde-Knape, K. Systemic bile acid sensing by G protein-coupled bile acid receptor 1 (GPBAR1) promotes PYY and GLP-1 release. *Br. J. Pharmacol.* **2013**, *169*, 671–684. [CrossRef]

48. Sasaki, T.; Kuboyama, A.; Mita, M.; Murata, S.; Shimizu, M.; Inoue, J.; Mori, K.; Sato, R. The exercise-inducible bile acid receptor Tgr5 improves skeletal muscle function in mice. *J. Biol. Chem.* **2018**, *293*, 10322–10332. [CrossRef]

49. Maruyama, T.; Tanaka, K.; Suzuki, J.; Miyoshi, H.; Harada, N.; Nakamura, T.; Miyamoto, Y.; Kanatani, A.; Tamai, Y. Targeted disruption of G protein-coupled bile acid receptor 1 (Gpbar1/M-Bar) in mice. *J. Endocrinol.* **2006**, *191*, 197–205. [CrossRef]

50. Sato, H.; Genet, C.; Strehle, A.; Thomas, C.; Lobstein, A.; Wagner, A.; Mioskowski, C.; Auwerx, J.; Saladin, R. Anti-hyperglycemic activity of a TGR5 agonist isolated from Olea europaea. *Biochem. Biophys. Res. Commun.* **2007**, *362*, 793–798. [CrossRef]

51. Pellicciari, R.; Gioiello, A.; Macchiarulo, A.; Thomas, C.; Rosatelli, E.; Natalini, B.; Sardella, R.; Pruzanski, M.; Roda, A.; Pastorini, E.; et al. Discovery of 6alpha-ethyl-23(S)-methylcholic acid (S-EMCA, INT-777) as a potent and selective agonist for the TGR5 receptor, a novel target for diabesity. *J. Med. Chem.* **2009**, *52*, 7958–7961. [CrossRef] [PubMed]

52. Hodge, R.J.; Lin, J.; Vasist Johnson, L.S.; Gould, E.P.; Bowers, G.D.; Nunez, D.J. Safety, Pharmacokinetics, and Pharmacodynamic Effects of a Selective TGR5 Agonist, SB-756050, in Type 2 Diabetes. *Clin. Pharmacol. Drug Dev.* **2013**, *2*, 213–222. [CrossRef]

53. Roden, M.; Bernroider, E. Hepatic glucose metabolism in humans—Its role in health and disease. *Best Pract. Res. Clin. Endocrinol. Metab.* **2003**, *17*, 365–383. [CrossRef]

54. Home, P.D.; Pacini, G. Hepatic dysfunction and insulin insensitivity in type 2 diabetes mellitus: A critical target for insulin-sensitizing agents. *Diabetes Obes. Metab.* **2008**, *10*, 699–718. [CrossRef] [PubMed]

55. Abdul-Ghani, M.A.; Jenkinson, C.P.; Richardson, D.K.; Tripathy, D.; DeFronzo, R.A. Insulin secretion and action in subjects with impaired fasting glucose and impaired glucose tolerance: Results from the Veterans Administration Genetic Epidemiology Study. *Diabetes* **2006**, *55*, 1430–1435. [CrossRef] [PubMed]

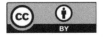

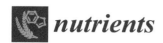

Article

No Effect of Diet-Induced Mild Hyperhomocysteinemia on Vascular Methylating Capacity, Atherosclerosis Progression, and Specific Histone Methylation

Courtney A. Whalen [1], Floyd J. Mattie [1], Cristina Florindo [2], Bertrand van Zelst [3], Neil K. Huang [1,4], Isabel Tavares de Almeida [2], Sandra G. Heil [3], Thomas Neuberger [5,6], A. Catharine Ross [1] and Rita Castro [1,2,7,*]

[1] Department of Nutritional Sciences, The Pennsylvania State University, University Park, PA 16802, USA; caw400@psu.edu (C.A.W.); fjm1311@gmail.com (F.J.M.); neil.huang@tufts.edu (N.K.H.); acr6@psu.edu (A.C.R.)
[2] Faculty of Pharmacy, Universidade de Lisboa, 1649-003 Lisbon, Portugal; cristinaflorindo@ff.ulisboa.pt (C.F.); italmeida@ff.ulisboa.pt (I.T.d.A.)
[3] Department of Clinical Chemistry, Medical Center Rotterdam, Erasmus MC University, 3015 GD Rotterdam, The Netherlands; b.vanzelst@erasmusmc.nl (B.v.Z.); s.heil@erasmusmc.nl (S.G.H.)
[4] Cardiovascular Nutrition Laboratory, Jean Mayer USDA Human Nutrition Research Center on Aging, Tufts University, Boston, MA 02111, USA
[5] Huck Institutes of the Life Sciences, The Pennsylvania State University, University Park, PA 16802, USA; tun3@psu.edu
[6] Biomedical Engineering, The Pennsylvania State University, University Park, PA 16802, USA
[7] Research Institute for Medicines (iMed. ULisboa), Universidade de Lisboa, 1649-003 Lisbon, Portugal
*   Correspondence: mum689@psu.edu; Tel.: +351-814-865-2938

Received: 6 June 2020; Accepted: 21 July 2020; Published: 23 July 2020

Abstract: Hyperhomocysteinemia (HHcy) is a risk factor for atherosclerosis through mechanisms which are still incompletely defined. One possible mechanism involves the hypomethylation of the nuclear histone proteins to favor the progression of atherosclerosis. In previous cell studies, hypomethylating stress decreased a specific epigenetic tag (the trimethylation of lysine 27 on histone H3, H3K27me3) to promote endothelial dysfunction and activation, i.e., an atherogenic phenotype. Here, we conducted a pilot study to investigate the impact of mild HHcy on vascular methylating index, atherosclerosis progression and H3K27me3 aortic content in apolipoprotein E-deficient ($ApoE^{-/-}$) mice. In two different sets of experiments, male mice were fed high-fat, low in methyl donors (HFLM), or control (HF) diets for 16 (Study A) or 12 (Study B) weeks. At multiple time points, plasma was collected for (1) quantification of total homocysteine (tHcy) by high-performance liquid chromatography; or (2) the methylation index of S-adenosylmethionine to S-adenosylhomocysteine (SAM:SAH ratio) by liquid chromatography tandem-mass spectrometry; or (3) a panel of inflammatory cytokines previously implicated in atherosclerosis by a multiplex assay. At the end point, aortas were collected and used to assess (1) the methylating index (SAM:SAH ratio); (2) the volume of aortic atherosclerotic plaque assessed by high field magnetic resonance imaging; and (3) the vascular content of H3K27me3 by immunohistochemistry. The results showed that, in both studies, HFLM-fed mice, but not those mice fed control diets, accumulated mildly elevated tHcy plasmatic concentrations. However, the pattern of changes in the inflammatory cytokines did not support a major difference in systemic inflammation between these groups. Accordingly, in both studies, no significant differences were detected for the aortic methylating index, plaque burden, and H3K27me3 vascular content between HF and HFLM-fed mice. Surprisingly however, a decreased plasma SAM: SAH was also observed, suggesting that the plasma compartment does not always reflect the vascular concentrations of these two metabolites, at least in this model. Mild HHcy in vivo was not be sufficient to induce vascular hypomethylating stress or the progression of atherosclerosis, suggesting that only higher accumulations of plasma tHcy will exhibit vascular toxicity and promote specific epigenetic dysregulation.

Keywords: homocysteine and vascular disease; H3K27me3; epigenetics; atherosclerosis; MRI (magnetic resonance imaging)

---

1. Introduction

Homocysteine (Hcy) is a sulfur-containing amino acid formed during the methionine metabolism. Mild hyperhomocysteinemia (HHcy), a condition defined by an accumulation of plasma tHcy between 15 and 25 μM, is highly prevalent in most Western populations, and may be an independent risk factor for atherosclerosis [1,2]. Nevertheless, the molecular basis of the association between Hcy and atherosclerosis is incompletely defined [1]; one possibility involves its impact on the cellular transmethylating reactions [3–5].

The intracellular concentration of Hcy is tightly regulated by several metabolic pathways, and it affects the cell methylating capacity, which is defined as the ratio of S-adenosylmethionine (SAM) to S-adenosylhomocysteine (SAH) in methionine metabolism [2,5]. SAM is the methyl donor to several methyltransferases that target innumerous biomolecules, including DNA and proteins. Importantly, excess SAH inhibits the activities of these SAM-dependent methyltransferases, which results in decreases in the SAM:SAH ratio and intracellular methylating capacity [6,7]. SAH is further converted into Hcy by a reaction that is reversible and strongly favors SAH synthesis rather than hydrolysis. Thus, if Hcy accumulates, SAH accumulates as well, decreasing the SAM: SAH ratio and causing hypomethylating stress [3,8,9].

Several observations from in vitro and in vivo studies support the concept that hypomethylating stress contributes to the adverse vascular consequences of HHcy [1–3,6–13]. This possibility has been also supported by several human studies. For example, one recent cohort study found that higher plasma SAH concentrations were positively associated with cardiovascular disease (CVD) risk in patients undergoing coronary angiography [14]. In another study, plasma concentration of SAH, but not of Hcy, was strongly associated with traditional CVD risk factors and subclinical atherosclerosis in subjects at low CVD risk [15]. Moreover, plasma SAH was found to be inversely associated with a measure of endothelial dysfunction (namely, endothelial nitric oxide synthase-dependent vasodilation) in a small sample of patients with coronary artery disease [16].

Several cell studies have documented the hypomethylating effect associated with decreased SAM: SAH ratios on epigenetically relevant targets that may contribute to the adverse vascular effects of Hcy accumulation [3,6,7]. Epigenetic modulators of gene expression include histone methylation [4]. Our prior study reported that hypomethylating stress contributes to a proatherogenic environment by down-regulating the activity of the SAM-dependent histone lysine methyltransferase known as an enhancer of zeste homolog 2 (EZH2) [17]. EZH2 silences gene expression by catalyzing the tri-methylation of histone H3 at lysine 27 (H3K27me3). EZH2 was identified as a new target affected by a hypomethylating environment, which caused a decrease in the endothelial content of H3K27me3 [17], promoting a pro-atherogenic phenotype [2,17]. Consistent with the involvement of this specific epigenetic modification in atherosclerosis progression, a reduction in H3K27me3 content in human plaques has been reported in two studies [18,19].

As aforementioned, mild HHcy is a condition highly prevalent in most populations and an independent risk factor for atherosclerosis by mechanisms which are incompletely defined. In light of these observations, we investigated whether a mild Hcy accumulation in vivo induces alterations in vascular methylating index and in the epigenetic marker, H3K27me3, to favor atherosclerosis progression. The remethylation of Hcy to methionine requires folate and vitamin B12 (cobalamin) as co-factors. Alternatively, Hcy can be remethylated to methionine by betaine, which is a choline metabolite. Moreover, the catabolism of Hcy to cysteine requires vitamin B6. Thus, dietary manipulation of the content of methyl donors and B vitamins is an established approach to produce the accumulation of tHcy in mice, especially in the presence of an excess of methionine [12,20,21]. With this purpose, we fed genetically susceptible apolipoprotein E-deficient (*ApoE* $^{-/-}$) mice [22] a high-fat diet hypomethylating (HFLM) diet, or a high-fat control diet (HF) with a normal content of methyl donors. After confirming the presence of mild HHcy only in the HFLM-fed mice, we measured systemic inflammation, the plasma and aortic SAM:SAH ratio, and compared the extent of atherosclerotic lesions formation. The volume of atherosclerosis in the aortas was quantified using advanced imaging techniques (high resolution magnetic resonance imaging, MRI). Lastly, following MRI analysis, the scanned aortas were subjected to the quantification of the epigenetic tag H3K27me3.

2. Methods

2.1. Animals and Diets

Seven-week-old *ApoE* $^{-/-}$ mice (Jackson Laboratory, Bar Harbor, ME, USA) were housed individually in cages with wire grid floors and fed diets that contained 1% sulfathiazole to ensure that the animal's only source of B vitamins was from the diet. Only male mice were included, to control for the known effect of gender on atherosclerosis in this strain [23]. The animals were maintained in a room at 22 ± 2 °C with a 12-h light–dark cycle with free access to water. Mice were fed ad libitum for 16 weeks (Study A) or 12 weeks (Study B), with one of the following diets prepared based on AIN 93M (Research Diets, New Brunswick, NJ, USA) [12,20]: a control diet (C, 11 Kcal% fat, 70 Kcal% carbohydrate, 19 Kcal% protein), an HF diet (HF, 40 Kcal% fat, 41 Kcal% carbohydrate, 19 Kcal% protein and 0.15% cholesterol), or an HFLM diet enriched in methionine and with decreased levels of methyl donors and vitamins (folate, choline, vitamin B6, and vitamin B12), as previously described [12,20]. The composition of the experimental diets is shown in the supplementary Table S1. Diets were replaced once a week, at which point animals and the remaining food were weighed. Food consumption was estimated as an average per mouse per day within each cage. All procedures were performed in compliance with the Institutional Animal Care and Use Committee of the Pennsylvania State University, which specifically approved this study.

2.2. Blood Collection

After mice were fed for 4, 8 and 12 weeks on each diet, blood was collected from the retroorbital cavity into heparinized tubes and immediately placed on ice. Plasma was isolated by centrifugation at 4 °C and immediately stored at −80 °C prior to further biochemical analyses.

2.3. Aorta Collection and Preparation of Lysates

After 16 (Study A) or 12 weeks (Study B) on each diet, mice were euthanized by carbon dioxide inhalation and, after the exposure of the aorta, 10 mL of cold phosphate saline buffer (PBS) was perfused using a syringe through the left ventricle of the heart. Approximately one third of the descending thoracic aorta was excised, transferred into 100 μL of a solution of acetonitrile, methanol, and water (2:2:1) containing 0.1M HCl (to preserve SAH during the subsequent lysate preparation), immediately immersed into liquid nitrogen, and stored at −80 °C until the preparation of the lysates for SAM and SAH quantification, described below. The remainders of the aorta (ascending aorta, aortic arch, and remaining descending thoracic aorta) was then perfused through the heart in situ via the left ventricle with 10% neutral buffered formalin (NBF) in PBS, and dissected from other tissues. The aortic tissue was fixed in 10% NBF overnight, washed with PBS, and subjected to Oil Red O staining, as described below.

Aorta lysates for SAM and SAH quantification were subsequently prepared by homogenization with 2.8 mm ceramic beads using a Bead Ruptor 12 (Omni, Kennesaw, GA, USA) with two cycles of

15 s at the maximum speed, with 30 s on ice in between. The lysate was cleared by centrifugation at 12,000 *g* and 4 °C for 10 min and immediately stored at −80 °C until SAH and SAM analysis.

2.4. Homocysteine and Methylating Index (SAM:SAH Ratio)

Plasma total Hcy (tHcy), defined as the total concentration of Hcy after the reductive cleavage of all disulfide bonds, was determined by high-performance liquid chromatography (HPLC) analysis according to an adapted method of Araki and Sako [24], and as previously described [11].

SAM and SAH levels were measured in plasma (after 8 weeks on each diet) and in aortic lysates (at the end point) using a liquid chromatography tandem-mass spectrometry (LC-MS/MS) method after the use of solid-phase extraction columns according to an adapted method of Gellekink et al. [25], and as previously described [26]. The stability of SAM and SAH in plasma was shown to be 100% if samples were stored immediately at −80 °C [23]. As aforementioned, to protect aortic lysates from degradation of SAM, we acidified the aortic lysates with 0.1M HCl, after which samples were stored at −80 °C [25]. Within-run precision was shown to be 2.9% and 2.4% for SAM and SAH, respectively.

2.5. Systemic Inflammation

Interleukin 6 (IL-6), interleukin 10 (IL-10), monocyte chemoattractant protein 1 (MCP-1), and tumor necrosis factor (TNF-α), previously identified in the pathogenesis of atherosclerosis [3], were measured in duplicate at two different time points (4 weeks and 12 weeks) in Study A, using MSD U-PLEX multiplex assay platforms (Meso Scale Diagnostics, Rockville, MD, U.S.) following the manufacturer's instructions.

2.6. Aorta Processing for MRI Analysis

Fixed aortas were stained with Oil Red O (EMD chemicals, Cat. #3125-12) to facilitate complete adventitial fat removal during dissection. Briefly, aortas were dehydrated in successive methanol–water solutions (25%, 50%, 78% methanol for 15 min each at room temperature, RT, with rocking). Aortas were then incubated in Oil Red O working solution (5 parts 2.8% Oil Red O in methanol: 2 parts 1 M sodium hydroxide) for 2 h at RT, with rocking. Subsequently, aortas were washed and rehydrated with successive PBS solutions with the following methanol concentrations (%): 78, 50, 25, or 0 (15 min each solution, RT, rocking). Connective tissues surrounding the aortas were dissected away under a stereomicroscope. Dissected aortas were then equilibrated in a solution of 0.1% Magnevist (Bayer), 0.25% sodium azide in PBS overnight at 4 °C, then placed into glass tubes (6 mm OD, 4 mm ID, 60 mmL) for MRI analysis.

2.7. MRI Analysis: Atherosclerotic Plaque Volume

Aortic plaque burden was determined by MRI, as previously described, but using an Agilent 14T micro imaging system and a home-built saddle coil with an inner diameter of 7 mm [27–29]. A previously validated [30] gradient echo imaging sequence with an imaging time of 9 h 48 min was used to generate 3D datasets of the aortas. Scan parameters included an echo time (TE) of 13 ms, a repetition time (TR) of 100.00 ms, eight averages, a field of view (FOV) of 12.6 × 4.2 × 4.2 mm^3 and a matrix size of 630 × 210 × 210, resulting in an isotropic resolution of 20 µm. After acquisition, MR data was reconstructed using Matlab (The MathWorks Inc., Natick, MA, USA). Zero-filling by a factor of 2 in each direction lead to a final isotropic pixel resolution of 10 µm.

Data segmentation was performed using Avizo 9.5 (Thermo Fisher Scientific, Waltham, MA, USA). The lumen of the aorta, the different plaques, and the aorta wall were manually segmented using the lasso tool. Quantification of plaque volume was determined using the material statistics function in Avizo 9.5 on the segmented aorta. The results were expressed as the percent of plaque area in relation to the total segmented area (plaque + lumen + wall).

2.8. Aorta Cryosectioning and Immunofluorescence Analysis: Specific Histone Methylation

Following MRI analysis, aortas were equilibrated in sucrose solution. Aortas were then cut into four regions, pinned out into arrays, embedded in Tissue-Tek Optimal Cutting Temperature compound (OCT, Sakura Finetek, Tokyo, Japan) and stored at −20 °C (Figure 1). Aorta arrays were sectioned at an angle generally perpendicular to the vessel into 12 μm thick sections using a Leica CM3050 S cryostat, at −20 °C, and attached to TruBond 380 microscope slides (Electron Microscopy Sciences, Hatfield, PA, USA). Slides were dried at least 1 h at 32 °C, then stored at −20 °C.

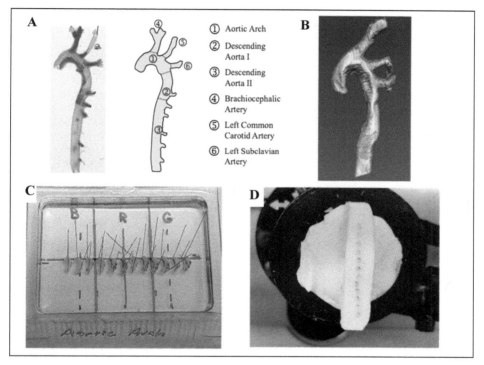

Figure 1. Aorta Cryosectioning (**A**) Example of one aorta from *ApoE* $^{-/-}$ mice and schematic representation of the different regions of the aorta including pre-embedding cut sites (dashed lines); (**B**) Example of the visualization of the aortic arteriosclerotic plaque (colored in yellow) using 14T-magnetic resonance imaging (MRI); (**C**) After MRI analysis, aortas from the same study were cut, each region was pinned into alignment, embedded in Optimal Cutting Temperature (OCT) compound and stored at −20 °C for 24 h. Blue letters B, R, and G only represent marks used as orientation and spacing guides. (**D**) The resulting cryoblock was then sectioned, creating arrays of aortic slices of similar orientation and position for immunofluorescence analysis.

Heat-Induced Epitope Retrieval (HIER) was conducted for 30 min at < 100 °C in a decloaking chamber (Biocare Medical, Pacheco, CA, USA), setting 9.5, using Rodent Decloaker solution (Biocare Medical, Pacheco, CA, USA) in accordance with manufacturer-provided protocols. Arrays were then encircled with an ImmEdge Hydropphobic Barrier PAP pen (Vector Laboratories, Burlingame, CA, USA), blocked with 2% BSA, 1% NGS, 0.05% Triton X-100, 0.05% Tween-20, 0.05% sodium azide in PBS (blocking buffer) for ≥ 1 h, and then incubated with primary antibodies in blocking buffer overnight at 4 °C. After washing, arrays were incubated with secondary antibodies in blocking buffer for ≥ 1 h at RT, washed, treated with Vector TrueVIEW Autofluorescence Quenching Kit (Vector Laboratories,

Burlingame, CA, USA), and mounted under coverslips in VECTASHIELD Vibrance Antifade Mounting Medium (Vector Laboratories). The antibodies used were: rabbit anti-histone H3K27me3 pAb (1:200, Cat.# A-4039, Epigentek, Farmingdale, NY, USA, Cat.# A-4039), mouse anti-histone H3 mAb 1B1-B2 (1:200, Cat.#819404, BioLegend, San Diego, CA, USA), Alexa Fluor 555 goat anti-rabbit IgG (1:250, Cat.# A-21428 Invitrogen, Carlsbad, CA, USA), Alexa Fluor 488 goat anti-mouse IgG3 (1:250, Cat.# A-21151, Invitrogen, Carlsbad, CA, USA). The residual Oil Red O in the slides did not interfere with the immunofluorescence detection (Figure S1), likely due to HIER or time since Oil Red O staining [31].

Immunofluorescence images were collected using an Olympus BX61 widefield fluorescence microscope at the Penn State Microscopy Facility (University Park, PA, USA). Images were segmented and quantified using FIJI [32]. Briefly, the aortic lumen, plaque, and outside of the aorta were segmented manually as Regions of Interest (ROIs). All other ROIs were calculated through additions of and/or subtractions from these initial segments. Histone H3 fluorescence images were used to define nuclei within these ROIs and fluorescence within these nuclei selections were measured in both the histone H3 and histone H3K27me3 immunofluorescence images. Autofluorescence from the elastic fibers within the vessel walls was suppressed using TrueVIEW® Autofluorescence Quenching Kit from Vector Laboratories. This allowed selection of the nuclei based on thresholding of the histone H3 fluorescence channel (green, Alexa488) image. Then, using only those areas selected as nuclei, the fluorescence of both the H3 (green, Alexa488) and H3K27me3 (red, Alexa555) channels could be quantified. Average fluorescence values from the nuclei contained in the various ROIs were collected for each aortic/vessel image. Average fluorescence intensity values within the nuclei represent the average pixel value over the whole group of selected nuclei (not the average intensity per nuclei). Those average fluorescence values were used to calculate the ratio of H3K27me3 to H3, which was used to assess relative changes in H3K27me3 content.

2.9. Statistical Analysis

Analyses were performed in GraphPad Prism 7 (GraphPad Software, La Jolla, CA, USA), with statistical significance set to $p < 0.05$. For comparison of two groups, an unpaired Student's *t*-test was used. For more than two groups, a one- or two-way analysis of variance (ANOVA) was performed and adjusted for multiple comparisons.

3. Results

3.1. General Characteristics

The mean food per week did not differ between HF and HFLM groups (data not shown). Nevertheless, after 16 weeks (Study A), HF mice gained more weight than HFLM mice ($p < 0.05$) or control mice ($p < 0.05$), while the latter two groups did not differ from each other (Figure 2). To exclude the causal role of secondary metabolic effects caused by an extended period of dietary treatment with suboptimal levels of micronutrients, a second group of mice was fed for a shorter period (12 weeks, Study B). Again, the HFLM-fed mice grew more poorly ($p < 0.05$) than the other two groups of mice.

3.2. Homocysteine and Methylating Index (SAM:SAH Ratio)

Mild HHcy was induced by the HFLM diet in both studies (A and B) (Figure 3) ($n = 5$–6 per study). In fact, in study A, and at week 4 and week 12, HFLB-fed mice had higher ($p < 0.05$) plasma tHcy concentration when compared to the HF-fed mice or control-fed mice (Figure 3A). These observations were further confirmed in study B, in which, equally after 4 or 12 weeks, HFLM-fed mice, but not those mice fed HF or control diets, accumulated mildly elevated tHcy plasmatic concentrations ($25\ \mu M > tHcy > 15\ \mu M$) (Figure 3B).

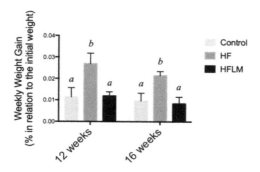

Figure 2. The effect of control, High-Fat (HF), or low in methyl donors (HFLM) diets on growth. Results are weekly weight gain (% of initial weight). Data shown are the mean ± SEM; n = 5–6/group, bars not sharing superscript letters differ from each other, $p < 0.05$.

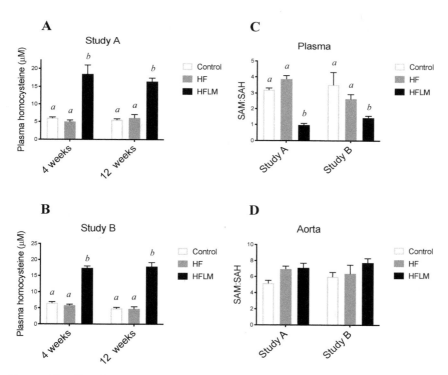

Figure 3. The effect of control, High-Fat (HF), or low in methyl donors (HFLM) diets on plasma tHcy concentrations (**A,B**), plasma SAM:SAH ratio (**C**), and aortic SAM:SAH ratio (**D**). Data shown are the mean ± SEM, n = 5–6/group; bars not sharing not sharing superscript letters differ by $p < 0.05$.

The ratio of SAM concentration divided by SAH concentration was used as an indicator of the methylating capacity, determined in plasma after 8 weeks of diet treatment, and in the aortas after 16 weeks (Study A) or 12 weeks (Study B) of diet treatment. In both studies ($n = 5$–6 per study), HFLM mice displayed a significantly lower plasma SAM: SAH ratio, when compared to HF or control mice (Figure 3C). In both studies, plasma SAM: SAH ratios were similar in HF and control mice (Figure 3C). Interestingly, however, the ratio of aortic concentrations of SAM: SAH in HFLM mice did not differ from HF or control mice either after 12 weeks or 16 weeks of diet (Figure 3D), thus showing the absence of an hypomethylating environment in the HFLM aortas.

3.3. Systemic Inflammation

Cytokines were measured at two different time points (4 weeks and 12 weeks) in Study A to evaluate the status of systemic inflammation, a key component of the atherosclerosis process. At both times, IL-6, IL-10, MCP1, and TNF α concentrations were significantly lower in control mice compared to mice fed either the HF or HFLB diet (Figure 4). Apart from this, mice fed HF diet, when compared at the same time to mice fed HFLM diet, had similar levels of all cytokines with few exceptions: TNF α was significantly elevated in HF mice at 4 weeks (but was similar after 12 weeks of diet); IL6 was elevated in the HFLB mice after 12 weeks; MCP-1 was higher in HF mice after 12 weeks (Figure 4).

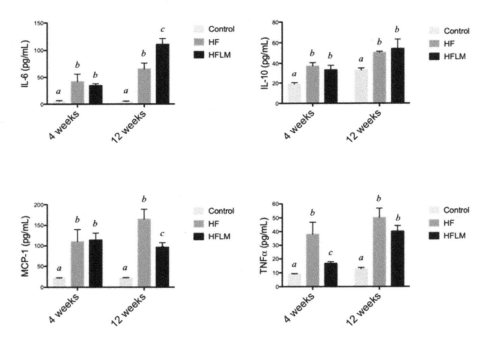

Figure 4. Systemic concentrations of interleukin 6 (IL-6), interleukin 10 (IL-10), monocyte chemoattractant protein 1 (MCP1) and tumor necrosis factor α (TNF- α) in mice fed- low in methyl donors (HFLM) diet, High-Fat (HF) diet or control diet during 16 weeks (study A). Results are mean ± SEM ($n = 4$ per group). Data not sharing superscript letters differ by $p < 0.05$.

3.4. Atherosclerotic Plaque Volume

A method based on ex vivo MR imaging was used to visualize and quantify the volume of atherosclerotic plaque. Distribution of the plaque was similar in all three diets, predominating in the aortic arch and BCA. Plaque volume was significantly increased in HF and HFLM groups compared to the control group, but no significant differences were detected (at the $p < 0.05$ level), between HF and HFLM groups, at either 16 weeks (Study A) or 12 weeks (Study B) (Figure 5). Moreover, this observation was independent of the segment of aorta analyzed (shown in Figure 1A): ascending aorta, aortic arch, or descending thoracic aorta. When mice fed the same diets were compared, there was a consistent increase in plaque burden over time, from 12 to 16 weeks, although the magnitude differed between mice fed the control and mice fed either of the HF diets.

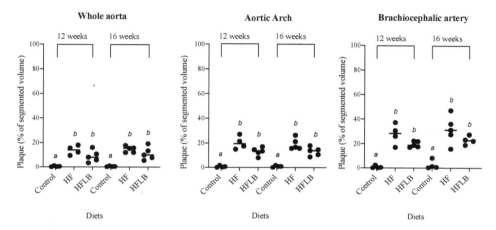

Figure 5. Ex vivo 14T-MRI volumetric assessment of the aortic atherosclerotic plaque in mice fed-hypomethylating (HFLM) and High-Fat (HF) diets, for 12 or 16 weeks. Plaque denotes the volume of plaque relative to the total segmented area. Data not sharing superscript letters differ by $p < 0.05$. Black circles represent individual values and horizontal lines represent the mean value for each group.

3.5. Specific Histone Methylation

Immunofluorescence was used to evaluate the content of H3K27me3 (in relation to total histone H3) in the HFLM aortas compared to the HF aortas (Figure 6), after 12 or 16 weeks of mild HHcy. Different aortic segments (aortic arch; brachiocephalic artery, BCA); and left common carotid artery, LCCA), and different ROIs (total vessel, plaque, and wall) were considered and, as shown in Figure 6D, no significant differences were detected (at the $p < 0.05$ level), for the content of the epigenetic tag H3K27me3.

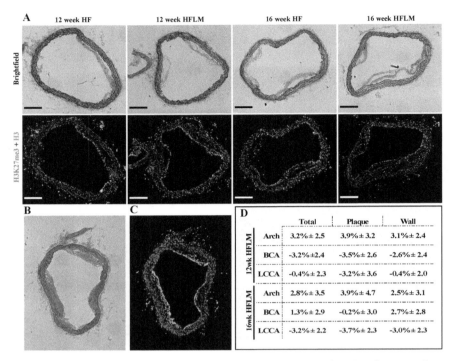

		Total	Plaque	Wall
12wk HFLM	Arch	3.2%± 2.5	3.9%± 3.2	3.1%± 2.4
	BCA	-3.2%±2.4	-3.5%± 2.6	-2.6%± 2.4
	LCCA	-0.4%± 2.3	-3.2%± 3.6	-0.4%± 2.0
16wk HFLM	Arch	2.8%± 3.5	3.9%± 4.7	2.5%± 3.1
	BCA	1.3%± 2.9	-0.2%± 3.0	2.7%± 2.8
	LCCA	-3.2%± 2.2	-3.7%± 2.3	-3.0%± 2.3

Figure 6. Immunofluorescent (IF) analysis (**A**) Brightfield and IF images of aortic arch cross sections from *ApoE* $^{-/-}$ mice fed either a High Fat (HF) or a High Fat Low Methyl donors (HFLM) diet for 12 or 16 weeks (wk) as indicated. Total Histone 3 (H3) in green, and Histone 3 trimethylated at lysine 27 (H3K27me3) in magenta. Scale bars = 200 μm. (**B**) Example of the manual segmentation using FIJI (ImageJ) to define Plaque (Red) and Wall (Yellow); (**C**) Example of the Plaque Nuclei (Cyan) and Wall Nuclei (Magenta) segments used to measure mean fluorescence ratios of H3K27me3:H3; (**D**) Variation of the relative H3K27me3 content in the HFLM aortas in relation to the corresponding HF aortas expressed as percent change; data are the mean ± SEM, *n* = 25. BCA, brachiocephalic artery; LCCA, left common carotid artery (localization shown in Figure 1A).

4. Discussion

The present study investigated in an in vivo model of atherogenesis whether mild HHcy alters aortic methylating index and the vascular epigenetic content of H3K27me3 to favor a pro-atherogenic phenotype.

SAH is the precursor of Hcy that may accumulate in the setting of HHcy to cause hypomethylating stress, and this, in turn, may contribute to the vascular toxicity [2,3,6,7]. This possibility is based on the ability of SAH, once its intracellular concentration reaches a certain threshold, to inhibit the methyltransferase reactions that rely on SAM. EZH2 is a SAM-dependent methyltransferase that participates in histone methylation and chromatin compaction, negatively regulating gene expression [33]. EZH2 establishes the epigenetic tag H3K27me3 that represses the expression of genes responsible for the establishment of a proatherogenic endothelial phenotype [34]. Accordingly, we have previously shown that, in endothelial cells, hypomethylating stress decreases H3K27me3 to promote inflammation and endothelial dysfunction and activation [17]. However, the in vivo effect of mild HHcy on the vascular methylating index and content of this epigenetic tag is elusive.

Dietary manipulation of the content of methyl donors and B vitamins is an established approach to produce the accumulation of tHcy in mice, especially in the presence of an excess of methionine [12,20,21].

Accordingly, in the present study, a mild but significant accumulation of circulating tHcy was achieved in the mice fed the HFLM diet [35].

Many studies have used dietary approaches similar to ours in *ApoE* $^{-/-}$ mice to explore the vascular phenotype associated with HHcy. Studies in which a moderate (25–50 µM) or severe (> 100 µM) accumulation of plasma tHcy was achieved reported that HHcy enhanced the development of atherosclerosis [21]. However, the findings associated with mild HHcy are inconsistent. For example, Liu et al. [36] reported that 8 weeks of severe HHcy with a concomitant decrease in SAM:SAH resulted in aggravated aortic plaque formation; however, a milder elevation of Hcy that did not alter plasma SAM:SAH did not alter the extent of atherosclerotic plaque development. More recently, Xiaoling et al. [37] reported that a similar mild elevation of Hcy increased aortic lesion area after 16 weeks of diet using a high-fat diet enriched in methionine, but no measures of methylating status were provided in this report. Interestingly, in a genetic model of mild HHcy achieved by crosses of *ApoE* $^{-/-}$ mice, with mice having a genetic defect in Hcy metabolism (cystathionine beta-synthase, CBS, deficiency), *ApoE* $^{-/-}$ *CBS* $^{-/-}$ mice developed more severe aortic root lesions than *ApoE*$^{-/-}$ mice at 12 months of age but not at earlier timepoints of 15 weeks or 6 months [38]. In the present study, a mildly elevated plasma Hcy for 16 weeks (Study A) (Figure 3A) did not significantly affect atherosclerosis progression (Figure 5) or aortic SAM: SAH values (Figure 3C). To the best of our knowledge, no previous murine studies have provided measures of the vascular methylating index under mild HHcy. Surprisingly however, a decreased plasma SAM: SAH, an indicator of systemic hypomethylating status, was also observed after 8 weeks of diet (Figure 3D), suggesting that the plasma compartment does not always reflect the vascular concentrations of these two metabolites. To confirm these observations, and to exclude the causal role of secondary metabolic effects due to an extended period of dietary treatment with suboptimal levels of micronutrients, a second group of mice was subjected to the same experimental design but for a shorter period (12 weeks, Study B). Again, plasma Hcy concentrations were in the range of mild HHcy (Figure 3B) and were not associated with aortic hypomethylation (Figure 3D) nor atherosclerosis progression (Figure 5). Moreover, and similarly to study A, lower plasma SAM:SAH was also observed in study B in HFLM mice when compared to both other groups (Figure 3C). In fact, it is known that methylation-regulating enzymes are differentially expressed in different murine tissues, which results in tissue-specific differences in SAM and SAH concentrations [12,13]. Our results suggest that, in this model, under mild HHcy, the systemic SAM:SAH ratio does not always reflect the vascular methylating capacity.

In the present study, ex vivo 14T-MR imaging was used to quantify the extent of atherosclerosis in the aortas of *ApoE* $^{-/-}$ mice enabling the visualization, and subsequent quantification of total plaque volume with sensitivity [27–29]. Moreover, this method preserved the aortic tissue that was further used to quantify histone methylation. Our observation that the volume of vascular lesions over the entire aorta was not higher in the hyperhomocysteinemic mice (HFLM) was further confirmed by evaluating plaque volume in segments of aorta that are more prone to develop atherosclerosis (BCA and aortic arch) (Figure 5). In these highly susceptible regions, no significant differences in the plaque burden were detected between HF and HFLM mice. Importantly, however, HFLM mice grew more slowly than HF animals, and this may have retarded the plaque progression in these animals explaining the observed absence of vascular toxicity. Previous studies have also noted a significant decrease in body weight in animals fed diets with high methionine and a lack of micronutrients [20,21]. Lastly, as anticipated, plaque volume in HF and HFLM mice was significantly increased compared to that in control mice (Figure 5), indicating a role of high-fat diet, regardless of B vitamin content, in the development of atherosclerosis.

The effect of diet on the circulating levels of cytokines previously implicated in the pathogenesis of atherosclerosis was also investigated previously [39]. IL-6 is an inflammatory cytokine that plays a central role in propagating the downstream inflammatory response that sustains atherosclerosis progression [40], whereas IL-10 is a prototypic anti-inflammatory cytokine released by activated macrophages that delays the growth of vascular lesions [41]. MCP1 is deeply implicated in the infiltration of immune cells into the vessel wall, an essential component of atherosclerosis progression [42]. Lastly, TNF-α is a key cytokine that facilitates the influx of inflammatory cells into the vessel wall, thus promoting the progression of the vascular lesions [43]. In the present study, both HF and HFLM diets promoted a significant systemic elevation of all the four cytokines, when compared to the control diet (Figure 4). This observation is in agreement with the positive effect of dietary fat on systemic inflammation [44]. Moreover, the increased systemic inflammation in HF and HFLM mice is consistent with the augmented arteriosclerotic plaque burden that was observed in these groups compared to control mice. Although some significant differences in plasma cytokines were present between HF and HFLM mice (Figure 4), the pattern of these changes does not support a major difference in disease mechanisms between these groups. Rather, the cytokine findings suggest comparable systemic inflammation in both the HF and HFLM groups, which is consistent with the plaque burden observed (Figure 5). Nevertheless, considering the systemic hypomethylation detected in the hyperhomocysteinemic animals, we are tempted to speculate that the up-regulation of IL6 expression observed in these animals after 12 weeks of diet when compared to the HF-fed mice (Figure 4) may result from the demethylation of the CpG islands in the promoter region of the gene encoding for this inflammatory cytokine [45,46]. In fact, DNA hypomethylation was previously observed under hypomethylating stress [3,4,8,9] and the decrease in promoter methylation status is a widely described mechanism associated with increased gene expression levels [3].

The ability of excess Hcy to disturb specific histone methylation has been demonstrated previously in murine models. Previously, we found that diet-induced moderate HHcy in rats decreased dimethylation of arginine 3 on histone H4 in a tissue-dependent manner [12]; however, in this study not all tissues analyzed showed a change in SAM: SAH ratio. Moreover, a severe accumulation of Hcy due to a genetic defect in Hcy metabolism (CBS deficiency) lessened the methylation of histone H3 at the arginine 8 position in the liver [13]. In a study in which the effect of excess SAH in *ApoE* ^{−/−} mice was explored in the absence of excess Hcy, plasma SAH was positively associated with increased atherosclerosis and negatively associated with the content of trimethylated histone H3 on lysine 9 in aortic lesions [47]. More recently, *ApoE* ^{−/−} mice were challenged with a high-fat high-methionine diet for 16 weeks to cause mild HHcy and, surprisingly, these HHcy mice had increased aortic levels of H3K27me3 [37], however, the SAM: SAH ratio was not measured in this model. As aforementioned, the epigenetic tag H3K27me3 is established by the SAM-dependent methyltransferase, EZH2, the activity of which is decreased by excess SAH, at least in endothelial cells under pharmacological treatments that cause a 6-fold reduction in the SAM: SAH ratio [17]. Thus, this paradoxical observation of increased levels of H3K27me3 under mild HHcy led us to investigate whether, in the aortas of our animals with mild HHcy, the same epigenetic tag was affected. To do so, we used a systematic immunofluorescence approach which revealed comparable amounts of this epigenetic tag in the HFLM and HF groups (Figure 6). This finding is consistent with the maintenance of the cell-methylating index in the aortas of HFLM mice when compared to HF mice, suggesting that, in this model under mild plasma HHcy, the concentrations of SAH accumulated in the tissue are below the Ki value for EZH2 [48].

5. Conclusions

In conclusion, in the present pilot study, two different sets of experiments were conducted, leading to the same observations: mildly elevated Hcy was associated with systemic hypomethylation but no differences between HLLM- and HF fed-mice were detected in vascular methylation status, specific epigenetic content and atherosclerosis progression. However, we do acknowledge that confirmatory studies with a higher number of animals may be needed to confirm these intriguing observations. Moreover, additional studies are being conducted using a diet promoting a more severe accumulation of Hcy to investigate the involvement of this phenotype on atherosclerosis progression via specific epigenetic dysregulation.

Nutrients **2020**, *12*, 2182

Supplementary Materials: The following are available online at http://www.mdpi.com/2072-6643/12/8/2182/s1, Table S1. Composition of the experimental diets (Control; HF, High Fat; HFLM, High Fat Low Methyl). Figure S1. Lack of fluorescence from Oil Red O post processing for IF detection.

Author Contributions: C.A.W. and F.J.M.: conceptualization, methodology, investigation, formal analysis, reviewing and editing; C.F. and B.v.Z.: methodology investigation, reviewing and editing; I.T.d.A. and N.K.H.: conceptualization, reviewing and editing; S.G.H. and T.N.: conceptualization, resources, formal analysis, reviewing and editing; A.C.R.: resources, supervision, conceptualization, and reviewing and editing of the final manuscript; and R.C.: resources, supervision, conceptualization, original draft preparation and reviewing and editing. All authors have read and agreed to the published version of the manuscript.

Funding: This work was supported by the Graduate Program in Nutritional Sciences, Penn State High-Field Magnetic Resonance Imaging Facility, and by the Huck Institutes of the Life Sciences of the Pennsylvania State University.

Acknowledgments: The authors wish to thank Diane E. Handy (Department of Medicine, Brigham and Women's Hospital, Harvard Medical School, Boston, MA) for her valuable comments.

Conflicts of Interest: The authors declared no potential conflict of interest with respect to the research, authorship, and/or publication of this article.

References

1. Joseph, J.; Handy, D.E.; Loscalzo, J. Quo vadis: Whither homocysteine research? *Cardiovasc. Toxicol.* **2009**, *9*, 53–63. [CrossRef]

2. Esse, R.; Barroso, M.; de Almeida, I.T.; Castro, R. The contribution of homocysteine metabolism disruption to endothelial dysfunction: State-of-the-art. *Int. J. Mol. Sci.* **2019**, *20*, 867. [CrossRef]

3. Handy, D.E.; Castro, R.; Loscalzo, J. Epigenetic modifications: Basic mechanisms and role in cardiovascular disease. *Circulation* **2011**, *123*, 2145–2156. [CrossRef]

4. Barroso, M.; Handy, D.E.; Castro, R. The link between hyperhomocysteinemia and hypomethylation: Implications for cardiovascular disease. *J. Inborn Errors Metab. Screen.* **2017**, *5*, 1–15. [CrossRef]

5. Castro, R.; Rivera, I.; Blom, H.J.; Jakobs, C.; de Almeida, I.T. Homocysteine metabolism, hyperhomocysteinaemia and vascular disease: An overview. *J. Inherit. Metab. Dis.* **2006**, *29*, 3–20. [CrossRef] [PubMed]

6. Balint, B.; Jepchumba, V.K.; Gueant, J.L.; Gueant-Rodriguez, R.M. Mechanisms of homocysteine-induced damage to the endothelial, medial and adventitial layers of the arterial wall. *Biochimie* **2020**. [CrossRef] [PubMed]

7. Perla-Kajan, J.; Jakubowski, H. Dysregulation of epigenetic mechanisms of gene expression in the pathologies of hyperhomocysteinemia. *Int. J. Mol. Sci.* **2019**, *20*, 3140. [CrossRef] [PubMed]

8. Castro, R.; Rivera, I.; Martins, C.; Struys, E.A.; Jansen, E.E.; Clode, N.; Graça, L.M.; Blom, H.J.; Jakobs, C.; de Almeida, I.T. Intracellular S-adenosylhomocysteine increased levels are associated with DNA hypomethylation in HUVEC. *J. Mol. Med.* **2005**, *83*, 831–836. [CrossRef] [PubMed]

9. Castro, R.; Rivera, I.; Struys, E.A.; Jansen, E.E.; Ravasco, P.; Camilo, M.E.; Blom, H.J.; Jakobs, C.; de Almeida, I.T. Increased homocysteine and S-adenosylhomocysteine concentrations and DNA hypomethylation in vascular disease. *Clin. Chem.* **2003**, *49*, 1292–1296. [CrossRef]

10. Barroso, M.; Florindo, C.; Kalwa, H.; Silva, Z.; Turanov, A.A.; Carlson, B.A.; de Almeida, I.T.; Blom, H.J.; Gladyshev, V.N.; Hatfield, D.L.; et al. Inhibition of cellular methyltransferases promotes endothelial cell activation by suppressing glutathione peroxidase 1 protein expression. *J. Biol. Chem.* **2014**, *289*, 15350–15362. [CrossRef]

11. Barroso, M.; Rocha, M.S.; Esse, R.; Goncalves, I., Jr.; Gomes, A.Q.; Teerlink, T.; Jakobs, C.; Blom, H.J.; Loscalzo, J.; Rivera, I.; et al. Cellular hypomethylation is associated with impaired nitric oxide production by cultured human endothelial cells. *Amino Acids* **2012**, *42*, 1903–1911. [CrossRef] [PubMed]

12. Esse, R.; Florindo, C.; Imbard, A.; Rocha, M.S.; de Vriese, A.S.; Smulders, Y.M.; Teerlink, T.; de Almeida, I.T.; Castro, R.; Blom, H.J. Global protein and histone arginine methylation are affected in a tissue-specific manner in a rat model of diet-induced hyperhomocysteinemia. *Biochim. Biophys. Acta* **2013**, *1832*, 1708–1714. [CrossRef] [PubMed]

13. Esse, R.; Imbard, A.; Florindo, C.; Gupta, S.; Quinlivan, E.P.; Davids, M.; Teerlink, T.; de Almeida, I.T.; Kruger, W.D.; Blom, H.J.; et al. Protein arginine hypomethylation in a mouse model of cystathionine beta-synthase deficiency. *FASEB J.* **2014**, *28*, 2686–2695. [CrossRef] [PubMed]

14. Xiao, Y.; Zhang, Y.; Wang, M.; Li, X.; Su, D.; Qiu, J.; Li, D.; Yang, Y.; Xia, M.; Ling, W. Plasma S-adenosylhomocysteine is associated with the risk of cardiovascular events in patients undergoing coronary angiography: A cohort study. *Am. J. Clin. Nutr.* **2013**, *98*, 1162–1169. [CrossRef]

15. Zawada, A.M.; Rogacev, K.S.; Hummel, B.; Berg, J.T.; Friedrich, A.; Roth, H.J.; Obeid, R.; Geisel, J.; Fliser, D.; Heine, G.H. S-adenosylhomocysteine is associated with subclinical atherosclerosis and renal function in a cardiovascular low-risk population. *Atherosclerosis* **2014**, *234*, 17–22. [CrossRef]

16. Xiao, Y.; Xia, J.; Cheng, J.; Huang, H.; Zhou, Y.; Yang, X.; Su, X.; Ke, Y.; Ling, W. Inhibition of s-adenosylhomocysteine hydrolase induces endothelial dysfunction via epigenetic regulation of p66shc-mediated oxidative stress pathway. *Circulation* **2019**, *139*, 2260–2277. [CrossRef]

17. Barroso, M.; Kao, D.; Blom, H.J.; de Almeida, I.T.; Castro, R.; Loscalzo, J.; Handy, D.E. S-adenosylhomocysteine induces inflammation through NFkB: A possible role for EZH2 in endothelial cell activation. *Biochim. Biophys. Acta* **2016**, *1862*, 82–92. [CrossRef]

18. Greissel, A.; Culmes, M.; Burgkart, R.; Zimmermann, A.; Eckstein, H.H.; Zernecke, A.; Pelisek, J. Histone acetylation and methylation significantly change with severity of atherosclerosis in human carotid plaques. *Cardiovasc. Pathol.* **2016**, *25*, 79–86. [CrossRef]

19. Greissel, A.; Culmes, M.; Napieralski, R.; Wagner, E.; Gebhard, H.; Schmitt, M.; Zimmermann, A.; Eckstein, H.-H.; Zernecke, A.; Pelisek, J. Alternation of histone and DNA methylation in human atherosclerotic carotid plaques. *Thromb. Haemost.* **2015**, *114*, 390–402. [CrossRef]

20. Troen, A.M.; Lutgens, E.; Smith, D.E.; Rosenberg, I.H.; Selhub, J. The atherogenic effect of excess methionine intake. *Proc. Natl. Acad. Sci. USA* **2003**, *100*, 15089–15094. [CrossRef]

21. Dayal, S.; Lentz, S.R. Murine models of hyperhomocysteinemia and their vascular phenotypes. *Arterioscler. Thromb. Vasc. Biol.* **2008**, *28*, 1596–1605. [CrossRef] [PubMed]

22. Getz, G.S.; Reardon, C.A. ApoE knockout and knockin mice: The history of their contribution to the understanding of atherogenesis. *J. Lipid. Res.* **2016**, *57*, 758–766. [CrossRef] [PubMed]

23. Caligiuri, G.; Nicoletti, A.; Zhou, X.; Tornberg, I.; Hansson, G.K. Effects of sex and age on atherosclerosis and autoimmunity in apoE-deficient mice. *Atherosclerosis* **1999**, *145*, 301–308. [CrossRef]

24. Araki, A.; Sako, Y. Determination of free and total homocysteine in human plasma by high-performance liquid chromatography with fluorescence detection. *J. Chromatogr.* **1987**, *422*, 43–52. [CrossRef]

25. Gellekink, H.; van Oppenraaij-Emmerzaal, D.; van Rooij, A.; Struys, E.A.; den Heijer, M.; Blom, H.J. Stable-isotope dilution liquid chromatography-electrospray injection tandem mass spectrometry method for fast, selective measurement of S-adenosylmethionine and S-adenosylhomocysteine in plasma. *Clin. Chem.* **2005**, *51*, 1487–1492. [CrossRef]

26. Heil, S.G.; Herzog, E.M.; Griffioen, P.H.; van Zelst, B.; Willemsen, S.P.; de Rijke, Y.B.; Steegers-Theunissen, R.P.M.; Steegers, E.A.P. Lower S-adenosylmethionine levels and DNA hypomethylation of placental growth factor (PlGF) in placental tissue of early-onset preeclampsia-complicated pregnancies. *PLoS ONE* **2019**, *14*, e0226969. [CrossRef]

27. Whalen, C.; Mattie, F.; Caamano, A.; Bach, E.; Huang, N.; Neuberger, T.; Ross, A.C.; Castro, R. Mild hyperhomocysteinemia induced by a hypomethylating diet does not favor aortic plaque formation in apoE knockout mice. *Curr. Dev. Nutr.* **2019**, *3*, P24–P37. [CrossRef]

28. Whalen, C.; Mattie, F.J.; Huang, K.-H.; Florindo, C.; Heil, S.G.; Ross, A.C.; Neuberger, T.; Castro, R. Mild hyperhomocysteinemia neither increased atherosclerotic plaque burden nor altered specific histone methylation in aortas from apolipoprotein E knockout mice. *Circulation* **2019**, *140*, A16327. [CrossRef]

29. McAteer, M.A.; Schneider, J.E.; Clarke, K.; Neubauer, S.; Channon, K.M.; Choudhury, R.P. Quantification and 3D reconstruction of atherosclerotic plaque components in apolipoprotein E knockout mice using ex vivo high-resolution MRI. *Arterioscler. Thromb. Vasc. Biol.* **2004**, *24*, 2384–2390. [CrossRef]

30. Schneider, J.E.; Bamforth, S.D.; Farthing, C.R.; Clarke, K.; Neubauer, S.; Bhattacharya, S. High-resolution imaging of normal anatomy, and neural and adrenal malformations in mouse embryos using magnetic resonance microscopy. *J. Anat.* **2003**, *202*, 239–247. [CrossRef]

31. Koopman, R.; Schaart, G.; Hesselink, M.K. Optimisation of oil red O staining permits combination with immunofluorescence and automated quantification of lipids. *Histochem. Cell Biol.* **2001**, *116*, 63–68. [CrossRef] [PubMed]
32. Schindelin, J.; Arganda-Carreras, I.; Frise, E.; Kaynig, V.; Longair, M.; Pietzsch, T.; Preibisch, S.; Rueden, C.; Saalfeld, S.; Schmid, B.; et al. Fiji: An open-source platform for biological-image analysis. *Nat. Methods* **2012**, *9*, 676–682. [CrossRef] [PubMed]
33. Margueron, R.; Reinberg, D. The Polycomb complex PRC2 and its mark in life. *Nature* **2011**, *469*, 343–349. [CrossRef] [PubMed]
34. Dreger, H.; Ludwig, A.; Weller, A.; Stangl, V.; Baumann, G.; Meiners, S.; Stangl, K. Epigenetic regulation of cell adhesion and communication by enhancer of zeste homolog 2 in human endothelial cells. *Hypertension* **2012**, *60*, 1176–1183. [CrossRef]
35. Wilson, K.M.; McCaw, R.B.; Leo, L.; Arning, E.; Lhotak, S.; Bottiglieri, T.; Austin, R.C.; Lentz, S.R. Prothrombotic effects of hyperhomocysteinemia and hypercholesterolemia in ApoE-deficient mice. *Arterioscler. Thromb. Vasc. Biol.* **2007**, *27*, 233–240. [CrossRef]
36. Liu, C.; Wang, Q.; Guo, H.; Xia, M.; Yuan, Q.; Hu, Y.; Zhu, H.; Hou, M.; Ma, J.; Tang, Z.; et al. Plasma S-adenosylhomocysteine is a better biomarker of atherosclerosis than homocysteine in apolipoprotein E-deficient mice fed high dietary methionine. *J. Nutr.* **2008**, *138*, 311–315. [CrossRef]
37. Yang, X.; Zhao, L.; Li, S.Q.; Ma, S.; Yang, A.; Ding, N.; Li, N.; Jia, Y.; Yang, X.; Li, G.; et al. Hyperhomocysteinemia in ApoE-/-mice leads to overexpression of enhancer of zeste homolog 2 via miR-92a regulation. *PLoS ONE* **2016**, *11*, e0167744. [CrossRef]
38. Wang, H.; Jiang, X.; Yang, F.; Gaubatz, J.W.; Ma, L.; Magera, M.J.; Yang, X.; Berger, P.B.; Durante, W.; Pownall, H.J.; et al. Hyperhomocysteinemia accelerates atherosclerosis in cystathionine beta-synthase and apolipoprotein E double knock-out mice with and without dietary perturbation. *Blood* **2003**, *101*, 3901–3907. [CrossRef]
39. Hansson, G.K. Inflammation, atherosclerosis, and coronary artery disease. *N. Engl. J. Med.* **2005**, *352*, 1685–1695. [CrossRef]
40. Hartman, J.; Frishman, W.H. Inflammation and atherosclerosis: A review of the role of interleukin-6 in the development of atherosclerosis and the potential for targeted drug therapy. *Cardiol. Rev.* **2014**, *22*, 147–151. [CrossRef]
41. Han, X.; Boisvert, W.A. Interleukin-10 protects against atherosclerosis by modulating multiple atherogenic macrophage function. *Thromb. Haemost.* **2015**, *113*, 505–512. [CrossRef] [PubMed]
42. Kennedy, A.; Gruen, M.L.; Gutierrez, D.A.; Surmi, B.K.; Orr, J.S.; Webb, C.D.; Hasty, A.H. Impact of macrophage inflammatory protein-1alpha deficiency on atherosclerotic lesion formation, hepatic steatosis, and adipose tissue expansion. *PLoS ONE* **2012**, *7*, e31508. [CrossRef] [PubMed]
43. Branen, L.; Hovgaard, L.; Nitulescu, M.; Bengtsson, E.; Nilsson, J.; Jovinge, S. Inhibition of tumor necrosis factor-alpha reduces atherosclerosis in apolipoprotein E knockout mice. *Arterioscler. Thromb. Vasc. Biol.* **2004**, *24*, 2137–2142. [CrossRef] [PubMed]
44. Duan, Y.; Zeng, L.; Zheng, C.; Song, B.; Li, F.; Kong, X.; Xu, K. Inflammatory links between high fat diets and diseases. *Front. Immunol.* **2018**, *9*, 2649. [CrossRef] [PubMed]
45. Tekpli, X.; Landvik, N.E.; Anmarkud, K.H.; Skaug, V.; Haugen, A.; Zienolddiny, S. DNA methylation at promoter regions of interleukin 1B, interleukin 6, and interleukin 8 in non-small cell lung cancer. *Cancer Immunol. Immunother.* **2013**, *62*, 337–345. [CrossRef] [PubMed]
46. Zuo, H.P.; Guo, Y.Y.; Che, L.; Wu, X.Z. Hypomethylation of Interleukin-6 Promoter is Associated with the Risk of Coronary Heart Disease. *Arq. Bras. Cardiol.* **2016**, *107*, 131–136. [CrossRef] [PubMed]
47. Xiao, Y.; Huang, W.; Zhang, J.; Peng, C.; Xia, M.; Ling, W. Increased plasma S-adenosylhomocysteine -accelerated atherosclerosis is associated with epigenetic regulation of endoplasmic reticulum stress in apoE-/-mice. *Arterioscler. Thromb. Vasc. Biol.* **2015**, *35*, 60–70. [CrossRef]
48. Schapira, M. Chemical inhibition of protein methyltransferases. *Cell Chem. Biol.* **2016**, *23*, 1067–1076. [CrossRef] [PubMed]

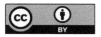

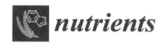

Review

TGR5 Signaling in Hepatic Metabolic Health

Marlena M. Holter, Margot K. Chirikjian, Viraj N. Govani and Bethany P. Cummings *

Department of Biomedical Sciences, Cornell University College of Veterinary Medicine, Ithaca, NY 14853, USA;
mmh277@cornell.edu (M.M.H.); mkc224@cornell.edu (M.K.C.); vng6@cornell.edu (V.N.G.)
* Correspondence: bpc68@cornell.edu; Tel.: +1-607-253-3552

Received: 30 July 2020; Accepted: 21 August 2020; Published: 26 August 2020

Abstract: TGR5 is a G protein-coupled bile acid receptor that is increasingly recognized as a key regulator of glucose homeostasis. While the role of TGR5 signaling in immune cells, adipocytes and enteroendocrine L cells in metabolic regulation has been well described and extensively reviewed, the impact of TGR5-mediated effects on hepatic physiology and pathophysiology in metabolic regulation has received less attention. Recent studies suggest that TGR5 signaling contributes to improvements in hepatic insulin signaling and decreased hepatic inflammation, as well as metabolically beneficial improvements in bile acid profile. Additionally, TGR5 signaling has been associated with reduced hepatic steatosis and liver fibrosis, and improved liver function. Despite the beneficial effects of TGR5 signaling on metabolic health, TGR5-mediated gallstone formation and gallbladder filling complicate therapeutic targeting of TGR5 signaling. To this end, there is a growing need to identify cell type-specific effects of hepatic TGR5 signaling to begin to identify and target the downstream effectors of TGR5 signaling. Herein, we describe and integrate recent advances in our understanding of the impact of TGR5 signaling on liver physiology and how its effects on the liver integrate more broadly with whole body glucose regulation.

Keywords: TGR5; liver; metabolic regulation

1. Introduction

TGR5 is a transmembrane G-protein coupled receptor (GPCR) for bile acids that is ubiquitously expressed in mouse and human tissues [1–6]. Bile acids are amphipathic steroid molecules, synthesized from cholesterol in the liver, that signal through the nuclear receptor, Farnesoid X receptor (FXR), and TGR5, to regulate lipid, glucose, and energy metabolism and to maintain metabolic homeostasis [7–9]. Dysregulated bile acid signaling has been implicated in the pathogenesis of insulin resistance and type 2 diabetes [10–12]. Initial studies revealed that TGR5 signaling regulates glucose tolerance, inflammation, and energy expenditure [9,13–15], such that TGR5 is now recognized as a potential target for the treatment of metabolic disorders. To this end, much metabolic research regarding TGR5 signaling has focused on TGR5-mediated effects on GLP-1 secretion from enteroendocrine L cells [9,16,17], mitochondrial thermogenesis in adipocytes [13,18,19], and decreased inflammatory cytokine secretion from immune cells [1,14,15].

While the role of TGR5 signaling in immune cells, adipocytes, and enteroendocrine L cells has been well described and extensively reviewed, the impact of TGR5 on hepatic physiology and pathophysiology has received less attention. TGR5 is highly expressed in the non-parenchymal cell-types of the liver [20–23] and has been recently identified in hepatocytes [24]. Examination of the role of TGR5 signaling in these various cell types has contributed to a growing body of literature highlighting TGR5 as a key contributor to liver physiology and pathophysiology. Genetic ablation of TGR5 has been shown to make mice more susceptible to impaired glucose tolerance, hepatic insulin resistance, hepatic steatosis and fibrosis, as well as altered bile acid metabolism [9,25,26]. Additionally, treatment of mice with TGR5-specific agonists has been shown to ameliorate many of these metabolic impairments, underscoring the potential therapeutic nature of TGR5 in treating metabolic disease [7,9,13,24,27–30]. However, the clinical development of TGR5 agonists is complicated by the breadth of effects associated with systemic TGR5 activation, particularly in regard to TGR5-specific effects on gallbladder filling and gallstone formation [22,24,30,31]. This review will summarize the currently available knowledge on the impact of TGR5 on hepatic physiology, its influences on metabolic regulation, and the knowledge gaps that need to be addressed to enable effective therapeutic targeting of the TGR5 signaling for the treatment of metabolic disease.

2. Hepatic TGR5 Signaling and Expression

TGR5 is a member of the rhodopsin-like family of GPCRs [2]. TGR5 is encoded by a single-exon gene and is widely conserved among vertebrates [2]. TGR5 is activated by several bile acids, with lithocholic acid (LCA) as the most potent natural agonist, followed by deoxycholic acid (DCA), chenodeoxycholic acid (CDCA) and cholic acid (CA) [2]. Further, taurine conjugation of bile acids increases the affinity for TGR5, as compared to unconjugated bile acids; however, conjugation with glycine has a negligible impact on TGR5 affinity [32]. Based on the robust metabolic effects of TGR5 signaling, multiple synthetic [3,9,13,30,33–35] and semi-synthetic [28] TGR5-specific agonists have been designed and synthesized, in addition to other natural ligands that have been identified [16,29].

In 2002, Maryuama et al., discovered TGR5 as a novel GPCR that, in response to bile acids, enhanced cAMP production in human cell lines [2]. Similarly, Kawamata et al., reported that treatment of a TGR5-expressing human monocytic cell line (THP-1) with taurolithocholic acid (TLCA), LCA, and DCA, dramatically increased cAMP production and suppressed cytokine production [1]. Together, these studies identified that, in most cell types, TGR5 is coupled to a stimulatory G-alpha-protein ($G\alpha_s$), whereby ligand binding to TGR5 results in the activation of adenylyl cyclase-cAMP-PKA signaling and the associated downstream effects, including the recruitment of cAMP response element-binding protein (CREB) to target genes [1,2]. However, further characterization of TGR5 expression and function in other cell types has demonstrated that TGR5 signaling activates multiple different kinase pathways in addition to PKA, including protein kinase B (AKT) [3], Rho kinase [4], mammalian target of rapamycin complex 1 (mTORC1) [3], as well as extracellular signal-related kinase 1/2 (ERK1/2) [5,6].

TGR5 is ubiquitously expressed in rodent and human tissues and has a well-defined role in many regulatory functions that affect whole body metabolism [9,13,15,20]. TGR5 is expressed in endocrine glands, the kidney, adipocytes, muscle, the central nervous system, immune cells, spleen, lung, the gastrointestinal tract (mainly in the ileum and colon), and the enteric nervous system [1,2,36]. TGR5 is also highly expressed in the liver, specifically within non-parenchymal cells, including Kupffer cells [20], sinusoidal endothelial cells [21], and cholangiocytes [22,23]. While it has been speculated that TGR5 is not expressed in hepatocytes, we are not aware of any previously published data demonstrating this. Recently, we reported that TGR5 is expressed in mouse hepatocytes [24], which is in line with previous work in which TGR5 expression was detected in a human hepatocellular carcinoma cell line [37] and in canine hepatocytes [38].

A growing body of literature suggests that TGR5 signaling plays an essential role in hepatic metabolic regulation. Our group recently identified a previously unknown role for hepatocyte TGR5 signaling in regulating whole body glucose homeostasis and insulin sensitivity; however, the underlying signaling pathway through which this occurs remains unresolved [24]. Moreover, other studies have characterized anti-inflammatory, choleretic, proliferative, and protective effects associated with TGR5 signaling in the nonparenchymal cell types of the liver. For instance, in Kupffer cells and resident macrophages, TGR5 activation dampens the hepatic inflammatory response through the attenuation of LPS-induced cytokine production, via the classical TGR5-cAMP-dependent pathway [20], and also through a reduction in NF-κB-dependent inflammatory responses [15] (Figure 1). TGR5 signaling antagonizes NF-κB by decreasing the phosphorylation of IκBα, the nuclear translocation of p65, and NF-κB DNA binding activity [15,39]. Through these separate pathways, TGR5 signaling functions to diminish hepatic inflammation.

The function of TGR5 signaling within the biliary tree has also been rigorously studied. Ligand binding to TGR5 in cholangiocytes induces CFTR-dependent chloride and bicarbonate secretion into bile, which enhances choleresis and forms a bicarbonate umbrella to protect the liver parenchyma from bile acid toxicity [23,40–42]. TGR5 signaling in cholangiocytes has also been shown to inhibit, as well as promote, cell proliferation depending on the subcellular localization of the TGR5 receptor. In non-ciliated cholangiocytes where TGR5 is localized to the apical membrane, TGR5 couples to $G\alpha_s$ to increase intracellular cAMP levels, resulting in increased ERK1/2 signaling and promotion of proliferation (Figure 1) [5]. In contrast, in ciliated cholangiocytes where TGR5 is localized to the cilia, TGR5 couples to $G\alpha_i$ to decrease intracellular cAMP levels, resulting in increased ERK1/2 signaling and inhibition of proliferation (Figure 1) [5]. TGR5 is also expressed in the smooth muscle cells of the gallbladder [43]. TGR5 signaling in these cells activates the cAMP-PKA pathway and causes hyperpolarization of smooth muscle cells by opening the K_{ATP} channels, ultimately leading to inhibition of gallbladder contractility and increased gallbladder filling [43] (Figure 1). Through these combined functions, TGR5 signaling protects the liver and biliary tree from the cytotoxic effects of bile acids. This is further underscored by the finding that whole body $Tgr5^{-/-}$ mice exhibit more severe liver damage, biliary injury, and impaired cholangiocyte proliferation in response to bile acid feeding, compared to wild-type mice [6,44].

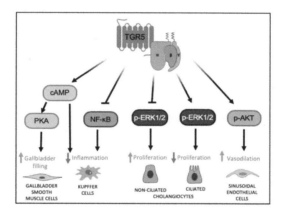

Figure 1. TGR5-mediated cell signaling pathways in different liver cell types. TGR5 activation leads to increased intracellular cAMP levels, followed by activation of PKA, ultimately leading to altered gene expression [1,2], resulting in relaxation of gallbladder smooth muscle cells and increased gallbladder filling. TGR5 signaling in Kupffer cells decreases LPS-induced cytokine production via a cAMP-dependent pathway [20] and antagonizes NF-κB, both resulting in a decreased hepatic inflammatory response [15,39]. TGR5 signaling in non-ciliated cholangiocytes inhibits ERK1/2 signaling, resulting in increased proliferation; whereas in ciliated cholangiocytes, TGR5 signaling increases ERK1/2 activity to decrease proliferation [5]. TGR5 signaling in liver sinusoidal endothelial cells enhances AKT phosphorylation and increases vasodilation [45,46].

Furthermore, in liver sinusoidal endothelial cells, TGR5 signaling increases the generation of vasodilatory molecules, nitrogen oxide and hydrogen sulfide. More specifically, TGR5 activation results in PKA-mediated phosphorylation of endothelial nitric oxide synthase leading to increased production of nitric oxide [21]. Additionally, ligand binding to TGR5 has been shown to activate AKT in these cells, resulting in serine phosphorylation of cystathionine γ-lyase and a subsequent increase in hydrogen sulfide production [45,46]. TGR5 signaling has also been shown to inhibit expression and secretion of endothelin-1, a potent vasoconstrictor [47]. Through TGR5 signaling, the generation of vasodilatory and inhibition of vasoconstrictor molecules serves to modulate liver microcirculation, mitigate portal hypertension and enable adaptation of hepatic blood flow to nutrient uptake [45,47].

3. TGR5 Regulation of Liver Health and Its Impact on Metabolic Disease

3.1. TGR5 and Glucose Regulation

Targeted disruption of TGR5 in mouse models of metabolic disease has identified a role for TGR5 signaling in the maintenance of whole body glucose homeostasis and insulin sensitivity. For instance, Thomas et al., have shown that mice with a gain-of-function of TGR5 have improved glucose tolerance, whereas whole body $Tgr5^{-/-}$ mice have impaired glucose tolerance during an oral glucose tolerance test as compared to weight-matched, high fat diet (HFD)-fed controls [9]. Previous work has also shown that whole body $Tgr5^{-/-}$ mice fed a HFD are more insulin-resistant than $Tgr5^{+/+}$ mice, as assessed by an insulin tolerance test [25]. Furthermore, TGR5 agonists have been shown to ameliorate glucose intolerance and improve insulin resistance in obese and diabetic mice [9,13,27–29,48]. Treatment of diet-induced obese (DIO) mice with INT-777, a semi-synthetic TGR5 agonist, has been shown to promote GLP-1 secretion from L-cells, improve insulin sensitivity in liver and muscle and decrease hepatic glucose production [9]. Compound 18, a potent and highly-specific TGR5 agonist, has been shown to robustly induce GLP-1 secretion and improve glucose tolerance in HFD-fed $Tgr5^{+/+}$ mice, but not in whole body $Tgr5^{-/-}$ mice [30]. Similarly, chronic treatment with oleanolic acid, an extract from *Olea europaea* and a TGR5 agonist, decreased fasting plasma insulin concentrations and improved glucose tolerance in mice [29]. These results also have translational relevance in humans, as a trend towards reduced hyperglycemia and elevated GLP-1 secretion was also seen in a group of patients with type 2 diabetes who received a high dose of the TGR5 agonist, SB-756050 [35]. Additionally, Potthoff et al., reported that treatment of DIO mice with the bile acid sequestrant, colesevelam, significantly reduced hyperinsulinemia and improved glucose tolerance through a decrease in hepatic glucose production, an effect that was absent in whole body $Tgr5^{-/-}$ mice [49]. Until recently, the effect of TGR5 signaling to improve glucose tolerance and insulin sensitivity has been attributed primarily to its effects on mitochondrial function in adipose tissue and GLP-1 secretion from enteroendocrine L cells, leading to insulin release from the pancreas (Figure 2A) [9,13,16,17,34,50].

However, since the liver is central to whole body glucose regulation, this suggests that hepatic TGR5 signaling may be a critical contributor to the overall metabolic benefits of TGR5. Therefore, we administered Compound 18 to hepatocyte-specific TGR5 knockout mice to assess the role of hepatocyte TGR5 on glucose regulation [30]. We found that administration of Compound 18 improves glucose tolerance and insulin sensitivity in HFD-fed $Tgr5^{HEP+/+}$ mice, but not in $Tgr5^{Hep-/-}$ mice. Furthermore, we found that this effect occurred independent of body weight and GLP-1 secretion [24]. Therefore, our findings demonstrate that TGR5 agonists improve glucose homeostasis through an additional, novel mechanism specific to hepatocyte TGR5 signaling (Figure 2A). However, the mechanisms through which hepatocyte TGR5 signaling improves glucose tolerance remain undefined. Further understanding of how liver TGR5 regulates glucose homeostasis is warranted but will necessitate further cell-type specific in vivo studies of hepatic TGR5 function.

3.2. TGR5 and Hepatic Bile Acid Metabolism

Alterations in bile acid homeostasis have been linked to the pathogenesis of insulin resistance and obesity [51–55]. Increased bile acid profile hydrophobicity and increased 12-α-hydroxylated bile acids [56], are associated with insulin resistance and type 2 diabetes in humans [57]. Conversely, administration of hydrophilic bile acids, such as ursodeoxycholic acid (UDCA), has been shown to improve insulin sensitivity in mouse models and patients with type 2 diabetes [58–60]. Therefore, understanding bile acid profile regulation may enable targeting of endogenous bile acid profile for the treatment of metabolic disease. To this end, a growing body of literature has highlighted the role of TGR5 in regulating bile acid profile. Mice with TGR5 ablation have a decreased total bile acid pool size [2,22,31], increased 12-α-hydroxylated bile acids and increased hydrophobic bile acids [26,31]. For example, Pean et al., found that whole body $Tgr5^{-/-}$ mice exhibited more hydrophobic biliary, circulating, and hepatic bile acid pool compositions, as well as decreased muricholic acid (MCA)/CA ratios in both the plasma and liver, as compared to wild-type controls [44]. Furthermore, Donepudi et al., previously found that whole body $Tgr5^{-/-}$ mice had an increased ratio of 12-α-hydroxylated bile acids to non-12-α-hydroxylated bile acids, which was specifically characterized by increased taurocholic acid (TCA) and decreased tauromuricholic acid (TMCA) [26]. Similarly, we reported that TGR5 signaling decreases circulating bile acid profile hydrophobicity following vertical sleeve gastrectomy (VSG) in mice, which was associated with a TGR5-dependent improvement in glucose tolerance [33]. The results of these studies suggest that TGR5 may play an important role in altering bile acid composition, specifically through a reduction in 12-α-hydroxylated bile acids. However, as bile acids are known to regulate lipid, glucose and energy homeostasis through activation of both FXR and TGR5, Pathak et al., administered INT-767, a dual FXR and TGR5 agonist, OCA, an FXR agonist, and INT-777, a TGR5 agonist, to HFD-fed mice to assess the effects of FXR and TGR5 signaling, alone and in combination, on hepatic bile acid metabolism [7]. INT-767 decreased TCA and CA, but increased TMCA, resulting in a decrease in hydrophobicity of the gallbladder bile acid pool [7]. Furthermore, INT-767 was most effective at improving hepatic insulin signaling and hepatic bile acid, lipid, and glucose metabolism [7]. Overall, these studies suggest that decreasing bile acid pool hydrophobicity through increased TGR5 signaling has the potential to improve hepatic glucose metabolism and hepatic insulin signaling; and further, that the most therapeutically efficacious way to do so may be the combinatorial targeting of TGR5 and FXR.

However, the mechanisms by which TGR5 regulates bile acid pool composition are not completely understood. Several studies have identified a role for TGR5 in modulating expression of the enzymes that regulate bile acid synthesis in the liver. CYP7A1 is the rate-limiting enzyme for hepatic bile acid synthesis and CYP8B1 is the hepatic enzyme required for the synthesis of 12-α-hydroxylated bile acids. Donepudi et al., reported that hepatic *Cyp7a1* expression was similar between whole body $Tgr5^{+/+}$ and $Tgr5^{-/-}$ mice, but that fasting induction of hepatic *Cyp8b1* was attenuated in whole body $Tgr5^{-/-}$ mice [26]. Similarly, we previously reported that the decrease in circulating bile acid profile hydrophobicity following VSG in mice was associated with a TGR5-dependent reduction in hepatic CYP8B1 protein expression, with no effect on CYP7A1 expression [33]. In line with this, Pathak et al., found that treatment of mice with OCA (an FXR-specific agonist) or INT-767 resulted in decreased hepatic *Cyp7a1* and *Cyp8b1* expression, whereas treatment with INT-777 only decreased hepatic *Cyp8b1* expression [7]. Together, these studies suggest that one mechanism through which TGR5 may regulate bile acid profile is through the selective downregulation of hepatic *Cyp8b1* expression (Figure 2B). Moreover, Donepudi et al., also reported a decrease in liver *Cyp7b1* and *Cyp27a1* levels, enzymes involved in the alternative pathway of bile acid synthesis, in whole body $Tgr5^{-/-}$ mice [26]. Similarly, Pathak et al., reported that treatment of DIO mice with INT-767 stimulates expression of *Cyp7b1* and *Cyp27a1* [7]. These findings suggest that TGR5 signaling may also upregulate the alternative pathway of bile acid synthesis, which reduces TCA and CA and increases TMCA, thereby decreasing the hydrophobicity of the bile acid pool (Figure 2B).

Another potential mechanism whereby TGR5 signaling regulates bile acid profile is through the selective reabsorption of hydrophobic bile acids through the biliary epithelium, a process called cholehepatic shunting. This hypothesis first gained traction when TGR5 was detected in colocalization with the apical sodium-dependent bile acid transporter (ABST) in gallbladder epithelial cells. Upon activation of TGR5, the subsequent increase in cAMP resulted in insertion of ABST into the apical membrane, leading to enhanced uptake of bile acids from bile into biliary epithelial cells [23]. Through this direct reabsorption into biliary epithelial cells, this shunt is hypothesized to restrict the hydrophobicity of the bile acid pool through the selective reabsorption of secondary bile acids [61]. To this end, Jourdainne et al., reported that through increased gallbladder dilation, TGR5 signaling may favor cholehepatic shunting, thereby increasing the ratio of primary to secondary bile acids [62]. However, the precise signaling and molecular mechanism operating this shunt remain to be explored. Overall, these studies provide ample evidence for a role of TGR5 signaling in the regulation of bile acid profile; however, the mechanisms through which this occurs remain incompletely understood and requires further study in tissue-specific knockout mouse models.

3.3. TGR5 and Hepatic Inflammation

Chronic inflammation is increasingly recognized as a key driver of insulin resistance [63]. Metabolic diseases are often characterized by abnormal cytokine production, increased acute-phase reactants, and activation of a network of inflammatory signaling pathways. Of note, the architectural organization of the liver is such that the metabolic cells, hepatocytes, are in close proximity to the immune cells, the Kupffer cells. This organization enables continuous and dynamic interactions between the metabolic and immune cells of the liver. Thus, the chronic inflammatory signaling associated with obesity promotes hepatic insulin resistance [64]. Moreover, under healthy conditions, hepatic insulin receptor signaling downregulates expression of key gluconeogenic enzymes. Therefore, in the presence of hepatic insulin resistance, endogenous hepatic glucose production is elevated, which contributes to whole body glucose dysregulation. As a therapeutic drug target for treating metabolic disease, TGR5 has been shown to have anti-inflammatory properties in the liver. For example, in response to liver injury, whole body $Tgr5^{-/-}$ mice experience exacerbated inflammatory responses and hepatic fibrosis compared to wild-type controls [65]. In line with this, various in vitro and in vivo studies have highlighted the role of TGR5 in the suppression of macrophage and Kupffer cell functions in response to bile acid treatment or stimulation by TGR5 agonists [1,15,20]. More specifically, in Kupffer cells and macrophages, TGR5 signaling leads to activation of a cAMP-dependent pathway that decreases LPS-induced cytokine expression and the NF-κB-dependent inflammatory response, thereby reducing hepatic inflammation [15,20]. This is particularly relevant to the therapeutic potential of TGR5 agonists as inhibition of NF-κB related inflammation has been shown to improve glucose tolerance in vivo [66]. Together, these studies suggest that the anti-inflammatory properties of hepatic TGR5 signaling may protect against the development and progression of hepatic insulin resistance to ultimately improve whole body glucose regulation (Figure 2C).

3.4. TGR5 and Bariatric Surgery

Bariatric surgery is currently the most effective treatment for obesity and is associated with high rates of T2DM remission [67,68]. Many of the early metabolic benefits of bariatric surgery, including improved insulin and glucose handling, occur prior to significant weight loss [67], which suggests that other hormonal or metabolic mediators may be driving these effects. Bariatric surgery has been shown to increase circulating bile acid concentrations in both humans and rodent models [33,69,70], which has led to the hypothesis that enhanced bile acid signaling may underlie the metabolic benefits of bariatric surgery. The role of bile acid signaling in bariatric surgery has been previously reviewed [71–73]. Here, however, we have focused on the role TGR5 in the effects of bariatric surgery on hepatic metabolism. Various studies have reported TGR5-dependent improvements in glucose tolerance following bariatric surgery, which was associated with improved hepatic insulin signaling (Figure 2D) [33,74]. For example, Ding et al., reported a TGR5-dependent improvement in whole body insulin sensitivity, as assessed by hyperinsulinemic-euglycemic clamp, as well as markedly suppressed hepatic glucose production following VSG in mice [74]. These results suggest that suppression of hepatic glucose production and elevation of peripheral glucose utilization both contributed to improved insulin sensitivity in their model. Similarly, our lab reported a TGR5-dependent improvement in hepatic insulin signaling following VSG in mice; and further, that this effect was associated with reduced hepatic inflammatory cytokine expression, suggesting that reduced inflammation improved hepatic insulin signaling to improve glucose tolerance [33]. Additionally, similar to the effect of TGR5 on the beneficial outcomes of VSG, Ryan et al., reported that FXR contributes to improvements in weight loss and glycemic control following VSG in mice [75], which provides further support for a combinatorial role of TGR5 and FXR in regulating whole body metabolism. However, additional studies in tissue-specific mouse models are needed to identify the cell-type(s) driving these metabolic benefits. Comparatively, Albaugh et al., detected a TGR5-independent improvement in glucose tolerance following bile diversion to the ileum (GB-IL) in mice, in which improvements in glucose tolerance following GB-IL was primarily due to a TGR5-independent effect of bile acids on improved hepatic insulin sensitivity [76]. Conversely, the results on the role of TGR5 in the metabolic benefits of Roux-en-Y gastric bypass (RYGB) have been mixed [77,78]. Zhai et al., suggest that ileal deoxycholic acid-TGR5-mTORC1 signaling contributes to increased GLP-1 production following RYGB in mice [78]. In contrast, Hao et al., reported similar improvements in glucose tolerance and insulin resistance, as assessed by insulin tolerance testing, in whole body $Tgr5^{+/+}$ and $Tgr5^{-/-}$ mice following RYGB [77]. Overall, the differential effects of whole body TGR5 signaling on hepatic metabolic outcomes following bariatric surgery could stem from differences in the underlying mechanisms through which surgery types improve metabolic regulation. Furthermore, this points to VSG as a particularly effective surgical model for the assessment of how liver TGR5 signaling contributes to whole body metabolic regulation (Figure 2D).

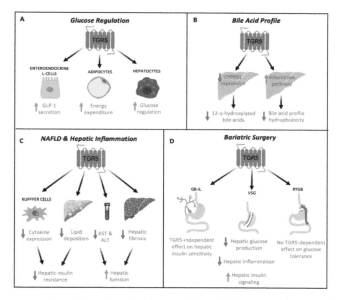

Figure 2. TGR5 signaling in hepatic metabolic regulation. (**A**) TGR5 signaling regulates glucose homeostasis by increasing GLP-1 secretion from enteroendocrine L cells [9,16] and energy expenditure in adipocytes [13]. TGR5 signaling also improves glucose tolerance through signaling in hepatocytes [24]. (**B**) TGR5 signaling decreases hepatic CYP8B1 expression, leading to a decrease in the production of 12-α-hydroxylated bile acids [26,33], and upregulates the alternative pathway of bile acid synthesis, thereby decreasing bile acid profile hydrophobicity [7,26]. (**C**) TGR5 signaling may protect against non-alcoholic fatty liver disease (NAFLD) by reducing hepatic cytokine expression in Kupffer cells [15,20] and decreasing hepatic lipid deposition [9,27], which together, attenuate hepatic insulin resistance. TGR5 signaling also decreases serum AST and ALT concentrations [9], as well as hepatic fibrosis [9], ultimately improving hepatic function. (**D**) TGR5-dependent improvements in glucose tolerance following bariatric surgery depend on surgery type. Vertical sleeve gastrectomy (VSG) results in decreased hepatic glucose production and inflammation, and increased hepatic insulin signaling [33,74]. Following gallbladder bile diversion to the ileum (GB-IL), there is no TGR5-dependent improvement in insulin sensitivity [76]. Roux-en-Y gastric bypass (RYGB) has no TGR5-dependent effect on glucose tolerance [77].

Nutrients **2020**, *12*, 2598

4. TGR5 and Hepatic Lipid Metabolism

Non-alcoholic fatty liver disease (NAFLD) is a common co-morbidity of obesity and develops due to an accumulation of lipid in the liver. NAFLD can progress to non-alcoholic steatohepatitis (NASH), characterized by inflammation, progressive fibrosis, and hepatocellular damage and can eventually progress to cirrhosis or hepatobiliary cancer. Loss of TGR5 signaling has been shown to promote liver lipid deposition in preclinical studies, suggesting that TGR5 signaling may protect against NAFLD. For example, HFD-fed male whole body $Tgr5^{-/-}$ mice exhibit increased liver lipid deposition compared with male wild-type mice. Furthermore, HFD-fed male whole body $Tgr5^{-/-}$ mice exhibit increased liver lipid deposition compared with female whole body $Tgr5^{-/-}$ mice, suggesting that the effect of TGR5 signaling on liver lipid deposition may be influenced by sex [25].

Studies investigating the effects of TGR5 agonists on NAFLD further demonstrate a role for TGR5 in protection against liver lipid deposition. Treatment of HFD-fed mice with INT-777 decreased plasma free fatty acids and liver steatosis, liver fibrosis and plasma AST and ALT levels [9]. Similarly, the TGR5 agonist, RDX8940, was shown to decrease liver weight and hepatic triglyceride and cholesterol levels in mice fed a Western diet [27]. Moreover, dual agonists of TGR5 and FXR protect against NAFLD. For example, treatment of DIO mice with INT-767 decreased hepatic and serum triglycerides and cholesterol levels in mice [7]. Similarly, long-term administration of INT-767 decreased serum AST and ALT concentrations, as well as decreased hypoxia, lipid accumulation, collagen deposition and mononuclear cell infiltrates in the livers of a rabbit model of HFD-induced metabolic syndrome [79]. Furthermore, INT-767 treatment reduced expression of liver pro-inflammatory genes, as well as genes related to *de novo* lipogenesis, and promoted expression of anti-inflammatory genes and genes related to lipid uptake [79]. In line with this, *ob/ob* mice on a HFD supplemented with trans-fat, cholesterol, and fructose treated with INT-767 exhibited a greater decrease in liver parenchymal fibrosis and inflammatory infiltrates compared to mice treated with OCA [80]. Moreover, treatment of mice on HFD supplemented with fructose with BAR502, another dual FXR and TGR5 agonist, reduced hepatic steatosis, inflammation and fibrosis [81]. Although we cannot discern the contribution of TGR5 to the beneficial metabolic effects of dual TGR5/FXR agonists on hepatic function, these findings suggest that the combinatorial targeting of FXR and TGR5 is a promising therapeutic modality for improving hepatic function.

Studies in mouse models of bariatric surgery report conflicting results on the role of TGR5 in the effect of bariatric surgery to reduce liver lipid deposition. Ding et al., reported that VSG decreased hepatic steatosis in wild-type but not in whole body $Tgr5^{-/-}$ mice [74]. In contrast, our lab reported TGR5-independent improvements in hepatic triglyceride content following VSG in mice [33]. The discrepancy between these findings could be explained by differences in the whole body $Tgr5^{-/-}$ mouse models used, duration of HFD-feeding, and variation in diet composition in each study [74].

Overall, these findings suggest that enhanced TGR5 signaling attenuates hepatic triglyceride accumulation and fibrosis, and improves liver function; however, the mechanisms through which this occurs remain unknown (Figure 2C). Further work is needed to address this limitation to more completely harness the therapeutic potential of TGR5 in patients with NAFLD. Moreover, these studies suggest that, similar to the regulation of bile acid profile, the combinatorial targeting of TGR5 and FXR may provide the most therapeutic utility.

5. Negative Side-Effects of Enhanced Hepatic TGR5 Signaling

Therapeutic targeting of TGR5 for the treatment of metabolic disease has been hindered by the wide range of effects associated with systemic TGR5 activation. In particular, a major side effect of TGR5 agonists is the inhibition of gallbladder emptying, leading to gallstone formation and cholestasis. TGR5 is highly expressed in the gallbladder and cholangiocytes [23]. TGR5 signaling stimulates relaxation of gallbladder smooth muscle cells to induce gallbladder filling [43]. Several studies have reported that the oral administration of the TGR5 agonists, such as INT-777, LCA, oleanolic acid, Compound 23g, Compound 18, and RO552739, increase biliary bile flow and gallbladder filling in wild type mice [24,28,29,31,82,83]. In line with this, several studies have reported reduced gallbladder volumes and reduced bile flow in whole body *Tgr5*$^{-/-}$ mice relative to wild-type controls [31,43]. However, whole body *Tgr5*$^{-/-}$ mice are protected against the formation of cholesterol crystals and gallstones when fed a lithogenic diet [22], which suggests that the continual build-up of bile in the biliary tract has the potential to cause cholestasis and indirect liver injury. Therefore, despite the robust metabolic benefits associated with hepatic TGR5 signaling, chronic stimulation of TGR5 within the biliary tract complicates the task of developing a safe and efficacious TGR5 agonist (Figure 3).

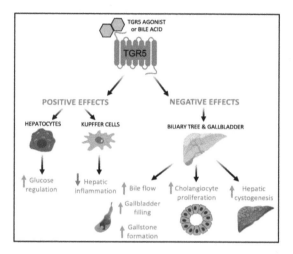

Figure 3. Positive and negative effects of elevated hepatic TGR5 signaling. Within the liver, TGR5 activation by TGR5-specific agonists and/or bile acids leads to beneficial metabolic outcomes, including improved glucose tolerance [24] and decreased hepatic inflammation [15,20]. However, TGR5 signaling in the biliary tract and gallbladder results in increased bile flow, gallbladder filling, and gallstone formation [22,24,28,29,31,82,83], as well as increased cholangiocyte proliferation and hepatic cystogenesis [84].

TGR5 expression in the biliary tract is also crucial for protection against bile acid overload. For example, TGR5 signaling strengthens the biliary epithelial barrier resulting in decreased hepatocyte necrosis in the presence of obstructive cholestasis in mice [42]. In contrast to this protective role, TGR5 activation in the biliary tract has been shown to contribute to the development of polycystic liver disease and cholangiocarcinoma [6,84]. Whole body *Tgr5*$^{-/-}$ mice exhibit decreased cholangiocyte and hepatocyte proliferation and increased liver injury in response to cholestatic stress [6]. In addition, taurolithocholic acid and oleanolic acid stimulation of TGR5 in vitro and in vivo have been shown to promote cholangiocyte proliferation through TGR5-dependent increases in cAMP production. However, this increased proliferation was accompanied by increased hepatic cystogenesis and the development of polycystic liver disease (Figure 3) [84]. Comparatively, treatment of cultured cystic cholangiocytes with the TGR5 antagonist, SBI-115, decreased proliferation, cholangiocyte spheroid growth and cAMP levels [84], suggesting that TGR5 inhibition may be a promising therapeutic approach to polycystic liver disease and treating malignant cholangiocytes. Therefore, while the proliferative and anti-apoptotic properties of TGR5 are crucial for hepatoprotection under conditions of bile acid toxicity, it also impedes the regulation of malignant cholangiocytes, which may lead to an increased risk of developing cholangiocarcinoma and liver cancer [6]. To this end, the negative effects of TGR5 agonists on cholestasis, cholangiocyte proliferation, and hepatic cystogenesis decreases the enthusiasm of therapeutically targeting TGR5 to treat liver disease (Figure 3).

6. Conclusions

In light of the ubiquitous expression of TGR5 throughout the liver, hepatic TGR5 signaling is increasingly recognized as a key contributor to whole body metabolic regulation. Nevertheless, the wide range of effects associated with liver TGR5 signaling complicates therapeutic targeting of TGR5. Further delineation of the downstream mediators of TGR5 signaling in the liver is needed to enable rational development of compounds targeting mediators of the metabolically beneficial actions of TGR5 in the liver. Such a compound could be coupled with an GLP-1 receptor agonist to develop a highly effective multimodal therapy for the treatment of type 2 diabetes.

Author Contributions: Conceptualization: M.M.H. and B.P.C.; Writing—Original Draft Preparation: M.M.H., M.K.C. and V.N.G.; Writing—Review and Editing: M.M.H., M.K.C., V.N.G. and B.P.C.; Supervision, Funding Acquisition: B.P.C. All authors have read and agreed to the published version of the manuscript.

Funding: This research was funded by Nutracia 2018-55 and NIH/NCI 5R21CA195002.

Conflicts of Interest: The authors declare no conflict of interest.

References

1. Kawamata, Y.; Fujii, R.; Hosoya, M.; Harada, M.; Yoshida, H.; Miwa, M.; Fukusumi, S.; Habata, Y.; Itoh, T.; Shintani, Y.; et al. AG protein-coupled receptor responsive to bile acids. *J. Biol. Chem.* **2003**, *278*, 9435–9440. [CrossRef]

2. Maruyama, T.; Miyamoto, Y.; Nakamura, T.; Tamai, Y.; Okada, H.; Sugiyama, E.; Nakamura, T.; Itadani, H.; Tanaka, K. Identification of membrane-type receptor for bile acids (M-BAR). *Biochem. Biophys. Res. Commun.* **2002**, *298*, 714–719. [CrossRef]

3. Perino, A.; Pols, T.W.; Nomura, M.; Stein, S.; Pellicciari, R.; Schoonjans, K. TGR5 reduces macrophage migration through mTOR-induced C/EBPbeta differential translation. *J. Clin. Investig.* **2014**, *124*, 5424–5436. [CrossRef] [PubMed]

4. Rajagopal, S.; Kumar, D.P.; Mahavadi, S.; Bhattacharya, S.; Zhou, R.; Corvera, C.U.; Bunnett, N.W.; Grider, J.R.; Murthy, K.S. Activation of G protein-coupled bile acid receptor, TGR5, induces smooth muscle relaxation via both Epac- and PKA-mediated inhibition of RhoA/Rho kinase pathway. *Am. J. Physiol. Gastrointest. Liver Physiol.* **2013**, *304*, G527–G535. [CrossRef] [PubMed]

5. Masyuk, A.I.; Huang, B.Q.; Radtke, B.N.; Gajdos, G.B.; Splinter, P.L.; Masyuk, T.V.; Gradilone, S.A.; LaRusso, N.F. Ciliary subcellular localization of TGR5 determines the cholangiocyte functional response to bile acid signaling. *Am. J. Physiol. Gastrointest. Liver Physiol.* **2013**, *304*, G1013–G1024. [CrossRef] [PubMed]

6. Reich, M.; Deutschmann, K.; Sommerfeld, A.; Klindt, C.; Kluge, S.; Kubitz, R.; Ullmer, C.; Knoefel, W.T.; Herebian, D.; Mayatepek, E.; et al. TGR5 is essential for bile acid-dependent cholangiocyte proliferation in vivo and in vitro. *Gut* **2016**, *65*, 487–501. [CrossRef] [PubMed]

7. Pathak, P.; Liu, H.; Boehme, S.; Xie, C.; Krausz, K.W.; Gonzalez, F.; Chiang, J.Y.L. Farnesoid X receptor induces Takeda G-protein receptor 5 cross-talk to regulate bile acid synthesis and hepatic metabolism. *J. Biol. Chem.* **2017**, *292*, 11055–11069. [CrossRef] [PubMed]

8. Cariou, B.; van Harmelen, K.; Duran-Sandoval, D.; van Dijk, T.H.; Grefhorst, A.; Abdelkarim, M.; Caron, S.; Torpier, G.; Fruchart, J.C.; Gonzalez, F.J.; et al. The farnesoid X receptor modulates adiposity and peripheral insulin sensitivity in mice. *J. Biol. Chem.* **2006**, *281*, 11039–11049. [CrossRef]

9. Thomas, C.; Gioiello, A.; Noriega, L.; Strehle, A.; Oury, J.; Rizzo, G.; Macchiarulo, A.; Yamamoto, H.; Mataki, C.; Pruzanski, M.; et al. TGR5-mediated bile acid sensing controls glucose homeostasis. *Cell Metab.* **2009**, *10*, 167–177. [CrossRef]

10. Erickson, S.K.; Lear, S.R.; Deane, S.; Dubrac, S.; Huling, S.L.; Nguyen, L.; Bollineni, J.S.; Shefer, S.; Hyogo, H.; Cohen, D.E.; et al. Hypercholesterolemia and changes in lipid and bile acid metabolism in male and female cyp7A1-deficient mice. *J. Lipid Res.* **2003**, *44*, 1001–1009. [CrossRef]

11. Ferslew, B.C.; Xie, G.; Johnston, C.K.; Su, M.; Stewart, P.W.; Jia, W.; Brouwer, K.L.; Barritt, A.S.t. Altered Bile Acid Metabolome in Patients with Nonalcoholic Steatohepatitis. *Dig. Dis. Sci.* **2015**, *60*, 3318–3328. [CrossRef] [PubMed]

12. Brufau, G.; Stellaard, F.; Prado, K.; Bloks, V.W.; Jonkers, E.; Boverhof, R.; Kuipers, F.; Murphy, E.J. Improved glycemic control with colesevelam treatment in patients with type 2 diabetes is not directly associated with changes in bile acid metabolism. *Hepatology* **2010**, *52*, 1455–1464. [CrossRef] [PubMed]

13. Watanabe, M.; Houten, S.M.; Mataki, C.; Christoffolete, M.A.; Kim, B.W.; Sato, H.; Messaddeq, N.; Harney, J.W.; Ezaki, O.; Kodama, T.; et al. Bile acids induce energy expenditure by promoting intracellular thyroid hormone activation. *Nature* **2006**, *439*, 484–489. [CrossRef] [PubMed]

14. Guo, C.; Qi, H.; Yu, Y.; Zhang, Q.; Su, J.; Yu, D.; Huang, W.; Chen, W.D.; Wang, Y.D. The G-Protein-Coupled Bile Acid Receptor Gpbar1 (TGR5) Inhibits Gastric Inflammation Through Antagonizing NF-kappaB Signaling Pathway. *Front. Pharmacol.* **2015**, *6*, 287. [CrossRef]

15. Wang, Y.D.; Chen, W.D.; Yu, D.; Forman, B.M.; Huang, W. The G-protein-coupled bile acid receptor, Gpbar1 (TGR5), negatively regulates hepatic inflammatory response through antagonizing nuclear factor kappa light-chain enhancer of activated B cells (NF-kappaB) in mice. *Hepatology* **2011**, *54*, 1421–1432. [CrossRef]

16. Katsuma, S.; Hirasawa, A.; Tsujimoto, G. Bile acids promote glucagon-like peptide-1 secretion through TGR5 in a murine enteroendocrine cell line STC-1. *Biochem. Biophys. Res. Commun.* **2005**, *329*, 386–390. [CrossRef]

17. Li, Y.; Cheng, K.C.; Niu, C.-S.; Lo, S.-H.; Cheng, J.-T.; Niu, H.-S. Investigation of triamterene as an inhibitor of the TGR5 receptor: Identification in cells and animals. *Drug Des. Dev. Ther.* **2017**, *11*, 1127–1134. [CrossRef]

18. Broeders, E.P.; Nascimento, E.B.; Havekes, B.; Brans, B.; Roumans, K.H.; Tailleux, A.; Schaart, G.; Kouach, M.; Charton, J.; Deprez, B. The bile acid chenodeoxycholic acid increases human brown adipose tissue activity. *Cell Metab.* **2015**, *22*, 418–426. [CrossRef]

19. Velazquez-Villegas, L.A.; Perino, A.; Lemos, V.; Zietak, M.; Nomura, M.; Pols, T.W.H.; Schoonjans, K. TGR5 signalling promotes mitochondrial fission and beige remodelling of white adipose tissue. *Nat. Commun.* **2018**, *9*, 1–13. [CrossRef]

20. Keitel, V.; Donner, M.; Winandy, S.; Kubitz, R.; Haussinger, D. Expression and function of the bile acid receptor TGR5 in Kupffer cells. *Biochem. Biophys. Res. Commun.* **2008**, *372*, 78–84. [CrossRef]

21. Keitel, V.; Reinehr, R.; Gatsios, P.; Rupprecht, C.; Gorg, B.; Selbach, O.; Haussinger, D.; Kubitz, R. The G-protein coupled bile salt receptor TGR5 is expressed in liver sinusoidal endothelial cells. *Hepatology* **2007**, *45*, 695–704. [CrossRef]

22. Vassileva, G.; Golovko, A.; Markowitz, L.; Abbondanzo, S.J.; Zeng, M.; Yang, S.; Hoos, L.; Tetzloff, G.; Levitan, D.; Murgolo, N.J.; et al. Targeted deletion of Gpbar1 protects mice from cholesterol gallstone formation. *Biochem. J.* **2006**, *398*, 423–430. [CrossRef]

23. Keitel, V.; Cupisti, K.; Ullmer, C.; Knoefel, W.T.; Kubitz, R.; Haussinger, D. The membrane-bound bile acid receptor TGR5 is localized in the epithelium of human gallbladders. *Hepatology* **2009**, *50*, 861–870. [CrossRef] [PubMed]

24. Holter, M.M.; Chirikjian, M.K.; Briere, D.A.; Maida, A.; Sloop, K.W.; Schoonjans, K.; Cummings, B.P. Compound 18 Improves Glucose Tolerance in a Hepatocyte TGR5-dependent Manner in Mice. *Nutrients* **2020**, *12*, 2124. [CrossRef]

25. Vassileva, G.; Hu, W.; Hoos, L.; Tetzloff, G.; Yang, S.; Liu, L.; Kang, L.; Davis, H.R.; Hedrick, J.A.; Lan, H.; et al. Gender-dependent effect of Gpbar1 genetic deletion on the metabolic profiles of diet-induced obese mice. *J. Endocrinol.* **2010**, *205*, 225–232. [CrossRef] [PubMed]

26. Donepudi, A.C.; Boehme, S.; Li, F.; Chiang, J.Y.L. G-protein-coupled bile acid receptor plays a key role in bile acid metabolism and fasting-induced hepatic steatosis in mice. *Hepatology* **2017**, *65*, 813–827. [CrossRef] [PubMed]

27. Finn, P.D.; Rodriguez, D.; Kohler, J.; Jiang, Z.; Wan, S.; Blanco, E.; King, A.J.; Chen, T.; Bell, N.; Dragoli, D.; et al. Intestinal TGR5 agonism improves hepatic steatosis and insulin sensitivity in Western diet-fed mice. *Am. J. Physiol. Gastrointest. Liver Physiol.* **2019**, *316*, G412–G424. [CrossRef]

28. Pellicciari, R.; Gioiello, A.; Macchiarulo, A.; Thomas, C.; Rosatelli, E.; Natalini, B.; Sardella, R.; Pruzanski, M.; Roda, A.; Pastorini, E.; et al. Discovery of 6alpha-ethyl-23(S)-methylcholic acid (S-EMCA, INT-777) as a potent and selective agonist for the TGR5 receptor, a novel target for diabesity. *J. Med. Chem.* **2009**, *52*, 7958–7961. [CrossRef]

29. Sato, H.; Genet, C.; Strehle, A.; Thomas, C.; Lobstein, A.; Wagner, A.; Mioskowski, C.; Auwerx, J.; Saladin, R. Anti-hyperglycemic activity of a TGR5 agonist isolated from Olea europaea. *Biochem. Biophys. Res. Commun.* **2007**, *362*, 793–798. [CrossRef]

30. Briere, D.A.; Ruan, X.; Cheng, C.C.; Siesky, A.M.; Fitch, T.E.; Dominguez, C.; Sanfeliciano, S.G.; Montero, C.; Suen, C.S.; Xu, Y.; et al. Novel Small Molecule Agonist of TGR5 Possesses Anti-Diabetic Effects but Causes Gallbladder Filling in Mice. *PLoS ONE* **2015**, *10*, e0136873. [CrossRef]

31. Li, T.; Holmstrom, S.R.; Kir, S.; Umetani, M.; Schmidt, D.R.; Kliewer, S.A.; Mangelsdorf, D.J. The G protein-coupled bile acid receptor, TGR5, stimulates gallbladder filling. *Mol. Endocrinol.* **2011**, *25*, 1066–1071. [CrossRef] [PubMed]

32. Sato, H.; Macchiarulo, A.; Thomas, C.; Gioiello, A.; Une, M.; Hofmann, A.F.; Saladin, R.; Schoonjans, K.; Pellicciari, R.; Auwerx, J. Novel potent and selective bile acid derivatives as TGR5 agonists: Biological screening, structure–activity relationships, and molecular modeling studies. *J. Med. Chem.* **2008**, *51*, 1831–1841. [CrossRef]

33. McGavigan, A.K.; Garibay, D.; Henseler, Z.M.; Chen, J.; Bettaieb, A.; Haj, F.G.; Ley, R.E.; Chouinard, M.L.; Cummings, B.P. TGR5 contributes to glucoregulatory improvements after vertical sleeve gastrectomy in mice. *Gut* **2017**, *66*, 226–234. [CrossRef] [PubMed]

34. Huang, S.; Ma, S.; Ning, M.; Yang, W.; Ye, Y.; Zhang, L.; Shen, J.; Leng, Y. TGR5 agonist ameliorates insulin resistance in the skeletal muscles and improves glucose homeostasis in diabetic mice. *Metabolism* **2019**, *99*, 45–56. [CrossRef] [PubMed]

35. Hodge, R.J.; Lin, J.; Vasist Johnson, L.S.; Gould, E.P.; Bowers, G.D.; Nunez, D.J. Safety, Pharmacokinetics, and Pharmacodynamic Effects of a Selective TGR5 Agonist, SB-756050, in Type 2 Diabetes. *Clin. Pharmacol. Drug Dev.* **2013**, *2*, 213–222. [CrossRef] [PubMed]

36. Poole, D.P.; Godfrey, C.; Cattaruzza, F.; Cottrell, G.S.; Kirkland, J.G.; Pelayo, J.C.; Bunnett, N.W.; Corvera, C.U. Expression and function of the bile acid receptor GpBAR1 (TGR5) in the murine enteric nervous system. *Neurogastroenterol. Motil.* **2010**, *22*, 814–825. [CrossRef] [PubMed]

37. Yang, J.I.; Yoon, J.H.; Myung, S.J.; Gwak, G.Y.; Kim, W.; Chung, G.E.; Lee, S.H.; Lee, S.M.; Kim, C.Y.; Lee, H.S. Bile acid-induced TGR5-dependent c-Jun-N terminal kinase activation leads to enhanced caspase 8 activation in hepatocytes. *Biochem. Biophys. Res. Commun.* **2007**, *361*, 156–161. [CrossRef]

38. Giaretta, P.R.; Suchodolski, J.S.; Blick, A.K.; Steiner, J.M.; Lidbury, J.A.; Rech, R.R. Distribution of bile acid receptor TGR5 in the gastrointestinal tract of dogs. *Histol. Histopathol.* **2018**, *34*, 18025.

39. Pols, T.W.; Nomura, M.; Harach, T.; Lo Sasso, G.; Oosterveer, M.H.; Thomas, C.; Rizzo, G.; Gioiello, A.; Adorini, L.; Pellicciari, R.; et al. TGR5 activation inhibits atherosclerosis by reducing macrophage inflammation and lipid loading. *Cell Metab.* **2011**, *14*, 747–757. [CrossRef]

40. Baghdasaryan, A.; Claudel, T.; Gumhold, J.; Silbert, D.; Adorini, L.; Roda, A.; Vecchiotti, S.; Gonzalez, F.J.; Schoonjans, K.; Strazzabosco, M.; et al. Dual farnesoid X receptor/TGR5 agonist INT-767 reduces liver injury in the Mdr2$^{-/-}$ (Abcb4$^{-/-}$) mouse cholangiopathy model by promoting biliary HCO(-)(3) output. *Hepatology* **2011**, *54*, 1303–1312. [CrossRef]

41. De Buy Wenniger, L.J.M.; Hohenester, S.; Maroni, L.; van Vliet, S.J.; Elferink, R.P.O.; Beuers, U. The Cholangiocyte Glycocalyx Stabilizes the 'Biliary HCO3-Umbrella': An Integrated Line of Defense against Toxic Bile Acids. *Dig. Dis.* **2015**, *33*, 397–407. [CrossRef] [PubMed]

42. Merlen, G.; Kahale, N.; Ursic-Bedoya, J.; Bidault-Jourdainne, V.; Simerabet, H.; Doignon, I.; Tanfin, Z.; Garcin, I.; Pean, N.; Gautherot, J.; et al. TGR5-dependent hepatoprotection through the regulation of biliary epithelium barrier function. *Gut* **2020**, *69*, 146–157. [CrossRef] [PubMed]

43. Lavoie, B.; Balemba, O.B.; Godfrey, C.; Watson, C.A.; Vassileva, G.; Corvera, C.U.; Nelson, M.T.; Mawe, G.M. Hydrophobic bile salts inhibit gallbladder smooth muscle function via stimulation of GPBAR1 receptors and activation of KATP channels. *J. Physiol.* **2010**, *588*, 3295–3305. [CrossRef] [PubMed]

44. Pean, N.; Doignon, I.; Garcin, I.; Besnard, A.; Julien, B.; Liu, B.; Branchereau, S.; Spraul, A.; Guettier, C.; Humbert, L.; et al. The receptor TGR5 protects the liver from bile acid overload during liver regeneration in mice. *Hepatology* **2013**, *58*, 1451–1460. [CrossRef] [PubMed]

45. Renga, B.; Cipriani, S.; Carino, A.; Simonetti, M.; Zampella, A.; Fiorucci, S. Reversal of Endothelial Dysfunction by GPBAR1 Agonism in Portal Hypertension Involves a AKT/FOXOA1 Dependent Regulation of H2S Generation and Endothelin-1. *PLoS ONE* **2015**, *10*, e0141082. [CrossRef]

46. Renga, B.; Bucci, M.; Cipriani, S.; Carino, A.; Monti, M.C.; Zampella, A.; Gargiulo, A.; d'Emmanuele di Villa Bianca, R.; Distrutti, E.; Fiorucci, S. Cystathionine γ-lyase, a H2S-generating enzyme, is a GPBAR1-regulated gene and contributes to vasodilation caused by secondary bile acids. *Am. J. Physiol. Heart Circ. Physiol.* **2015**, *309*, H114–H126. [CrossRef]

47. Klindt, C.; Reich, M.; Hellwig, B.; Stindt, J.; Rahnenführer, J.; Hengstler, J.G.; Köhrer, K.; Schoonjans, K.; Häussinger, D.; Keitel, V. The G Protein-Coupled Bile Acid Receptor TGR5 (Gpbar1) Modulates Endothelin-1 Signaling in Liver. *Cells* **2019**, *8*, 1467. [CrossRef]

48. Brighton, C.A.; Rievaj, J.; Kuhre, R.E.; Glass, L.L.; Schoonjans, K.; Holst, J.J.; Gribble, F.M.; Reimann, F. Bile Acids Trigger GLP-1 Release Predominantly by Accessing Basolaterally Located G Protein-Coupled Bile Acid Receptors. *Endocrinology* **2015**, *156*, 3961–3970. [CrossRef]

49. Potthoff, M.J.; Potts, A.; He, T.; Duarte, J.A.; Taussig, R.; Mangelsdorf, D.J.; Kliewer, S.A.; Burgess, S.C. Colesevelam suppresses hepatic glycogenolysis by TGR5-mediated induction of GLP-1 action in DIO mice. *Am. J. Physiol. Gastrointest. Liver Physiol.* **2013**, *304*, G371–G380. [CrossRef]

50. Kumar, D.P.; Rajagopal, S.; Mahavadi, S.; Mirshahi, F.; Grider, J.R.; Murthy, K.S.; Sanyal, A.J. Activation of transmembrane bile acid receptor TGR5 stimulates insulin secretion in pancreatic β cells. *Biochem. Biophys. Res. Commun.* **2012**, *427*, 600–605. [CrossRef]

51. Sun, W.; Zhang, D.; Wang, Z.; Sun, J.; Xu, B.; Chen, Y.; Ding, L.; Huang, X.; Lv, X.; Lu, J.; et al. Insulin Resistance is Associated with Total Bile Acid Level in Type 2 Diabetic and Nondiabetic Population: A Cross-Sectional Study. *Medicine* **2016**, *95*, e2778. [CrossRef]

52. Bennion, L.J.; Grundy, S.M. Effects of diabetes mellitus on cholesterol metabolism in man. *N. Engl. J. Med.* **1977**, *296*, 1365–1371. [CrossRef]

53. Li, T.; Francl, J.M.; Boehme, S.; Ochoa, A.; Zhang, Y.; Klaassen, C.D.; Erickson, S.K.; Chiang, J.Y. Glucose and insulin induction of bile acid synthesis: Mechanisms and implication in diabetes and obesity. *J. Biol. Chem.* **2012**, *287*, 1861–1873. [CrossRef]

54. Suhre, K.; Meisinger, C.; Döring, A.; Altmaier, E.; Belcredi, P.; Gieger, C.; Chang, D.; Milburn, M.V.; Gall, W.E.; Weinberger, K.M.; et al. Metabolic footprint of diabetes: A multiplatform metabolomics study in an epidemiological setting. *PLoS ONE* **2010**, *5*, e13953. [CrossRef]

55. Hyogo, H.; Roy, S.; Paigen, B.; Cohen, D.E. Leptin promotes biliary cholesterol elimination during weight loss in ob/ob mice by regulating the enterohepatic circulation of bile salts. *J. Biol. Chem.* **2002**, *277*, 34117–34124. [CrossRef]

56. Lefebvre, P.; Cariou, B.; Lien, F.; Kuipers, F.; Staels, B. Role of bile acids and bile acid receptors in metabolic regulation. *Physiol. Rev.* **2009**, *89*, 147–191. [CrossRef]

57. Haeusler, R.A.; Astiarraga, B.; Camastra, S.; Accili, D.; Ferrannini, E. Human insulin resistance is associated with increased plasma levels of 12alpha-hydroxylated bile acids. *Diabetes* **2013**, *62*, 4184–4191. [CrossRef]

58. Mahmoud, A.A.; Elshazly, S.M. Ursodeoxycholic acid ameliorates fructose-induced metabolic syndrome in rats. *PLoS ONE* **2014**, *9*, e106993. [CrossRef]

59. Özcan, U.; Yilmaz, E.; Ozcan, L.; Furuhashi, M.; Vaillancourt, E.; Smith, R.O.; Gorgun, C.Z.; Hotamisligil, G.S. Chemical chaperones reduce ER stress and restore glucose homeostasis in a mouse model of type 2 diabetes. *Science* **2006**, *313*, 1137–1140. [CrossRef]

60. Shima, K.R.; Ota, T.; Kato, K.I.; Takeshita, Y.; Misu, H.; Kaneko, S.; Takamura, T. Ursodeoxycholic acid potentiates dipeptidyl peptidase-4 inhibitor sitagliptin by enhancing glucagon-like peptide-1 secretion in patients with type 2 diabetes and chronic liver disease: A pilot randomized controlled and add-on study. *BMJ Open Diabetes Res. Care* **2018**, *6*, e000469. [CrossRef]

61. Debray, D.; Rainteau, D.; Barbu, V.; Rouahi, M.; El Mourabit, H.; Lerondel, S.; Rey, C.; Humbert, L.; Wendum, D.; Cottart, C.H.; et al. Defects in gallbladder emptying and bile Acid homeostasis in mice with cystic fibrosis transmembrane conductance regulator deficiencies. *Gastroenterology* **2012**, *142*, 1581–1591.e1586. [CrossRef]

62. Jourdainne, V.; Péan, N.; Doignon, I.; Humbert, L.; Rainteau, D.; Tordjmann, T. The Bile Acid Receptor TGR5 and Liver Regeneration. *Dig. Dis.* **2015**, *33*, 319–326. [CrossRef]

63. Yoshizaki, T.; Schenk, S.; Imamura, T.; Babendure, J.L.; Sonoda, N.; Bae, E.J.; Oh, D.Y.; Lu, M.; Milne, J.C.; Westphal, C.; et al. SIRT1 inhibits inflammatory pathways in macrophages and modulates insulin sensitivity. *Am. J. Physiol. Endocrinol. Metab.* **2010**, *298*, E419–E428. [CrossRef]

64. Cai, D.; Yuan, M.; Frantz, D.F.; Melendez, P.A.; Hansen, L.; Lee, J.; Shoelson, S.E. Local and systemic insulin resistance resulting from hepatic activation of IKK-beta and NF-kappaB. *Nat. Med.* **2005**, *11*, 183–190. [CrossRef]

65. Rao, J.; Yang, C.; Yang, S.; Lu, H.; Hu, Y.; Lu, L.; Cheng, F.; Wang, X. Deficiency of TGR5 exacerbates immune-mediated cholestatic hepatic injury by stabilizing the β-catenin destruction complex. *Int. Immunol.* **2020**, *32*, 321–334. [CrossRef]

66. Yin, J.; Zuberi, A.; Gao, Z.; Liu, D.; Liu, Z.; Ye, J. Shilianhua extract inhibits GSK-3beta and promotes glucose metabolism. *Am. J. Physiol. Endocrinol. Metab.* **2009**, *296*, E1275–E1280. [CrossRef]

67. Buchwald, H.; Avidor, Y.; Braunwald, E.; Jensen, M.D.; Pories, W.; Fahrbach, K.; Schoelles, K. Bariatric surgery: A systematic review and meta-analysis. *JAMA* **2004**, *292*, 1724–1737. [CrossRef]

68. Schauer, P.R.; Kashyap, S.R.; Wolski, K.; Brethauer, S.A.; Kirwan, J.P.; Pothier, C.E.; Thomas, S.; Abood, B.; Nissen, S.E.; Bhatt, D.L. Bariatric surgery versus intensive medical therapy in obese patients with diabetes. *N. Engl. J. Med.* **2012**, *366*, 1567–1576. [CrossRef]

69. Patti, M.E.; Houten, S.M.; Bianco, A.C.; Bernier, R.; Larsen, P.R.; Holst, J.J.; Badman, M.K.; Maratos-Flier, E.; Mun, E.C.; Pihlajamaki, J.; et al. Serum bile acids are higher in humans with prior gastric bypass: Potential contribution to improved glucose and lipid metabolism. *Obesity (Silver Spring)* **2009**, *17*, 1671–1677. [CrossRef]

70. Steinert, R.E.; Peterli, R.; Keller, S.; Meyer-Gerspach, A.C.; Drewe, J.; Peters, T.; Beglinger, C. Bile acids and gut peptide secretion after bariatric surgery: A 1-year prospective randomized pilot trial. *Obesity (Silver Spring)* **2013**, *21*, E660–E668. [CrossRef]

71. Zaborska, K.E.; Cummings, B.P. Rethinking Bile Acid Metabolism and Signaling for Type 2 Diabetes Treatment. *Curr. Diab. Rep.* **2018**, *18*, 109. [CrossRef]

72. Wang, W.; Cheng, Z.; Wang, Y.; Dai, Y.; Zhang, X.; Hu, S. Role of Bile Acids in Bariatric Surgery. *Front. Physiol.* **2019**, *10*, 374. [CrossRef]

73. Albaugh, V.L.; Banan, B.; Ajouz, H.; Abumrad, N.N.; Flynn, C.R. Bile acids and bariatric surgery. *Mol. Asp. Med.* **2017**, *56*, 75–89. [CrossRef]

74. Ding, L.; Sousa, K.M.; Jin, L.; Dong, B.; Kim, B.W.; Ramirez, R.; Xiao, Z.; Gu, Y.; Yang, Q.; Wang, J. Vertical sleeve gastrectomy activates GPBAR-1/TGR5 to sustain weight loss, improve fatty liver, and remit insulin resistance in mice. *Hepatology* **2016**, *64*, 760–773. [CrossRef]

75. Ryan, K.K.; Tremaroli, V.; Clemmensen, C.; Kovatcheva-Datchary, P.; Myronovych, A.; Karns, R.; Wilson-Pérez, H.E.; Sandoval, D.A.; Kohli, R.; Bäckhed, F.; et al. FXR is a molecular target for the effects of vertical sleeve gastrectomy. *Nature* **2014**, *509*, 183–188. [CrossRef]

76. Albaugh, V.L.; Banan, B.; Antoun, J.; Xiong, Y.; Guo, Y.; Ping, J.; Alikhan, M.; Clements, B.A.; Abumrad, N.N.; Flynn, C.R. Role of Bile Acids and GLP-1 in Mediating the Metabolic Improvements of Bariatric Surgery. *Gastroenterology* **2019**, *156*, 1041–1051.e1044. [CrossRef]

77. Hao, Z.; Leigh Townsend, R.; Mumphrey, M.B.; Gettys, T.W.; Yu, S.; Munzberg, H.; Morrison, C.D.; Berthoud, H.R. Roux-en-Y Gastric Bypass Surgery-Induced Weight Loss and Metabolic Improvements Are Similar in TGR5-Deficient and Wildtype Mice. *Obes. Surg.* **2018**. [CrossRef]

78. Zhai, H.; Li, Z.; Peng, M.; Huang, Z.; Qin, T.; Chen, L.; Li, H.; Zhang, H.; Zhang, W.; Xu, G. Takeda G Protein-Coupled Receptor 5-Mechanistic Target of Rapamycin Complex 1 Signaling Contributes to the Increment of Glucagon-Like Peptide-1 Production after Roux-en-Y Gastric Bypass. *EBioMedicine* **2018**, *32*, 201–214. [CrossRef]

79. Comeglio, P.; Cellai, I.; Mello, T.; Filippi, S.; Maneschi, E.; Corcetto, F.; Corno, C.; Sarchielli, E.; Morelli, A.; Rapizzi, E.; et al. INT-767 prevents NASH and promotes visceral fat brown adipogenesis and mitochondrial function. *J. Endocrinol.* **2018**, *238*, 107–127. [CrossRef]

80. Roth, J.D.; Feigh, M.; Veidal, S.S.; Fensholdt, L.K.; Rigbolt, K.T.; Hansen, H.H.; Chen, L.C.; Petitjean, M.; Friley, W.; Vrang, N.; et al. INT-767 improves histopathological features in a diet-induced ob/ob mouse model of biopsy-confirmed non-alcoholic steatohepatitis. *World J. Gastroenterol.* **2018**, *24*, 195–210. [CrossRef]

81. Carino, A.; Cipriani, S.; Marchiano, S.; Biagioli, M.; Santorelli, C.; Donini, A.; Zampella, A.; Monti, M.C.; Fiorucci, S. BAR502, a dual FXR and GPBAR1 agonist, promotes browning of white adipose tissue and reverses liver steatosis and fibrosis. *Sci. Rep.* **2017**, *7*, 42801. [CrossRef] [PubMed]

82. Duan, H.; Ning, M.; Chen, X.; Zou, Q.; Zhang, L.; Feng, Y.; Zhang, L.; Leng, Y.; Shen, J. Design, synthesis, and antidiabetic activity of 4-phenoxynicotinamide and 4-phenoxypyrimidine-5-carboxamide derivatives as potent and orally efficacious TGR5 agonists. *J. Med. Chem.* **2012**, *55*, 10475–10489. [CrossRef] [PubMed]

83. Ullmer, C.; Alvarez Sanchez, R.; Sprecher, U.; Raab, S.; Mattei, P.; Dehmlow, H.; Sewing, S.; Iglesias, A.; Beauchamp, J.; Conde-Knape, K. Systemic bile acid sensing by G protein-coupled bile acid receptor 1 (GPBAR1) promotes PYY and GLP-1 release. *Br. J. Pharmacol.* **2013**, *169*, 671–684. [CrossRef] [PubMed]

84. Masyuk, T.V.; Masyuk, A.I.; Lorenzo Pisarello, M.; Howard, B.N.; Huang, B.Q.; Lee, P.Y.; Fung, X.; Sergienko, E.; Ardecky, R.J.; Chung, T.D.Y.; et al. TGR5 contributes to hepatic cystogenesis in rodents with polycystic liver diseases through cyclic adenosine monophosphate/Gαs signaling. *Hepatology* **2017**, *66*, 1197–1218. [CrossRef] [PubMed]

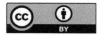

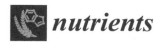

Review

Micronutrient Deficiencies in Laparoscopic Sleeve Gastrectomy

Omar Jamil [1], Raquel Gonzalez-Heredia [2], Pablo Quadri [3], Chandra Hassan [4], Mario Masrur [4], Reed Berger [5], Karen Bernstein [6] and Lisa Sanchez-Johnsen [7,*]

[1] Department of Internal Medicine, University of Chicago, Chicago, IL 60637, USA; Omar.Jamil@uchospitals.edu

[2] Department of Surgery, University of Illinois at Mount Sinai Hospital, Chicago, IL 60609, USA; r.gheredia82@gmail.com

[3] Department of Surgery, Saint Louis University, St. Louis, MO 63104, USA; pablo.quadri@health.slu.edu

[4] Department of Surgery, Division of General, Minimally Invasive & Robotic Surgery, University of Illinois at Chicago, Chicago, IL 60612, USA; chandrar@uic.edu (C.H.); mmasrur@uic.edu (M.M.)

[5] Departments of Surgery and Medicine, University of Illinois at Chicago, Chicago, IL 60612, USA; rberger@uic.edu

[6] Department of Pediatrics, Division of Adolescent Medicine, University of Illinois at Chicago, Chicago, IL 60612, USA; kbernste@uic.edu

[7] Department of Family Medicine, Rush University Medical Center, Chicago, IL 60612, USA

* Correspondence: Lisa_Sanchez-Johnsen@rush.edu; Tel.: +1-312-563-1290

Received: 17 August 2020; Accepted: 18 September 2020; Published: 22 September 2020

Abstract: The purpose of this study was to conduct a literature review to examine micronutrient deficiencies in laparoscopic sleeve gastrectomy. We conducted a literature review using PubMed and Cochrane databases to examine micronutrient deficiencies in SG patients in order to identify trends and find consistency in recommendations. Seventeen articles were identified that met the defined criteria. Iron, vitamin B12 and vitamin D were the primary micronutrients evaluated. Results demonstrate the need for consistent iron and B12 supplementation, in addition to a multivitamin, while vitamin D supplementation may not be necessary. Additional prospective studies to establish a clearer picture of micronutrient deficiencies post-SG are needed.

Keywords: laparoscopic sleeve gastrectomy; micronutrients; deficiency

1. Introduction

Sleeve Gastrectomy (SG) represented the most frequently performed bariatric procedure in the U.S. in 2017, with rates of bariatric surgery as follows: 59.4% SG, 17.8% Roux-en Y Gastric Bypass (RYGB), 2.8% Laparoscopic Adjustable Gastric Banding (LAGB) and 0.7% Biliopancreatic Diversion with Duodenal Switch (BPD-DS) [1]. SG was previously considered a purely restrictive procedure which was used as a first stage surgery before BPD-DS [2]. A study from 2015 demonstrated that SG resulted in the same level of micronutrient deficiency as gastric banding, a purely restrictive procedure [3]. Since becoming a standalone procedure, SG has quickly become a preferred treatment option. In addition to being a restrictive procedure, sleeve gastrectomy is hypothesized to reduce the hormone ghrelin, which increases hunger [4]. SG is now considered a safe procedure that results in substantial and sustained weight loss, reduction of comorbidities and improvements in quality of life [4]. Moreover, the risk associated with SG is considered to be lower than RYGB [5].

In SG, a gastric tube (sleeve) between 50 and 200 cc in volume is created while the remainder of the stomach is excised [6]. SG has the advantage over other operations of preserving the pylorus of the stomach, thereby avoiding dumping syndrome [7,8]. By eluding the intestinal bypass of the DS and

Nutrients 2020, 12, 2896; doi:10.3390/nu12092896
www.mdpi.com/journal/nutrients

RYGB, many complications are avoided, resulting in a lower mortality rate [8–10]. The procedure is safer than other complicated malabsorptive surgeries such as RYGB and BPD-DS and more effective than purely restrictive procedures such as LAGB [11]. Early studies suggested that, unlike RYGB, SG presented no risk for micronutrient deficiency [8,9,12]. More recently, many studies have noted measurable postoperative deficiencies in vitamin B12, vitamin D, iron and folate [9,13–20]. However, disagreements exist about the extent of the postoperative micronutrient deficiencies, the benefits and timing of supplementation and their correlation with preoperative health. Prior to surgery, patients with obesity have a higher incidence of micronutrient deficiencies than the population at large due to the reduced bioavailability of nutrients associated with obesity [21].

Several factors contribute to micronutrient deficiencies in patients who have undergone SG: the reduction in stomach size which results in decreased food intake, a decrease in ghrelin and other gastrointestinal (GI) hormones that reduce appetite, a decreased tolerance of some foods and a reduced metabolism of certain micronutrients, in part due to the loss of intrinsic factor [22]. Moreover, the recommendations for supplementation for SG patients that currently exist are not consistent and often based on data from patients who underwent RYGB and are not unique to SG patients [23]. As such, the purpose of this paper is to review and analyze the findings on micronutrient deficiencies in patients undergoing SG, as a comprehensive review of micronutrient deficiencies for this procedure is lacking.

2. Materials and Methods

A literature review was conducted to examine micronutrient deficiencies in SG patients in order to identify trends and determine consistency in recommendations. PubMed and Cochrane database searches were conducted from January 2009 to March 2020 to locate the relevant literature. The key words used were the following: "Sleeve Gastrectomy", "Micronutrient Deficiency", "Vitamin D deficiency", "Vitamin B12 deficiency", "Iron deficiency" "Bariatric" and "Deficiencies". Studies that explicitly focused on micronutrient deficiencies while examining a cohort of patients were selected. Studies often included data from patients undergoing RYGB, but only the data from SG patients were extracted and included in the results. Review articles were excluded so that primary studies from review articles could be examined. All values were expressed as mean (standard deviation). All studies in the review cited below prescribed a daily multivitamin postoperatively. Specific postoperative supplementation is described in each relevant section below.

A deficiency was defined as a serum plasma level measured below the reference range for normal. Excess was defined as a serum plasma level above the reference range for normal. Normal levels were defined based on the American Society for Metabolic and Bariatric Surgery Integrated Health Nutritional Guidelines for the Surgical Weight Loss Patient 2016 Update: Micronutrients [24]. Normal limits were as follows: iron (μg/dL) 60–170, ferritin (ng/mL) 12–300 (male) and 12–150 (female), Hb (g/dL) 12–17, B12 (pg/mL) 200–1000, folate (ng/mL) 2.5–20 and vitamin D (ng/mL) 25–65. There was some variation in the definition of the "normal" limits between studies; in some cases, these are either described or discussed within the tables. The percent of patients with deficiencies were described based on the parameters within each respective study.

3. Results

As shown in Table 1, 17 studies examined micronutrient deficiencies in SG patients. Sixteen out of the 17 studies were conducted outside of the U.S., with approximately half ($n = 9$) being prospective and half being retrospective ($n = 8$). The mean number of patients included in studies was 84.9 ranging from 30 to 336 patients.

Table 1. Articles reviewed.

Article Number	Year	Authors	Reference #	Prospective vs. Retrospective	Country	# Patients
1	2009	Hakeam et al.	[9]	Prospective	Saudi Arabia	61
2	2010	Gehrer et al.	[11]	Prospective	Switzerland	50
3	2010	Aarts et al.	[14]	Prospective	Netherlands	60
4	2011	Ruiz-Tovar et al.	[25]	Retrospective	Spain	30
5	2011	Kehagias et al.	[26]	Prospective	Greece	30
6	2012	Damms-Machado et al.	[15]	Prospective	Germany	54
7	2012	Moize et al.	[16]	Prospective	Spain	61
8	2012	Saif et al.	[17]	Retrospective	USA	35
9	2012	Capoccia et al.	[27]	Prospective	Italy	138
10	2013	Eltweri et al.	[13]	Retrospective	UK	41
11	2013	Gjessing et al.	[28]	Retrospective	Norway	125
12	2015	Belfiore et al.	[29]	Retrospective	Italy	47
13	2015	Ben-Porat et al.	[30]	Retrospective	Israel	77
14	2015	Lanzarini al.	[31]	Prospective	Spain	96
15	2016	Al-Mulhim	[18]	Prospective	Saudi Arabia	112
16	2016	Gillon et al.	[19]	Retrospective	Norway	336
17	2016	Zarshenas et al.	[20]	Retrospective	Australia	91

3.1. Iron and Ferritin

As shown in Table 2, individuals with obesity are frequently noted to be iron deficient prior to bariatric surgery [9,11] Obesity can result in both an anemia of chronic disease and dysregulation of iron uptake at the level of the enterocytes [32]. Studies have also found that iron deficiency anemia is most likely due to a lack of gastric hydrochloric acid production and the inability to convert iron to a more absorbable form postoperatively [19,23]. The presence of a postoperative iron deficiency could be partially explained by a preoperative deficiency. Eleven of the 17 studies specifically examined iron levels, and, of those, five studies revealed deficiencies in iron levels over time [9,11,14,15,17]. The majority of the studies reviewed did not describe additional iron supplementation, although four studies specifically mentioned supplementation was provided beyond a multivitamin with iron [11,16,17,29]. In the absence of iron supplementation, the operation itself can result in new deficiencies, by either exacerbating those of deficient patients or creating new deficiencies in patients who did not previously have them [33]. These deficiencies were not seen in later studies due to the benefit of iron supplementation in those studies.

Table 2. Iron (%): Percentage (%) of patients with deficiencies at each postoperative visit.

Study	Preop (%)	3 Months (%)	6 Months (%)	12 Months (%)	24 Months (%)	36 Months (%)
Hakeam et al.	0		4.9	4.9		
Gehrer et al.	3	2	12	16	18	
Aarts et al.				43		
Kehagias et al.	20					17.8
Damms-Machado et al.	29	39.3	37.9			
Moize et al.	30.8		4.3	10.3	9.4	
Saif et al.	6.6			3		10.5
Belfiore et al.	14.9	11.4	8.8			
Ben-Porat et al.	40.4			27.7		
Al-Mulhim	11.6		5.4	7.1		
Zarshenas et al.	0		0	1	0	1

As shown in Table 2, the three studies that have the largest numbers of patients with iron deficiencies do not describe a targeted approach to iron supplementation beyond multivitamins [14,15,26]. There was no evidence to suggest that any of these studies had a larger number of women of childbearing age who were menstruating (a group more likely to be iron deficient due to menstruation) versus post-menopausal women, as these data were not reported. The supplementation regimens for these studies are further described in Appendix A [14,15,26]. Out of the three studies that found the fewer patients with iron deficiency post-surgery [16–18], two clearly describe an iron supplementation regimen, either with 160 mg of iron with 100% compliance or with iron supplementation in addition to the multivitamin regimen described in other studies [16,17]. Notably, studies that demonstrate a dedicated iron supplementation regimen and demonstrate lower levels of iron deficiency come in later years after the American Society for Metabolic & Bariatric Surgery in 2013 recommended iron supplementation for all bariatric patients [34].

Serum ferritin is an acute phase reactant that is a marker of decreased iron storage and iron deficiency. Table 3 demonstrates that those studies which reported on serum ferritin found declining serum ferritin levels post-surgery, and a number of studies reported that patients had ferritin deficiencies [13,16,19,20,26,30]. An exception to this is Zarshenas and colleagues' study [20], which was also the only study that did not reveal an iron deficiency. When assessed, ferritin deficiency is much more apparent in SG patients than iron deficiency. This may suggest that, even with normal iron levels, these patients are still iron deficient, as serum ferritin gives a more accurate assessment of the body's total iron storage [35].

Table 3. Ferritin (%): Percentage (%) of patients with deficiencies at each postoperative visit.

Study	Preop (%)	3 Months (%)	6 Months (%)	12 Months (%)	24 Months (%)	36 Months (%)	60 Months (%)
Kehagias et al.	3.3					17.8	
Moize et al.	8.3		0	6.5	20.6		
Eltweri et al.				8			
Ben-Porat et al.	8.3			11.1			
Gillon et al.	3.3			11.6	20		36.2
Zarshenas et al.	8		11	15	18	24	

3.2. B12 and Folate

Fourteen studies examined B12 levels (Table 4) and demonstrated notable deficiencies in post-bariatric surgery patients that increased over time. Folate, an important DNA precursor, was examined in 13 studies (Table 5). Several studies treated patients with in-office intramuscular B12 injections postoperatively and dosages ranged 1000–3000 mcg. These studies [16,26,29] had a lower rate of patients with B12 deficiencies compared to the other studies without a comparable supplementation regimen. In-office intramuscular injection appeared to eliminate issues related to adherence to vitamin regimens. Moreover, those with poor adherence to a supplementation regimen demonstrated higher levels of vitamin B12 deficiencies at 12 months postoperatively [19]. Patients who received aggressive folic acid regimens had fewer vitamin B12 deficiencies over time [30]. Appendix A also lists additional notes from the studies that were reviewed.

Table 4. Vitamin B12: Percentage (%) of patients with deficiencies at each postoperative visit.

Study	Preop (%)	3 Months (%)	6 Months (%)	12 Months (%)	24 Months (%)	36 Months (%)	60 Months (%)
Hakeam et al.	8.1		19.6	26.2			
Gehrer et al.	3	2	12	14	14		
Aarts et al.				9			
Ruiz-Tovar et al.	0	0	0	0	0		
Kehagias et al.	3.3						3.5
Damms-Machado et al.	9.3	4.8	9.8	17.2			
Moize et al.	2.7		3.7	3.2	5.9		12.5
Saif et al.				2.9			
Eltweri et al.				20			
Belfiore et al.	10.7	9	6				
Ben-Porat et al.	11.7			16.7			
Al-Mulhim	1.8		7.1	14.3			
Gillon et al.	6.5			19	12.8		3.8
Zarshenas et al.	1		3	0	0	0	

Table 5. Folate: Percentage (%) of patients with deficiencies at each postoperative visit.

Study	Preop (%)	3 Months (%)	6 Months (%)	12 Months (%)	24 Months (%)	36 Months (%)	60 Months (%)
Hakeam et al.	0		6.5	9.8			
Gehrer et al.	3	10	16		20		
Aarts et al.				15			
Ruiz-Tovar et al.	3.3	0	0	0	0		
Kehagias et al.	0					0	
Damms-Machado et al.	5.5	9.5	9.8	13.8			
Saif et al. [1]				8.8	0	5.5	
Gjessing et al.	23			8			
Belfiore et al. [1]	19.1	29.6	11.8				
Ben-Porat et al. [1]	40.5			21.4			
Al-Mulhim	0.9			5.4	6.25		
Gillon et al.	8.8			12.3	7.6		10.6
Zarshenas et al.	0		0	0	0	0	

[1] Additional iron supplementation for patients, further described in Appendix A.

3.3. Vitamin D and Calcium

As seen in Table 6, almost all of the studies report a decrease in the proportion of patients with vitamin D deficiencies postoperatively as early as six months postoperatively, sustained until 24 months [11,14,25]. Results from studies with a longer follow up period reveal an increased number of patients with vitamin D deficiencies at 24- and 36-month follow-up [16,17]. It is not clear why more two- and three-year follow-ups demonstrated an increase in deficiencies, but patients with SG often begin regaining weight at the 24-month mark [36]. Notably, the three studies with the largest declines in the number of patients with vitamin D deficiencies postoperatively did not show dedicated vitamin D supplementation regimens beyond a multivitamin postoperatively [18,19,29]. For example, in one intervention, Lanzarini and colleagues provided 16,000 IU calcifediol to patients with preoperative vitamin D deficiencies and no additional supplementation for patients without preoperative deficiencies [31]. Their results reveal that, by 24-month postoperative follow-up, the intervention group (16,000 IU calcifediol for deficient patients) and non-intervention group (baseline multivitamin supplementation for all patients) had similar levels of vitamin D deficiency. In other words, as long as patients did not have a vitamin D deficiency preoperatively, additional vitamin D supplementation was not necessary to achieve satisfactory results. Notably, this is in contrast to RYGB patients where the intervention group benefitted significantly [31]. However, in a study where appropriate supplementation was given, fewer patients were deficient at four-year follow-up in both SG and RYGB groups [37]. Appendix A also lists additional notes regarding supplementation from the studies that were reviewed.

Table 6. Vitamin D: Percentage (%) of patients with deficiencies at each postoperative visit.

Study	Preop (%)	3 Months (%)	6 Months (%)	12 Months (%)	24 Months (%)	36 Months (%)	60 Months (%)
Gehrer et al.	23		6	22	28		
Aarts et al.				39			
Ruiz-Tovar et al.	96.7	13.2	3.3	3.3	3.3		
Kehagias et al.							
Damms-Machado et al.	83	76.2	70.7	70.4			
Moize et al.	90		22.7	37	66.7		
Saif et al.	75			34		55	
Capoccia et al.							
Eltweri et al.				81			
Gjessing et al.	47			49			
Belfiore et al.	31.9	20.5	11.8				
Ben-Porat et al.	97.9			93.6			
Lanzarini al.	100			40.9	13.6		
Lanzarini al. [1]	0			28.1	15		
Al-Mulhim	60		21	8.9			
Gillon et al.	20.4			4.9	8.2		6.7
Zarshenas et al.	46		25	14	19	20	

[1] Vitamin D intervention group.

4. Discussion

The purpose of this study was to conduct a comprehensive review of the literature on micronutrient deficiencies in post-SG patients. Past reviews have focused on other bariatric procedures, and, to our knowledge, this is the first review to focus exclusively on SG [38]. In terms of iron supplementation, based on the results from these 17 studies, it appears that post-bariatric surgery supplementation with iron beyond a multivitamin resulted in the fewest deficiencies [9,18,20]. This is due to the prevalence of postoperative proton pump inhibitor (PPI) use and a reduction in hydrochloric acid production after the SG, which prevents conversion of the iron supplement to the absorbable ferrous form [14,23]. Iron supplementation can be optimized when taken with vitamin C or citrus fruit to allow the conversion of iron to its most absorbable form [39]. Postoperatively, patients have decreased inflammatory markers and a hypothesized upregulation of iron uptake in the small bowel [40]. As such, based on the studies that were reviewed [11,16,30], it appears that supplementation with iron will aid in decreasing iron deficiencies post-SG.

Vitamin B12 deficiencies are expected post-SG due to the resection of the fundus and the loss of intrinsic factor produced by parietal cells, which are essential in the absorption of B12 [11,14,15,40]. Vitamin B12 and folic acid both need gastric acid to be properly released from food [14]. Gastric acid is reduced by means of the gastrectomy and also proton pump inhibitors use postoperatively. While evidence to suggest a link between bariatric surgery and adverse neonatal outcomes is weak and inconclusive, women of childbearing age should optimize folate levels, as deficiencies may be related to neural tube defects [9,15,41]. Folate deficiencies are possibly caused by food choices rather than a mechanism related to surgery [14,42]. Folate stores are depleted within months unlike vitamin B12, which can be stored in the liver for 1–2 years [14,15,19]. As such, folate deficiencies are likely to appear earlier than B12 deficiencies due to the difference in the body's storage capacity. Studies with aggressive B12 and folic acid regimens postoperatively, as well as the use of large dose intra-muscular doses for vitamin B12 deficiencies demonstrate the most beneficial outcomes for patients [9,16,26]. Intramuscular dosing of B12 allows direct uptake into the blood stream and avoids the problems of absorption created by post-SG anatomy. Additionally, when deficiencies were corrected preoperatively, there were lower rates of deficiency postoperatively [18].

Patients with obesity may suffer from vitamin D deficiency due to the sequestration of vitamin D in the fat, decreased sun exposure, sedentary lifestyle and the psychological component of covering more skin [18,20,28,43]. Sufficient sunlight is important for adequate levels of vitamin D, and patients with more adipose tissue are less likely to engage in activities such as sunbathing where skin is exposed [44]. Vitamin D is a fat-soluble vitamin that requires lipids absorption for proper uptake into the body and poor lipid absorption can result in vitamin D deficiencies. The vitamin D deficiencies found in postoperative patients may also explain secondary hyperparathyroidism, which was found in 39% of patients [14,15]. Vitamin D is negatively correlated with body fat, as patients with obesity have difficulty metabolizing and storing this nutrient properly [45]. As such, many of these issues seem to resolve with postoperative weight loss. Overall, additional research regarding the benefits of vitamin D supplementation is warranted to determine whether aggressive vitamin D supplementation beyond a multivitamin is indicated in SG patients. Studies that demonstrated very high rates of vitamin D deficiency postoperatively also had high rates preoperatively, and studies in which vitamin D deficiencies were corrected through supplementation preoperatively did not show high rates of deficiency postoperatively [18]. Since vitamin D levels can vary based on skin tone and environmental sunlight exposure [46], it is essential that health care providers are aware of patients' race/ethnic background and geographic location when making vitamin D supplementation recommendations. Overall, the majority of the studies found vitamin D deficiencies did not develop de-novo postoperatively and improved with supplementation [15,25,31,37]. Vitamin D has been observed as the vitamin most often deficient prior to surgery in patients with obesity [47].

As demonstrated in this review, there is a dearth of research examining micronutrient deficiencies post-SG. Moreover, the efficacy of multivitamin supplementation post-SG, although nearly universally utilized, seems to be poor in short-term follow up [48]. This may be partially due to poor patient adherence in the long term [49], but lack of specific and targeted interventions appear to also play a role. Overall, results from this review indicate that there is a need for prospective, longitudinal studies to better understand how various interventions impact postoperative deficiencies. As both vitamin B12 and vitamin D deficiencies decrease when corrected preoperatively, clear guidelines for preoperative supplementation and prospective studies to affect their efficacy should be explored.

For vitamin B12 supplementation, intramuscular injections should be examined. Such in-office injections reduce issues related to adherence to vitamin regimens and avoid the need for intrinsic factor that is lost during bariatric surgery. Related to this is that there is a need to develop guidelines related to decision-making about the feasibility and efficacy of in-office versus at-home supplementation for vitamin B12 and folate. Results from the studies that were reviewed reveal that vitamin D supplementation regimens beyond a multivitamin postoperatively were not needed to reduce postoperative deficiencies [18,19,29]. As such, additional studies examining the need for aggressive vitamin D supplementation postoperatively should be conducted. In a recent study, a specialized vitamin resulted in fewer de-novo micronutrient deficiencies in long-term follow-up than a more basic multivitamin, and recommendations about the type of specialized multivitamin that is best suited for patients who undergo SG should be explored [50]. Overall, there is a need to conduct additional research studies regarding micronutrient supplementation post-SG in order to develop and augment current guidelines about the timing, dosage and type of supplementation recommended.

Limitations of this review include the fact that the majority of these studies were conducted outside of the U.S. and that many of them had a short follow-up period. In addition, there were variations between the studies in the study design, vitamin supplementation and location that, at times, made it difficult to compare outcomes across studies.

5. Conclusions

Current micronutrient supplementation guidelines published by the British Obesity and Metabolic Surgery Society and the American Society for Metabolic & Bariatric Surgery in 2020 and 2019, respectively, will be augmented by this comprehensive review of micronutrient deficiencies in SG patients [51,52]. Between these sets of guidelines, only the latter focuses on recommendations specifically for SG patients and notes weakness in evidence of vitamin recommendations for these patients when compared to other procedures. We hope this review can help support future revisions of guidelines and highlight the need for prospective studies. In particular, we hope that prospective studies can be conducted within the U.S. to appropriately address this patient population. This is critically important because utilizing data from other countries with regards to micronutrient deficiencies may lead to inaccurate recommendations due to the tremendous variation in diet and eating habits between countries, as well as regions of the world with different environments that may also affect micronutrient intake and absorption.

Author Contributions: Conceptualization, O.J. and R.G.-H.; methodology, O.J.; investigation, O.J.; writing—original draft preparation, O.J.; writing—review and editing, R.G.-H., P.Q., C.H., M.M., R.B., K.B., and L.S.-J.; visualization, O.J. and L.S.-J.; and supervision, C.H. and L.S.-J. All authors have read and agreed to the published version of the manuscript.

Funding: This research received no external funding.

Conflicts of Interest: The authors declare no conflict of interest.

Appendix A

Table A1. Additional information describing supplementation regimens for each study cited above.

Article #	Authors	Iron and Ferritin	B12	Folate	Vitamin D
1	Hakeam et al.	All patients who received omeprazole postop developed iron deficiency.	Patients with preop B12 deficiency given 1000 mcg intramuscular injection 1 day postop. 6 months postop, 6 patients received 1000 mcg IM for two months. 9 of 16 patients who developed B12 deficiency used omeprazole for at least 6 months postop.	0.2 mg folic acid, 12 mcg cyanocobalamin. No notes on compliance	
2	Gehrer et al.	100% of iron deficiency treated with IV injection of iron-III-hydroxide	Postop, 80% of B12 deficiency successfully treated with IM.		100% of Vitamin D deficiency treated with 300,000 IE of oily suspension cholecalciferol. Secondary hyperparathyroidism treated with normal Vitamin D supplementation. Multivitamin 3× daily. No notes on compliance.
3	Aarts et al.				
4	Ruiz-Tovar et al.				Multivitamin daily. No notes on compliance.
5	Kehagias et al.		B12 supplement IM 1000–3000 if deficient preop.		

Table A1. *Cont.*

Article #	Authors	Iron and Ferritin	B12	Folate	Vitamin D
6	Damms-Machad et al.		11% B12 injections		Vitamin D supplementation was protective for Vit D deficiency.
7	Moize et al.	160 mg of iron.	1000 mcg B12 IM monthly		880 IU Vitamin D.
8	Saif et al.	Iron + 1200 mg calcium citrate. No significant difference noted in Iron deficiencies based on supplementation compliance.			Vitamin D additionally prescribed based on need. No significant difference noted in Vitamin D deficiency based on supplementation compliance.
9	Capoccia et al.				
10	Eltweri et al.				Vitamin D daily. No notes on compliance.
11	Gjessing et al.				Vitamin D 10 mcg/day. No notes on compliance.
12	Belfiore et al.	Patients with iron deficiency given 329.7 mg ferrous sulfate.	Vitamin B12 deficiency treated orally or by 1000 mcg IM. Folate deficiency treated with 105 mg folate daily for 3 months.	Patients with folate deficiency given 20 mg folate.	
13	Ben-Porat et al.	Iron deficiency treated with 200 mg iron supplementation daily.		Folate deficiency treated with 105 mg folate daily for 3 months.	400 IU Vitamin D and 500 mg Calcium. No notes on compliance.
14	Lanzarini al.				16,000 IU calcifediol for patients with deficiency in intervention group. No notes on compliance. Intervention groups compared.
15	Al-Mulhim				Multivitamin daily. No notes on compliance.
16	Gillon et al.		B12 supplementation based on deficiency. Compliance well documented.	Folic acid supplementation based on deficiency. Compliance well documented.	Vitamin D supplementation based on deficiency. Compliance well documented. 1200 mg calcium daily. No notes on compliance.
17	Zarshenas et al.	Deficiencies corrected as needed.			50,000 IU prescribed for patients with preop Vitamin D deficiency. Other deficiencies corrected as needed.

References

1. Estimate of Bariatric Surgery Numbers, 2011–2017. Available online: https://asmbs.org/resources/estimate-of-bariatric-surgery-numbers (accessed on 15 November 2019).
2. Alvarez-Leite, J. Nutrient deficiencies secondary to bariatric surgery. *Curr. Opin. Clin. Nutr. Metab. Care* **2004**, *7*, 569–575. [CrossRef] [PubMed]
3. De Barros, F.; Setúbal, S.; Martinho, J.M.; Monteiro, A.B.S. Early Endocrine and Metabolic Changes After Bariatric Surgery in Grade III Morbidly Obese Patients: A Randomized Clinical Trial Comparing Sleeve Gastrectomy and Gastric Bypass. *Metab. Syndr. Relat. Disord.* **2015**, *13*, 264–271. [CrossRef] [PubMed]
4. Bohdjalian, A.; Langer, F.B.; Shakeri-Leidenmühler, S.; Gfrerer, L.; Ludvik, B.; Zacherl, J.; Prager, G. Sleeve Gastrectomy as Sole and Definitive Bariatric Procedure: 5-Year Results for Weight Loss and Ghrelin. *Obes. Surg.* **2010**, *20*, 535–540. [CrossRef]
5. ASMBS Clinical Issues Committee. Updated position statement on sleeve gastrectomy as a bariatric procedure. *Surg. Obes. Relat. Dis.* **2012**, *8*, e21–e26. [CrossRef] [PubMed]
6. Vidal, P.; Moros, J.M.R.; Busto, M.; Domínguez-Vega, G.; Goday, A.; Pera, M.; Grande, L. Residual Gastric Volume Estimated with a New Radiological Volumetric Model: Relationship with Weight Loss After Laparoscopic Sleeve Gastrectomy. *Obes. Surg.* **2013**, *24*, 359–363. [CrossRef] [PubMed]
7. Elli, E.F.; Gonzalez-Heredia, R.; Sarvepalli, S.; Masrur, M. Laparoscopic and Robotic Sleeve Gastrectomy: Short- and Long-Term Results. *Obes. Surg.* **2014**, *25*, 967–974. [CrossRef]
8. Baltasar, A.; Serra, C.; Pérez, N.; Bou, R.; Bengochea, M.; Ferri, L. Laparoscopic Sleeve Gastrectomy: A Multi-purpose Bariatric Operation. *Obes. Surg.* **2005**, *15*, 1124–1128. [CrossRef]
9. Hakeam, H.A.; O'Regan, P.J.; Salem, A.M.; Bamehriz, F.Y.; Eldali, A.M. Impact of Laparoscopic Sleeve Gastrectomy on Iron Indices: 1 Year Follow-Up. *Obes. Surg.* **2009**, *19*, 1491–1496. [CrossRef]
10. Melissas, J.; Koukouraki, S.; Askoxylakis, J.; Stathaki, M.; Daskalakis, M.; Perisinakis, K.; Karkavitsas, N. Sleeve Gastrectomy—A Restrictive Procedure? *Obes. Surg.* **2007**, *17*, 57–62. [CrossRef]
11. Gehrer, S.; Kern, B.; Peters, T.; Christoffel-Courtin, C.; Peterli, R. Fewer Nutrient Deficiencies After Laparoscopic Sleeve Gastrectomy (LSG) than After Laparoscopic Roux-Y-Gastric Bypass (LRYGB)—A Prospective Study. *Obes. Surg.* **2010**, *20*, 447–453. [CrossRef]
12. Fuks, D.; Verhaeghe, P.; Brehant, O.; Sabbagh, C.; Dumont, F.; Riboulot, M.; Delcenserie, R.; Regimbeau, J.-M. Results of laparoscopic sleeve gastrectomy: A prospective study in 135 patients with morbid obesity. *Surgery* **2009**, *145*, 106–113. [CrossRef] [PubMed]
13. Eltweri, A.M.; Bowrey, D.J.; Sutton, C.D.; Graham, L.; Williams, R.N. An audit to determine if vitamin b12 supplementation is necessary after sleeve gastrectomy. *SpringerPlus* **2013**, *2*, 218. [CrossRef]
14. Aarts, E.O.; Janssen, I.M.C.; Berends, F.J. The Gastric Sleeve: Losing Weight as Fast as Micronutrients? *Obes. Surg.* **2010**, *21*, 207–211. [CrossRef]
15. Damms-Machado, A.; Friedrich, A.; Kramer, K.M.; Stingel, K.; Meile, T.; Küper, M.A.; Königsrainer, A.; Bischoff, S.C. Pre- and Postoperative Nutritional Deficiencies in Obese Patients Undergoing Laparoscopic Sleeve Gastrectomy. *Obes. Surg.* **2012**, *22*, 881–889. [CrossRef]
16. Moize, V.; Andreu, A.; Flores, L.; Torres, F.; Ibarzabal, A.; Delgado, S.; Lacy, A.; Rodríguez, L.; Vidal, J. Long-Term Dietary Intake and Nutritional Deficiencies following Sleeve Gastrectomy or Roux-En-Y Gastric Bypass in a Mediterranean Population. *J. Acad. Nutr. Diet.* **2013**, *113*, 400–410. [CrossRef] [PubMed]
17. Saif, T.; Strain, G.W.; Dakin, G.; Gagner, M.; Costa, R.; Pomp, A. Evaluation of nutrient status after laparoscopic sleeve gastrectomy 1, 3, and 5 years after surgery. *Surg. Obes. Relat. Dis.* **2012**, *8*, 542–547. [CrossRef] [PubMed]
18. Al-Mulhim, A.S. Laparoscopic Sleeve Gastrectomy and Nutrient Deficiencies. *Surg. Laparosc. Endosc. Percutan. Tech.* **2016**, *26*, 208–211. [CrossRef]
19. Gillon, S.; Jeanes, Y.M.; Andersen, J.R.; Våge, V. Micronutrient Status in Morbidly Obese Patients Prior to Laparoscopic Sleeve Gastrectomy and Micronutrient Changes 5 years Post-surgery. *Obes. Surg.* **2016**, *27*, 606–612. [CrossRef]
20. Zarshenas, N.; Nacher, M.; Loi, K.W.; Jorgensen, J.O. Investigating Nutritional Deficiencies in a Group of Patients 3 Years Post Laparoscopic Sleeve Gastrectomy. *Obes. Surg.* **2016**, *26*, 2936–2943. [CrossRef]
21. Kaidar-Person, O.; Person, B.; Szomstein, S.; Rosenthal, R. Nutritional Deficiencies in Morbidly Obese Patients: A New Form of Malnutrition? *Obes. Surg.* **2008**, *18*, 1028–1034. [CrossRef]

22. Mans, E.; Serra-Prat, M.; Palomera, E.; Suñol, X.; Clavé, P. Sleeve gastrectomy effects on hunger, satiation, and gastrointestinal hormone and motility responses after a liquid meal test. *Am. J. Clin. Nutr.* **2015**, *102*, 540–547. [CrossRef] [PubMed]

23. Snyder-Marlow, G.; Taylor, D.; Lenhard, M.J. Nutrition Care for Patients Undergoing Laparoscopic Sleeve Gastrectomy for Weight Loss. *J. Am. Diet. Assoc.* **2010**, *110*, 600–607. [CrossRef] [PubMed]

24. Parrott, J.; Frank, L.; Rabena, R.; Craggs-Dino, L.; Isom, K.A.; Greiman, L. American Society for Metabolic and Bariatric Surgery Integrated Health Nutritional Guidelines for the Surgical Weight Loss Patient 2016 Update: Micronutrients. *Surg. Obes. Relat. Dis.* **2017**, *13*, 727–741. [CrossRef] [PubMed]

25. Rúiz-Tovar, J.; Oller, I.; Tomás, A.; Llavero, C.; Arroyo, A.; Calero, A.; Martínez-Blasco, A.; Calpena, R. Mid-term Effects of Sleeve Gastrectomy on Calcium Metabolism Parameters, Vitamin D and Parathormone (PTH) in Morbid Obese Women. *Obes. Surg.* **2011**, *22*, 797–801. [CrossRef]

26. Kehagias, I.; Karamanakos, S.N.; Argentou, M.; Kalfarentzos, F. Randomized Clinical Trial of Laparoscopic Roux-en-Y Gastric Bypass Versus Laparoscopic Sleeve Gastrectomy for the Management of Patients with BMI <50 kg/m^2. *Obes. Surg.* **2011**, *21*, 1650–1656. [CrossRef]

27. Capoccia, D.; Coccia, F.; Paradiso, F.; Abbatini, F.; Casella, G.; Basso, N.; Leonetti, F. Laparoscopic Gastric Sleeve and Micronutrients Supplementation: Our Experience. *J. Obes.* **2012**, *2012*, 1–5. [CrossRef]

28. Gjessing, H.R.; Nielsen, H.J.; Mellgren, G.; Gudbrandsen, O.A. Energy intake, nutritional status and weight reduction in patients one year after laparoscopic sleeve gastrectomy. *SpringerPlus* **2013**, *2*, 352. [CrossRef] [PubMed]

29. Belfiore, A.; Cataldi, M.; Minichini, L.; Aiello, M.L.; Trio, R.; Rossetti, G.; Guida, B. Short-Term Changes in Body Composition and Response to Micronutrient Supplementation After Laparoscopic Sleeve Gastrectomy. *Obes. Surg.* **2015**, *25*, 2344–2351. [CrossRef]

30. Ben-Porat, T.; Elazary, R.; Yuval, J.B.; Wieder, A.; Khalaileh, A.; Weiss, R.; Abed, K. Nutritional deficiencies after sleeve gastrectomy: Can they be predicted preoperatively? *Surg. Obes. Relat. Dis.* **2015**, *11*, 1029–1036. [CrossRef]

31. Lanzarini, E.; Nogués, X.; Goday, A.; Benaiges, D.; De Ramón, M.; Villatoro, M.; Pera, M.; Grande, L.; Ramón, J.M. High-Dose Vitamin D Supplementation is Necessary After Bariatric Surgery: A Prospective 2-Year Follow-up Study. *Obes. Surg.* **2015**, *25*, 1633–1638. [CrossRef]

32. Tussing-Humphreys, L.; Pustacioglu, C.; Nemeth, E.; Braunschweig, C. Rethinking Iron Regulation and Assessment in Iron Deficiency, Anemia of Chronic Disease, and Obesity: Introducing Hepcidin. *J. Acad. Nutr. Diet.* **2012**, *112*, 391–400. [CrossRef] [PubMed]

33. Mason, M.E.; Jalagani, H.; Vinik, A.I. Metabolic Complications of Bariatric Surgery: Diagnosis and Management Issues. *Gastroenterol. Clin. N. Am.* **2005**, *34*, 25–33. [CrossRef] [PubMed]

34. Mechanick, J.I.; Youdim, A.; Jones, D.B.; Garvey, W.T.; Hurley, D.L.; McMahon, M.M.; Heinberg, L.J.; Kushner, R.; Adams, T.D.; Shikora, S.; et al. Clinical Practice Guidelines for the Perioperative Nutritional, Metabolic, and Nonsurgical Support of the Bariatric Surgery Patient—2013 Update: Cosponsored by American Association of Clinical Endocrinologists, The Obesity Society, and American Society for Metabolic & Bariatric Surgery. *Endocr. Pract.* **2013**, *19*, 337–372. [CrossRef] [PubMed]

35. Arosio, P.; Elia, L.; Poli, M. Ferritin, cellular iron storage and regulation. *IUBMB Life* **2017**, *69*, 414–422. [CrossRef]

36. Berry, M.; Urrutia, L.; Lamoza, P.; Molina, A.; Luna, E.; Parra, F.; Domínguez, M.J.; Alonso, R. Sleeve Gastrectomy Outcomes in Patients with BMI Between 30 and 35-3 Years of Follow-Up. *Obes. Surg.* **2018**, *28*, 649–655. [CrossRef]

37. Fox, A.; Slater, C.; Ahmed, B.; Ammori, B.J.; Senapati, S.; Akhtar, K.; Ellison, J.; Summers, L.K.M.; Robinson, A.; New, J.P.; et al. Vitamin D Status After Gastric Bypass or Sleeve Gastrectomy over 4 Years of Follow-up. *Obes. Surg.* **2019**, *30*, 1473–1481. [CrossRef] [PubMed]

38. Shankar, P.; Boylan, M.; Sriram, K. Micronutrient deficiencies after bariatric surgery. *Nutrients* **2010**, *26*, 1031–1037. [CrossRef] [PubMed]

39. 39. McColl, K.E. Effect of Proton Pump Inhibitors on Vitamins and Iron. *Am. J. Gastroenterol.* **2009**, *104* Suppl 2, S5–S9. [CrossRef]

40. Tussing-Humphreys, L.; Nemeth, E.; Fantuzzi, G.; Freels, S.; Holterman, A.-X.L.; Galvani, C.; Ayloo, S.; Vitello, J.; Braunschweig, C. Decreased Serum Hepcidin and Improved Functional Iron Status 6 Months After Restrictive Bariatric Surgery. *Obesity (Silver Spring)* **2010**, *18*, 2010–2016. [CrossRef]

41. Jans, G.; Matthys, C.; Bogaerts, A.; Lannoo, M.; Verhaeghe, J.; Van Der Schueren, B.; Devlieger, R. Maternal micronutrient deficiencies and related adverse neonatal outcomes after bariatric surgery: A systematic review. *Adv. Nutr.* **2015**, *6*, 420–429. [CrossRef]

42. Bloomberg, R.D.; Fleishman, A.; Nalle, J.E.; Herron, D.M.; Kini, S. Nutritional Deficiencies following Bariatric Surgery: What Have We Learned? *Obes. Surg.* **2005**, *15*, 145–154. [CrossRef]

43. VanLint, S. Vitamin D and Obesity. *Nutrients* **2013**, *5*, 949–956. [CrossRef]

44. Kull, M.; Kallikorm, R.; Lember, M. Body mass index determines sunbathing habits: Implications on vitamin D levels. *Intern. Med. J.* **2009**, *39*, 256–258. [CrossRef] [PubMed]

45. Shapses, S.A.; Pop, L.C.; Schneider, S.H. Vitamin D in Obesity and Weight Loss. *Nutr. Influ. Bone Health* **2016**, 185–196. [CrossRef]

46. Clemens, T.; Adams, J.; Henderson, S.; Holick, M. increased skin pigment reduces the capacity of skin to synthesise vitamin D3. *Lancet* **1982**, *319*, 74–76. [CrossRef]

47. Sherf-Dagan, S.; Zelber-Sagi, S.; Webb, M.; Keidar, A.; Raziel, A.; Sakran, N.; Goitein, D.; Shibolet, O. Nutritional Status Prior to Laparoscopic Sleeve Gastrectomy Surgery. *Obes. Surg.* **2016**, *26*, 2119–2126. [CrossRef] [PubMed]

48. Rúiz-Tovar, J.; OBELCHE Group; Llavero, C.; Zubiaga, L.; Boix, E. Maintenance of Multivitamin Supplements After Sleeve Gastrectomy. *Obes. Surg.* **2016**, *26*, 2324–2330. [CrossRef] [PubMed]

49. Ben-Porat, T.; Elazary, R.; Goldenshluger, A.; Dagan, S.S.; Mintz, Y.; Weiss, R. Nutritional deficiencies four years after laparoscopic sleeve gastrectomy—Are supplements required for a lifetime? *Surg. Obes. Relat. Dis.* **2017**, *13*, 1138–1144. [CrossRef]

50. Smelt, H.; Van Loon, S.; Pouwels, S.; Boer, A.-K.; Smulders, J.F.; Aarts, E.O. Do Specialized Bariatric Multivitamins Lower Deficiencies After Sleeve Gastrectomy? *Obes. Surg.* **2019**, *30*, 427–438. [CrossRef]

51. O'Kane, M.; Parretti, H.M.; Pinkney, J.; Welbourn, R.; Hughes, C.A.; Mok, J.; Walker, N.; Thomas, D.; Devin, J.; Coulman, K.D.; et al. British Obesity and Metabolic Surgery Society Guidelines on perioperative and postoperative biochemical monitoring and micronutrient replacement for patients undergoing bariatric surgery—2020 update. *Obes. Rev.* **2020**. [CrossRef]

52. Mechanick, J.I.; Apovian, C.; Brethauer, S.; Garvey, W.T.; Joffe, A.M.; Kim, J.; Kushner, R.F.; Lindquist, R.; Pessah-Pollack, R.; Seger, J.; et al. Clinical practice guidelines for the perioperative nutrition, metabolic, and nonsurgical support of patients undergoing bariatric procedures-2019 update: Cosponsored by american association of clinical endocrinologists/american college of endocrinology, the obesity society, american society for metabolic & bariatric surgery, obesity medicine association, and american society of anesthesiologists-executive summary. *Endocr. Pract.* **2019**, *25*, 1346–1359. [CrossRef] [PubMed]

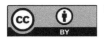

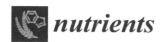

Article

The Cardiotonic Steroid Marinobufagenin Is a Predictor of Increased Left Ventricular Mass in Obesity: The African-PREDICT Study

Michél Strauss-Kruger [1], Ruan Kruger [1,2], Wayne Smith [1,2], Lebo F. Gafane-Matemane [1,2], Gontse Mokwatsi [1,2], Wen Wei [3], Olga V. Fedorova [3] and Aletta E. Schutte [1,2,4,*]

[1] Hypertension in Africa Research Team (HART), North-West University, Potchefstroom 2520, South Africa; Straussmichel1@gmail.com (M.S.-K.); Ruan.kruger@g.nwu.ac.za (R.K.); wayne.smith@nwu.ac.za (W.S.); lebo.gafane@nwu.ac.za (L.F.G.-M.); 22368590@nwu.ac.za (G.M.)
[2] MRC Research Unit for Hypertension and Cardiovascular Disease, North-West University, Potchefstroom 2520, South Africa
[3] National Institute on Aging, NIH, Baltimore, MD 212242, USA; wen.wei@nih.gov (W.W.); fedorovo@grc.nia.nih.gov (O.V.F.)
[4] School of Population Health, University of New South Wales, The George Institute for Global Health, Sydney 2052, Australia
* Correspondence: a.schutte@unsw.edu.au; Tel.: +61-(0)450-315-918

Received: 29 September 2020; Accepted: 15 October 2020; Published: 18 October 2020

Abstract: The endogenous Na^+/K^+-ATPase inhibitor, marinobufagenin (MBG), strongly associates with salt intake and a greater left ventricular mass index (LVMi) in humans and was shown to promote cardiac fibrosis and hypertrophy in animals. The adverse effects of MBG on cardiac remodeling may be exacerbated with obesity, due to an increased sensitivity of Na^+/K^+-ATPase to MBG. This study determined whether MBG is related to the change in LVMi over time in adults with a body mass index (BMI) ≥ 30 kg/m^2 (obese) and <30 kg/m^2 (non-obese). The study followed 275 healthy participants (aged 20–30 years) from the African-Prospective study on the Early Detection and Identification of Cardiovascular disease and Hypertension (African-PREDICT) study over 4.5 years. At baseline, we measured 24 h urine MBG excretion. MBG levels were positively associated with salt intake. LVMi was determined by two-dimensional echocardiography at baseline and after >4.5 years. With multivariate adjusted analyses in obese adults ($N = 56$), we found a positive association of follow-up LVMi (Adjusted (Adj.) $R^2 = 0.35$; Std. $\beta = 0.311$; $p = 0.007$) and percentage change in LVMi (Adj. $R^2 = 0.40$; Std. $\beta = 0.336$; $p = 0.003$) with baseline MBG excretion. No association of LVMi (Adj. $R^2 = 0.37$; $p = 0.85$) or percentage change in LVMi (Adj. $R^2 = 0.19$; $p = 0.68$) with MBG excretion was evident in normal weight adults ($N = 123$). These findings suggest that obese adults may be more sensitive to the adverse cardiac effects of MBG and provide new insight into the potential role of dietary salt, by way of MBG, in the pathogenesis of cardiac remodeling in obese individuals.

Keywords: body mass index; cardiotonic steroids; left ventricular mass; marinobufagenin; obesity; dietary salt intake; young adults

1. Introduction

Obesity affects 671 million adults globally [1] and contributes significantly to the pathogenesis of cardiovascular disease (CVD) [2]. Obesity is associated with hypertension [3], left ventricular hypertrophy [4], and an overall greater risk of incident CVD [5]. Adipose tissue exerts an array of effects on the cardiovascular system through adipokines and low-grade inflammation [2] but also hemodynamically through volume loading [6]. Increased sodium retention observed in obese individuals [7] promotes extracellular volume expansion and concurrently causes a rightward shift in the renal function curve, ultimately elevating mean arterial pressure [6]. The latter mechanism is proposed to contribute to the development of hypertension [6] and cardiac remodeling [8] associated with obesity.

Obese individuals are also more likely to have poor dietary habits, such as higher caloric intake accompanied by excessive salt intake, which is the leading dietary risk factors associated with cardiovascular and all-cause mortality [9]. While the adverse effects of excess salt intake on the cardiovascular system is well known [10], more attention has been brought to the role of cardiotonic steroids, which are associated with increased salt intake in the development of CVD. This includes the biomarker marinobufagenin (MBG) [11], which is synthesized and secreted by the adrenal cortex in response to sodium loading [12]. Indeed, our group has previously demonstrated a strong positive correlation between MBG and estimated salt intake in young healthy adults [13].

MBG is an endogenous sodium-potassium adenosine triphosphatase (Na^+/K^+-ATPase) inhibitor that primarily promotes natriuresis in response to volume loading, acting as a compensatory mechanism to lower blood pressure [14]. However, during sustained periods of high salt intake, MBG levels continue to increase so that it ultimately evokes a pathophysiological response in the cardiovascular system. The latter occurs via the MBG inhibition of cardiovascular Na^+/K^+-ATPase [14]. Elevated MBG promotes cardiac fibrosis and hypertrophy in animals by way of the Na^+/K^+-ATPase-Src and/or Na^+/K^+-ATPase-SMAD-transforming growth factor beta (TGFβ) signaling cascades [15–17], which may involve oxidative stress initiated via Na^+/K^+-ATPase [18]. In humans with excessive MBG excretion, an independent cross-sectional association of MBG with increased left ventricular mass index (LVMi) [19] was demonstrated, but it is unknown whether obesity would further exacerbate this relationship.

In animal studies, obese rats were previously shown to have attenuated cardiac Na^+/K^+-ATPase expression when compared to lean controls [20]. In non-obese Na/K-ATPase α1 heterozygote knock-out mice ($α1^{+/-}$) (displaying suppressed Na^+/K^+-ATPase expression), the effects of MBG were potentiated as shown by increased myocyte apoptosis and left ventricular dilation compared to wild-type mice in response to MBG infusion [21]. This may suggest that an attenuated expression of cardiomyocyte Na^+/K^+-ATPase with obesity [20] could increase the sensitivity of cardiac tissue to the pathological effects of MBG [22]. Therefore, it is likely that elevated MBG in obese individuals with a high habitual dietary salt intake may contribute to early cardiac remodeling. The female sex hormone estradiol has been shown to restore Na^+/K^+-ATPase activity in obese male Wistar rats, and it may play a cardioprotective role with obesity [20].

The aim of this study was to determine whether MBG is related to changes in LVMi over time in obese compared to non-obese individuals, and whether MBG predicts an increase in LVMi over time. The 4.5-year baseline and follow-up data of 275 young adults, aged 20–30 years at baseline, with no previous history of diagnosed CVD was analyzed. We hypothesize that obese participants will demonstrate an adverse association of MBG with follow-up LVMi as well as with the change in LVMi over 4.5 years. These associations were not expected to be seen in participants with a healthy body composition.

2. Results

Table 1 presents the basic characteristics of 275 participants at baseline (mean age 25.4 ± 3.16) and follow-up (mean age 30.0 ± 3.21), with an even distribution between sex and black and white ethnic groups (black: 50.2% and men 45.5%). The median time from baseline to follow-up was 1639 days (4.49 years). There was a marked increase in the body weight, body mass index (BMI), and waist/height ratio (WHtR) (all $p < 0.001$) from baseline to follow-up. In addition, there was an increase in the number of participants who were classified as obese using BMI ($N_{baseline} = 60$ to $N_{follow-up} = 82$) or a composite obesity score of BMI, waist circumference (WC), and WHtR criteria ($N_{baseline} = 55$ to $N_{follow-up} = 74$) ($p < 0.001$). Participants' systolic blood pressure (SBP) ($p < 0.001$) and left ventricular mass index (LVMi, $p < 0.001$) increased significantly from baseline to follow-up, while the end diastolic volume index (EDVi) and stroke volume index (SVi) decreased ($p < 0.001$). There were 26 obese participants at baseline that had masked hypertension. When comparing the baseline characteristics of participants followed up in this sub-study ($N = 275$) with those not yet followed up ($N = 927$), the ethnic and sex distributions, blood pressure (BP), 24 h MBG excretion, and estimated salt intake were similar (Table S1). However, the sub-group included in this study had higher BMI (0.99 kg/m^2 mean difference) but lower LVMi (2.93 kg/m^2 mean difference).

Table 1. Characteristics of 275 participants followed over 4.5 years.

	Baseline	Follow-Up	Difference	p
Men, N (%)	125 (45.5)	125 (45.5)		
Black, N (%)	138 (50.2)	138 (50.2)		
Age (years)	25.4 ± 3.16	30.0 ± 3.21	4.60 (4.49; 4.70)	<0.001
Anthropometric measurements				
Height (m)	1.68 ± 0.09	1.68 ± 0.09	0.00 (−0.001; 0.001)	0.68
Weight (kg)	73.3 ± 18.3	77.9 ± 20.2	4.64 (3.51; 5.77)	<0.001
Waist circumference (cm)	81.5 ± 14.2	83.2 ± 14.5	1.66 (0.91; 2.41)	<0.001
BMI (kg/m^2)	25.8 ± 5.79	27.3 ± 6.57	1.51 (1.21; 1.82)	<0.001
WHtR	0.48 ± 0.08	0.49 ± 0.09	0.01 (0.01; 0.01)	<0.001
Frequency of obesity based on:				
BMI, N (%)	60 (21.8)	82 (29.8)	22 (36.7)	<0.001
WC, N (%)	95 (34.5)	109 (39.6)	14 (14.7)	0.014
WHtR, N (%)	94 (34.2)	103 (37.5)	9 (0.9)	0.11
Composite obesity criteria, N (%) *	55 (20.0)	74 (26.9)	19 (34.5)	<0.001
Blood pressure				
Clinic SBP (mmHg)	120 ± 12.4	116 ± 12.7	−3.76 (−4.97; −2.55)	<0.001
Clinic DBP (mmHg)	78.9 ± 8.07	79.3 ± 9.45	0.30 (−0.63; 1.24)	0.52
Central SBP (mmHg)	109 ± 9.48	110 ± 10.4	0.87 (−0.12; 1.86)	0.085
Hypertension, N (%) #	39 (14.2)	42 (15.3)	3 (7)	0.76
Hypertension medication, N (%)	0 (0.0)	3 (1.0)		0.25
Echocardiography				
LVMi (g/m^2)	70.7 ± 15.7	77.8 ± 18.7	7.02 (5.03; 9.00)	<0.001
IVSd (cm/m)	0.47 ± 0.10	0.53 ± 0.09	0.06 (0.05; 0.08)	<0.001
LVIDd (cm/m)	2.84 ± 0.25	2.78 ± 0.24	−0.07 (−0.09; −0.04)	<0.001
PWTd (cm/m)	0.50 ± 0.09	0.54 ± 0.01	0.05 (0.03; 0.06)	<0.001
EDVi (mL/m)	64.0 ± 13.7	60.3 ± 13.0	−3.70 (−4.94; −2.46)	<0.001
SVi (ml/m$^{2.04}$)	25.1 ± 5.52	23.1 ± 4.96	−2.03 (−2.61; −1.45)	<0.001
Urinary profile				
eGFR (ml/min/1.73 m^2)	111 ± 16.4	108 ± 16.6	−3.15 (−4.90; −1.39)	<0.001
24 h MBG excretion (nmol/day)	3.38 (1.12; 9.13)	-		
Estimated salt intake (g/day) [1]	7.73 (2.80; 19.4)	7.13 (1.61; 24.4)	−0.22 (10.3)	0.47
Biochemical profile				
Glucose (mmol/L)	4.63 ± 0.76	4.08 ± 0.65	−0.55 (−0.66; −0.44)	<0.001
HDL-C (mmol/L)	1.34 ± 0.39	1.25 ± 0.34	−0.09 (−0.12; −0.05)	<0.001
LDL-C (mmol/L)	2.80 ± 0.92	2.66 ± 0.91	−0.14 (−0.22; −0.06)	0.001
C-reactive protein (mg/L)	1.04 (0.11; 9.38)	1.07 (0.15; 10.3)	0.01 (1.46)	0.56
γ-glutamyl transferase (U/L)	21.9 (8.74; 61.1)	21.4 (7.21; 63.5)	−0.48 (9.12)	0.46

Data presented as mean ± SD and geometric mean (5th and 95th percentiles). Difference from baseline to follow-up represented as mean (95% Confidence intervals (CI)) for normally distributed data and median (Inter quartile range (IQR)) for non-parametric data. * Obesity: BMI > 30 kg/m^2 [23] and WC > 94 cm for white men; >81.2 cm for black men; >80 cm for white women and >81 cm for black women [24] and WHtR >0.5 [23] # Hypertension: Clinic SBP ≥ 140 mmHg and/or DBP ≥ 90 mmHg [1] Estimated salt intake based on 24 h sodium excretion. BMI, body mass index; DBP, diastolic blood pressure; EDVi: end diastolic volume index; eGFR: estimated glomerular filtration rate; HDL-C: high density lipoprotein cholesterol; IVSd: interventricular septum at end-diastole; LDL-C: low density lipoprotein cholesterol; LVIDd: LV internal diameter at end-diastole; LVMi, left ventricular mass index; MBG, marinobufagenin; PWTd: posterior wall thickness at end-diastole SBP, systolic blood pressure; SVi, stroke volume index; WC, waist circumference; WHtR, waist/height ratio.

Baseline and follow-up characteristics of participants were compared, with participants stratified as non-obese (BMI < 30 kg/m^2) and obese (BMI ≥ 30 kg/m^2) (Table S2A,B). In both non-obese (p < 0.001) and obese (p = 0.029) participants, clinic SBP decreased significantly from baseline to follow-up, although central SBP (cSBP) increased only in obese adults (mean diff. 2.58 mmHg, 95%CI 0.17; 4.99) (p = 0.037). Non-obese and obese adults had an increase in LVMi and a decrease in EDVi and SVi (p < 0.001). Still, obese adults had a significantly greater increase in LVMi when compared to non-obese adults (mean diff. 5.81 g/m^2, 95% CI 3.67; 7.95 vs. mean diff. 11.3 g/m^2, 95%CI 6.43; 16.2; p = 0.024).

When comparing the LVMi of participants within different BMI categories at baseline, only underweight adults had a significantly smaller LVMi when compared to obese participants (p = 0.033). However, obese adults had significantly greater EDVi (71.8 mL/m) when compared to underweight (57.4 mL/m), normal weight (60.8 mL/m), and overweight participants (64.7 mL/m) at baseline (p < 0.001). At follow-up, we found that participants who were obese at baseline had a significantly greater percentage change in LVMi over time as well as follow-up LVMi when compared to participants with a normal BMI (p = 0.001), when adjusting for sex, ethnicity, age, and baseline LVMi (Figure 1A,B). However, follow-up EDVi in obese adults (61.4 mL/m) was similar to that of normal weight (59.6 mL/m) (p = 1.00) and overweight participants (61.7 mL/m) (p = 1.00), when adjusting for sex, ethnicity, age, and baseline EDVi. There were no significant differences in the estimated salt intake of obese adults (8.17 g/day) when compared to overweight (7.93 g/day) (p = 0.77), normal weight (7.64 g/day) (p = 0.45), or underweight participants (6.04 g/day) (p = 0.070). Despite no significant difference in the baseline estimated salt intake of participants between different BMI categories (p = 0.32) (Figure 1C), underweight adults had a lower MBG excretion when compared to overweight (p = 0.037) or obese adults (p = 0.024) (Figure 1D). MBG correlated positively with estimated salt intake (underweight: r = 0.494, p = 0.061; normal weight: r = 0.553, p < 0.001; overweight: r = 0.514, p < 0.001; obese: r = 0.470, p < 0.001).

2.1. Pearson, Partial, and Multiple Regression Analyses

Pearson correlations were performed between follow-up LVMi as well as the percentage change in LVMi with MBG excretion within non-obese and obese participants at baseline (Figure 2A,B). In non-obese adults, a positive correlation was found between follow-up LVMi and MBG excretion at baseline (r = 0.166; p = 0.015) and a negative correlation between percentage change in LVMi and MBG excretion (r = −0.139; p = 0.042), but these relationships lost significance with multivariate adjusted analysis (p > 0.05). In addition, when the non-obese group was additionally stratified as normal weight and overweight (Table S3), there was no association between LVMi or the percentage change in LVMi and MBG excretion (all p > 0.05). However, in obese adults, follow-up LVMi (r = 0.392; p = 0.002), as well as the percentage change in LVMi (r = 0.352; p = 0.006) correlated positively with baseline MBG excretion. The association of LVMi (Adj. R^2 = 0.35; Std. β = 0.311: p = 0.007) and percentage change in LVMi (Adj. R^2 = 0.40; Std. β = 0.336: p = 0.003) with MBG excretion in obese participants remained significant after multivariate adjusted analyses (Table 2). The present results remained robust when repeating analyses in a sub-group (N = 51) with stringently defined obesity based on three composite criteria (BMI ≥ 30 kg/m^2 and WC > 94 cm for white men; >81.2 cm for black men; >80 cm for white women; and >81 cm for black women and WHtR >0.5; LVMi: Adj. R^2 = 0.36; Std. β = 0.310: p = 0.009; percentage change in LVMi: Adj. R^2 = 0.37; Std. β = 0.350: p = 0.003; see Table S4).

Table 2. Multiple regression analyses with follow-up LVMi and percentage change in LVMi as dependent variables and baseline MBG excretion as the main independent variable.

Dependent Variable	MBG Excretion (nmol/Day)					
	Non-Obese 18.6–29.9 kg/m^2 N = 211			Obese BMI > 30 kg/m^2 N = 56		
	Adj R^2	Std. β	p	Adj R^2	Std. β	p
LVMi (g/m^2)	0.39	NS		0.35	0.311	0.007
% Δ LVMi	0.21	NS		0.4	0.336	0.003
	Sensitivity analysis additionally adjusted for estimated salt intake					
LVMi (g/m^2)	0.39	NS		0.35	0.311	0.008
% Δ LVMi	0.21	NS		0.4	0.337	0.003
	Sensitivity analysis additionally adjusted for estradiol					
LVMi (g/m^2)	0.39	NS		0.47	0.305	0.007
% Δ LVMi	0.21	NS		0.5	0.344	0.002

Adjusted for sex, ethnicity, age, clinic SBP, eGFR, glucose, HDL, c-reactive protein (CRP), gamma-glutamyl transferase (GGT), and baseline LVMi. NS refers to $p > 0.05$.

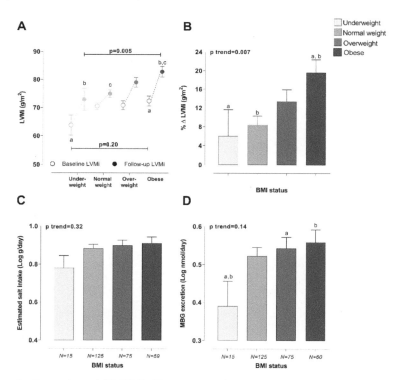

Figure 1. Comparison of (**A**) LVMi, (**B**) percentage change in LVMi, (**C**) baseline estimated salt intake, and (**D**) baseline MBG excretion levels of participants with different BMI categories at baseline. Adjusted for sex, ethnicity, and age (follow-up LVMi and percentage change in LVMi additionally adjusted for baseline LVMi). [a,b,c] Indicate significant difference between BMI categories, where data points or bars with the same superscript letter differ significantly ($p < 0.05$).

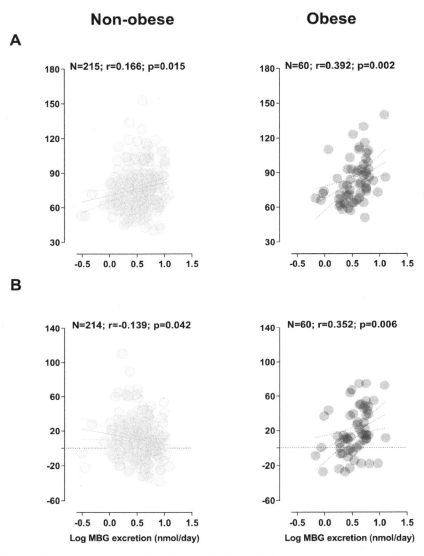

Figure 2. Pearson correlations of (**A**) follow-up LVMi and (**B**) the percentage change in LVMi with baseline MBG excretion in non-obese and obese participants.

2.2. Sensitivity Analyses

2.2.1. Estimated Salt Intake

We additionally adjusted for estimated salt intake to determine whether salt intake influences the relationship between LVMi and MBG excretion. The relationship with both LVMi and percentage change in LVMi remained robust in obese participants (Adj. R^2 = 0.35; Std. β = 0.311: p = 0.008; Adj. R^2 = 0.40; Std. β = 0.337: p = 0.003; see Table 2). When performing backward stepwise regression analysis with salt as the main independent variable (Table S5), there was no association between estimated salt intake and LVMi.

2.2.2. Estradiol

Estradiol was previously reported to increase Na^+/K^+-ATPase activity in obese animals [20], and it is suggested to play a cardiac protective role in obesity [22]. As expected, women from this study had higher levels of estradiol when compared to men (54.3 pg/mL vs. 37.0 pg/mL; $p < 0.001$; see Table S6). Pearson correlations were performed to demonstrate the correlation of estradiol and the percentage change in LVMi in men and women (Table S7). When performing multiple regression analyses with the additional adjustment for estradiol (Table 2), LVMi was negatively associated with estradiol in obese adults (Adj. $R^2 = 0.47$; Std. β $= -0.220$: $p = 0.045$). Nonetheless, the positive relationship of LVMi and MBG excretion remained robust (Adj. $R^2 = 0.47$; Std. β $= 0.305$: $p = 0.007$). In the non-obese group, the association of LVMi and percentage change in LVMi with MBG was not significant ($p > 0.05$). When analyses were repeated in normal weight and overweight adults, respectively, a significant negative association between MBG and percentage change in LVMi was evident in overweight adults (Adj. $R^2 = 0.32$; Std. β $= -0.221$: $p = 0.035$; Table S3).

3. Discussion

This is the first study to our knowledge that investigated the relationship of the cardiotonic steroid, MBG, with longitudinal cardiovascular data in a young human population with no previous history of CVD. The main finding from the present study was that baseline MBG excretion levels were associated with increased LVMi over 4.5 years in obese but not in normal weight individuals. These results support the hypothesis that the adverse effects of MBG in cardiac remodeling may be potentiated in obese adults, despite having similar MBG excretion levels when compared to normal weight adults.

A positive association of follow-up LVMi with MBG excretion in obese but not underweight, normal weight, or overweight adults supports the notion that an increased sensitivity of cardiotonic steroids may play a role in the pathogenesis of CVD in individuals with obesity [22]. A recent review by Obradovic et al. highlighted the potential adverse role of reduced Na^+/K^+-ATPase in the development of CVD with obesity [22], which is associated with the downregulation of Na^+/K^+-ATPase in animals [20] and humans [25]. The attenuated levels of Na^+/K^+-ATPase likely contribute to the deleterious effect of MBG on the heart. Indeed, non-obese α1-Na^+/K^+-ATPase knockout mice (α1$^{+/-}$) with lower Na^+/K^+-ATPase levels (-38% lower Na^+/K^+-ATPase) were shown to have an increased myocardial Na^+/K^+-ATPase sensitivity to MBG infusion when compared to wild-type mice [21]. It is via the inhibition of cardiac Na^+/K^+-ATPase and the concurrent downward Src signaling cascade that MBG promotes cardiac remodeling [15,16]. Similarly, in the Dahl-S model of salt-sensitive hypertension, MBG-activated cardiovascular TGF-β pro-fibrotic signaling via Na^+/K^+-ATPase resulted in an increase in LVMi while also promoting the development of fibrosis and cardiac remodeling [17].

In contrast with our findings in obese adults, a negative association was observed between percentage change in LVMi and MBG excretion in overweight adults when including estradiol into the model. Estradiol can activate Na/K-ATPase in the cardiovascular system [20,26] and counterbalance an inhibitory effect of MBG on the cardiovascular Na/K-ATPase enzymatic activity. In addition, estradiol may exhibit its cardiac protective effect by means of attenuated vasoconstriction and tissue fibrosis by binding to other estrogen receptors (ER), including, ER-α, ER-β, and GPR−30 [27]. It is also known that estradiol, i.e., estrogen, can activate atrial natriuretic peptide (ANP) receptors and increase ANP levels [28,29]. It was demonstrated that ANP can counterbalance the pro-fibrotic and pro-hypertensive effects of MBG in the cardiovascular system and exhibit a synergistic effect with MBG on renal natriuretic function [30]. It might only be with the shift from an overweight to an obese phenotype that this natriuretic function of MBG is overridden by the pathophysiological effects thereof. The beneficial effect of estradiol in association with MBG in subjects with normal weight and moderately overweight subjects is an important observation and will merit further investigation. It is likely that in the obese subjects, the positive impact of estradiol is similar to the observation made in age-associated salt sensitivity in the animal model [30]. In addition, the increased sensitivity of Na^+/K^+-ATPase to MBG can underlie the pathophysiological function of MBG, as it was previously demonstrated in Dahl-S rats, which exhibited an increased sensitivity of the cardiovascular Na^+/K^+-ATPase to MBG [31,32]. Acute salt loading of the normotensive Sprague–Dawley rats and salt-sensitive Dahl-S rats was accompanied by a similar stimulation of MBG in both strains and by the inhibition of an aortic Na pump in Dahl-S rats only [32], which was likely due to the higher sensitivity of cardiovascular Na^+/K^+-ATPase to cardiotonic steroids in Dahl-S rats. Dahl-S rats on a high salt intake also developed left ventricular hypertrophy, which was accompanied by an increased sensitivity of cardiac Na^+/K^+-ATPase to MBG [31]. An increased sensitivity of cardiovascular Na^+/K^+-ATPase to the endogenous inhibitors may contribute to the exaggerated effect of MBG on the Na^+/K^+-ATPase-initiated down-stream pro-fibrotic signaling [15,17].

Taken together, the activation of the Na^+/K^+-ATPase-Src signaling cascade may be promoted with obesity and contribute to early cardiac remodeling. The inhibition of cardiac Na^+/K^+-ATPase as a result of MBG is associated with oxidative stress [33], cardiac myocyte apoptosis [21], collagen synthesis [15,17], and cardiac myocyte hypertrophy [17], which are all factors of overall structural cardiac changes. Meanwhile, the endocytosis of Na^+/K^+-ATPase with obesity is proposed to play an important role in promoting a pro-inflammatory environment [34]; further studies are needed to investigate the role of MBG on macrophage adhesion and cytokines activation in the cardiac remodeling of obese individuals.

While young obese adults had a similar LVMi to normal weight or overweight adults at baseline, the greater LVMi at follow-up in obese participants of this study, when compared to underweight and normal weight adults, is in accordance with previous reports [4]. In addition, the greater EDVi observed in obese adults at baseline suggests a volume-loading phenotype in this population associated with obesity [35]. Since this study made use of LVM indexed to body surface area (BSA), the present findings are independent of cardiac structural changes as a result of increased body weight with obesity [36]. Considering the young age of this study population, the findings of the present study highlight the importance of creating a greater awareness regarding the substantial impact of modifiable risk factors, such as obesity and diet, on cardiovascular health. Indeed, the estimated salt intake of this study population (7.73 g/day) exceeded the daily recommendation of the World Health Organization (5 g/day) [37]. In the present study, behavioral lifestyle choices such as high salt intake from a young age in the obese condition is already associated with changes in cardiac structure.

In a recent review by He et al., the authors highlighted the diverse mechanisms whereby a high dietary salt intake may contribute to a greater risk of CVD [10]. Eminently, of the 10 million CVD-related deaths attributed to dietary risk factors in 2017, a high dietary salt intake was the leading risk factor [9]. However, excessive dietary salt intake may also indirectly contribute to early CVD development as a result of elevated MBG [11], which is strongly related to estimated salt intake [13]. MBG was firstly described as a natriuretic hormone; it increased with sodium-induced volume loading [38]. Subsequent investigations into the pathophysiological role of MBG have yielded strong evidence of an adverse effect of excessive MBG on the cardiovascular system. In animal and experimental studies, MBG was shown to promote cardiac myocyte apoptosis [21], cardiovascular fibrosis, and cardiac hypertrophy [15–17,39]. While in humans, MBG was found to be associated with autonomic activity [40], microvascular dysfunction [41], arterial stiffness [13,42], and increased LVMi [19]. Given that obesity is known to be associated with left ventricular hypertrophy [4], these findings may help reiterate the importance of lowering salt intake in obese individuals who are already more susceptible to early CVD development due to a harmful cardiometabolic profile.

In animals [20,25] and humans [25], hyperinsulinemia, which is associated with obesity, has been implicated in the downregulation of Na^+/K^+-ATPase. Additionally, insulin resistance in Dahl-S animals consuming a high salt intake [43] may increase the sensitivity of Na^+/K^+-ATPase to CTS. Obesity is one of the facets of metabolic syndrome, and it is often accompanied by insulin resistance [2]. This creates an "ideal" condition for MBG, which can activate the vicious pro-fibrotic circle without being elevated to a pathologic level. Therefore, obese individuals may be predisposed to early cardiac remodeling due to insulin resistance, which sensitizes cardiovascular Na^+/K^+-ATPase to CTS. The estimation of the insulin sensitivity and its association with cardiovascular parameters and cardiovascular markers in young obese and non-obese individuals merits future investigation. Furthermore, a high-fat diet has also been shown to stimulate MBG synthesis in hyperlipidemic states [34]. Further studies are also necessary to determine the role of a habitual high dietary intake of sugar and trans fats in the adverse effects of MBG on the heart and vasculature of obese adults.

4. Strengths and Limitations

A major strength of the present study was the inclusion of longitudinal data of young black and white adults, free of CVD at baseline with complete baseline data on 24-h MBG and sodium excretion. However, the study included volunteers without random selection. The main limitation of this study was the small group of obese adults included in the analyses. Given that the present study only included $N = 275$ from the larger African-PREDICT study population ($N = 1202$), it is possible that selection bias may have contributed to the findings. The follow-up studies, which will be performed in a larger sample to substantiate these results, will merit future investigation. The small sample size was a limitation factor in performing sex-specific analyses, which is recommended for future studies.

5. Materials and Methods

5.1. Study Design and Methodology

This study included the data of the first 275 (50% black; 44% men) participants from the African-Prospective study on the Early Detection and Identification of Cardiovascular disease and Hypertension (African-PREDICT) with baseline MBG excretion and follow-up LVMi data.

The African-PREDICT study is a longitudinal study that aims to track and monitor the cardiovascular health profile of young black and white adults. Details on the study design, recruitment, and baseline measurements were previously published [44]. Participant recruitment for the study started in 2012 and was conducted in communities living in proximity to the Potchefstroom area in the northwest province of South Africa. Apparently healthy volunteers were screened at baseline for eligibility to be included into the study based on the following criteria: black or white ethnicity; aged 20–30 years; clinic blood pressure (BP) < 140/90; HIV uninfected; had no previous diagnosis of chronic illness (self-reported) or using any chronic medications; not pregnant or lactating.

Ultimately, $N = 1202$ (606 black and 596 white) eligible participants were enrolled in the baseline phase of the African-PREDICT study (February 2013 to November 2017). Follow-up data collection started in February 2018 and remains ongoing. This analysis made use of the follow-up data collected between 2018 and 2019. At the point of statistical analyses for this study, 430 participants had been successfully contacted and participated in follow-up measurements. Of the 430 participants who had taken part in follow-up measurements, we excluded 88 participants with missing MBG data and a further 67 with missing follow-up echocardiography data. Therefore, this study analyzed the data of 275 participants. Baseline and follow-up data collection were performed under controlled conditions, using good clinical practice at the Hypertension Research and Training Clinic at North-West University.

Written informed consent was obtained from all participants at baseline and follow-up, and all procedures adhered to Institutional Guidelines and the Declaration of Helsinki of 1975, which were revised in 2013. The African-PREDICT study was approved by the Health Research Ethics Committee of the North-West University, South Africa (NWU-00001-12-A1). The study is registered at ClinicalTrials.gov (identifier: NCT03292094). Assignable to the informed consent given by participants, the data for this study, which is centrally managed by the data manager using REDCap, can be obtained by means of the necessary arrangements with Prof Aletta E Schutte or Prof Carina Mels from the Hypertension in Africa Research Team (HART) [44]. Potential collaborators are invited to contact the principal investigator of African-PREDICT for further information.

5.2. Questionnaire and Anthropometric Data

Participants completed a General Health and Demographic Questionnaire at baseline and follow-up to obtain detailed information (self-reported) on demographics (age, sex, ethnicity, and socio-economic status) and medical history (medication use).

Anthropometric measurements including weight (kg; SECA 813 Electronic Scales), height (m; SECA 213 Portable Stadiometer; SECA, Hamburg, Germany), and WC (cm) (Lufkin Steel Anthropometric Tape; W606PM; Lufkin, Apex, NC, USA) were measured in triplicate, according to the guidelines of the International Society for the Advancement of Kinanthropometry. We subsequently calculated the BMI (weight (kg)/height (m^2)), BSA ($\sqrt{\text{height (cm)} \times \text{weight (kg)}/3600}$), and WHtR of participants. Participants were classified as underweight (BMI < 18.5 kg/m^2), normal weight (BMI 18.5–24.9 kg/m^2), overweight (25–29.9 kg/m^2), or obese (BMI ≥ 30 kg/m^2) according to baseline BMI [23]. As a sensitivity measure, we additionally identified participants who would be classified as obese based on baseline BMI > 30 kg/m^2, WC (WC > 94 cm for white men; >81.2 cm for black men; >80 cm for white women, and >81 cm for black women) [23,24] and WHtR cut points (>0.5) [45] (i.e., participants who met all three criteria for obesity—BMI, WC, and WHtR—were classified as being obese).

5.3. Cardiovascular Measurements

The Dinamap Procare 100 Vital Signs Monitor (GE Medical Systems, Milwaukee, WI, USA) was used to measure SBP and diastolic (DBP) BP with an appropriately sized brachial blood pressure cuff. Participants were seated with their arm rested at heart level. Measurements were performed in duplicate on the left and right arm (with a five-minute resting period between measures). The mean SBP and DBP from the right arm was calculated [46]. Hypertension was defined as SBP ≥ 140 mmHg and or DBP ≥ 90 mmHg [47]. We made use of the SphygmoCor XCEL device (AtCor Medical Pty. Ltd., Sydney, Australia) to measure cSBP in duplicate by means of pulse wave analysis, while participants lay rested in a supine position with an appropriately sized brachial BP cuff fitted to the right upper arm. cSBP is determined using a general transfer function.

Two-dimensional echocardiography was done using the General Electric Healthcare Vivid E9 device (GE Vingmed Ultrasound A/S, Horten, Norway), a 2.5 to 3.5 MHz transducer, and a single electrocardiogram (ECG) lead. A medical clinical technician performed echocardiographic imaging according to standardized procedures outlined by the American Society of Echocardiography [36]. Left ventricular mass was calculated from dimensions using the Devereaux "cube" formula (LVM = 0.8×1.04 ((IVSd + LVIDd + PWTd)^3 − LVIDd^3) + 0.6 g), where IVS is the interventricular septum at end diastole, LVID is the LV internal diameter at end diastole, and PWT is the inferolateral wall thickness at end diastole. Left ventricular mass and LV volumes were determined using the biplane method. Since LVM is strongly influenced by body size, LVMi was indexed to BSA to minimize obesity-related changes in LVM. Reporting LVM indexed to BSA is recommended by the American Society of Echocardiography [36]. Stroke volume was indexed for height to the power 2.04 (SVi) and end diastolic volume (EDV) (calculated using the Teichholz formula) was indexed to height.

5.4. Biochemical Sampling and Biochemical Analyses

Participants were instructed to refrain from eating or drinking (except water) from at least 22:00 the night before measurements took place. A trained research nurse performed early morning biological sampling (before 09:30) using a sterile winged infusion set and syringes. Samples were immediately moved to an onsite laboratory, centrifuged, and aliquoted into cryovials. A detailed description on sample preparation was published elsewhere [19]. All biological samples were stored in onsite bio freezers at −80 °C.

Then, 24 h urine sampling was performed in accordance with protocols of the Pan American Health Organization/World Health Organization (PAHO/WHO), with participants being given instructions on how to ensure accurate collection [48]. All participants had a urinary volume >300 mL. Baseline MBG was analyzed from 24 h urine samples using a solid-phase Dissociation-Enhanced Lanthanide Fluorescent Immunoassay, which was based on a 4G4 anti-MBG mouse monoclonal antibody described in detail by Fedorova et al. [49]. Twenty-four-hour urinary sodium excretion was measured (Cobas Integra 400plus, Roche, Basel Switzerland) to calculate estimated salt intake. Estimated glomerular filtration rate was calculated using the Chronic Kidney Disease Epidemiology Collaboration Equation (CKD-EPI) no race equation [50].

From serum samples, total cholesterol, high-density lipoprotein cholesterol (HDL-C), low-density lipoprotein cholesterol (LDL-C), creatinine, C-reactive protein (CRP), and γ-glutamyl transferase (GGT) were measured (Cobas Integra 400plus, Roche, Basel Switzerland). Glucose was determined from sodium fluoride plasma (Cobas Integra 400plus, Roche, Switzerland).

5.5. Statistical Analyses

Statistical analyses were performed using SPSS version 26 (IBM; Armonk, New York, NY, USA) and created figures using GraphPad Prism version 5.0 (GraphPad Software Inc., La Jolla, CA, USA). Data following a normal distribution were presented as the arithmetic mean ± standard deviation, and variables with a non-Gaussian distribution were logarithmically transformed and presented as geometric mean (5th and 95th percentiles). Differences in the basic characteristics of participants from baseline to follow-up were determined using a paired t-test or Wilcoxon Signed-Ranks Test for parametric or non-parametric continuous variables, and McNemar tests for categorical variables. Baseline estimated salt intake and MBG excretion of participants were compared within different BMI statuses (underweight, normal weight, overweight, and obese) using ANCOVA, adjusting for sex, ethnicity, and age. Scatterplots demonstrating Pearson correlations between LVMi as well as the percentage change in LVMi overtime and MBG excretion are shown for different BMI statuses. The relationship of LVMi and the percentage change LVMi with MBG excretion was further explored using backward stepwise multiple regression analyses, considering the limited number of participants who were classified as obese and having follow-up LVMi data ($N = 56$). Backward stepwise regression models were adjusted for sex, ethnicity, age, clinic SBP, eGFR, glucose, HDL-C, CRP, GGT, and baseline LVMi. Sensitivity analyses were performed for estimated salt intake and estradiol to determine whether the latter had an influence on the relationship between MBG and LVMi. Backward stepwise regression analyses were repeated, whereby obesity was stringently defined as not only having a BMI >30 kg/m^2 but also according to WC (WC > 94 cm for white men; >81.2 cm for black men; >80 cm for white women; and >81 cm for black women) [23,24] and WHtR cut points (>0.5) [45] (i.e., participants who met all three criteria for obesity—BMI, WC, and WHtR—were classified as being obese $N = 51$).

6. Conclusions

The findings from the present study indicate that obese adults may be more vulnerable to the adverse cardiac effects of excessive salt intake by means of increased MBG sensitivity. This was demonstrated by an independent positive association between follow-up LVMi and MBG excretion in obese adults only. An increased sensitivity to MBG may exacerbate the vulnerability of obese adults to the harmful effects of excessive salt intake on cardiac remodeling, besides volume loading. These findings encourage cardioprotective strategies such as the targeting of modifiable risk factors (a healthy diet, low salt intake, weight reduction).

Supplementary Materials: The following are available online at http://www.mdpi.com/2072-6643/12/10/3185/s1. Table S1: Characteristics of 275 participants followed over 4.5 years compared with 927 participants from the African-PREDICT cohort. Table S2A: Characteristics of 215 participants with a BMI < 30 kg/m^2 (non-obese) followed over 4.5 years. Table S2B: Characteristics of 60 participants with a BMI ≥ 30 kg/m^2 (obese) followed over 4.5 years. Table S3: Multiple regression analyses with follow-up LVMi and percentage change in LVMi as dependent variables and baseline MBG excretion as the main independent variable. Table S4: Backward stepwise regression model with obesity defined according to BMI, WC, and WHtR criteria. Table S5. Backward stepwise multiple regression analyses with follow-up LVMi and percentage change in LVMi as dependent variables, and baseline estimated NaCl intake as the main independent variable. Table S6: Estradiol levels of men and women in the African-PREDICT study. Table S7: Pearson correlations between the percentage change in LVMi and estradiol in men and women.

Author Contributions: Conceptualization, M.S.-K.; methodology, M.S.-K., R.K., L.F.G.-M., G.M., W.S., W.W., O.V.F. and A.E.S.; validation, R.K., L.F.G.-M., G.M., W.S., W.W., O.V.F. and A.E.S.; formal analysis, M.S.-K.; investigation, M.S.-K.; resources, M.S.-K., R.K., L.F.G.-M., G.M., W.S., O.V.F. and A.E.S.; data curation, M.S.-K.; writing—original draft preparation, M.S.-K.; writing—review and editing, R.K., L.F.G.-M., G.M., W.S., O.V.F. and A.E.S.; visualization, M.S.-K.; supervision, R.K., L.F.G.-M., G.M., W.S., O.V.F. and A.E.S.; project administration, A.E.S.; funding acquisition, A.E.S. All authors have read and agreed to the published version of the manuscript.

Funding: The research funded in this manuscript is part of an ongoing research project financially supported by the South African Medical Research Council (SAMRC) with funds from National Treasury under its Economic Competitiveness and Support Package; the South African Research Chairs Initiative (SARChI) of the Department of Science and Technology and National Research Foundation (NRF) of South Africa (GUN 86895); SAMRC with funds received from the South African National Department of Health, GlaxoSmithKline R&D (Africa Non-Communicable Disease Open Lab grant), the UK Medical Research Council and with funds from the UK Government's Newton Fund; as well as corporate social investment grants from Pfizer (South Africa), Boehringer-Ingelheim (South Africa), Novartis (South Africa), the Medi Clinic Hospital Group (South Africa) and in kind contributions of Roche Diagnostics (South Africa). Any opinion, findings, and conclusions or recommendations expressed in this material are those of the authors, and therefore, the NRF does not accept any liability in this regard. This research was supported in part by National Institute on Aging, NIH Intramural Research Program (USA).

Acknowledgments: The authors are grateful toward all individuals participating voluntarily in the study. The dedication of the support and research staff as well as students at the Hypertension Research and Training Clinic at the North-West University are also duly acknowledged.

Conflicts of Interest: All authors declared no conflict of interest.

Abbreviations

Na$^+$/K$^+$-ATPase	sodium-potassium adenosine triphosphatase
PAHO/WHO	Pan American Health Organization/World Health Organization
CKD-EPI	Chronic Kidney Disease Epidemiology Collaboration
LVMi	Left ventricular mass index
WHtR	Waist/height ratio
EDVi	End diastolic volume index
TGF-β	Transforming growth factor beta
ANP	Atrial natriuretic peptide
BMI	Body mass index
BSA	Body surface area
CRP	C-reactive protein
CVD	Cardiovascular disease
ECG	Echocardiogram
GGT	Gamma glutamyl transferase
HDL	High density lipoprotein
LDL	Low density lipoprotein
MBG	Marinobufagenin
SBP	Systolic blood pressure
SVi	Stroke volume index
ER	Estradiol receptor
WC	Waist circumference

References

1. Non-communicable Disease Risk Factor Collaboration. Worldwide trends in body-mass index, underweight, overweight, and obesity from 1975 to 2016: A pooled analysis of 2416 population-based measurement studies in 128·9 million children, adolescents, and adults. *Lancet* **2017**, *390*, 2627–2642. [CrossRef]
2. Koliaki, C.; Liatis, S.; Kokkinos, A. Obesity and cardiovascular disease: Revisiting an old relationship. *Metab. Clin. Exp.* **2019**, *92*, 98–107. [CrossRef] [PubMed]
3. Kotsis, V.; Stabouli, S.; Bouldin, M.; Low, A.; Toumanidis, S.; Zakopoulos, N. Impact of obesity on 24-hour ambulatory blood pressure and hypertension. *Hypertension* **2005**, *45*, 602–607. [CrossRef] [PubMed]
4. Ahmad, M.I.; Li, Y.; Soliman, E.Z. Association of obesity phenotypes with electrocardiographic left ventricular hypertrophy in the general population. *J. Electrocardiol.* **2018**, *51*, 1125–1130. [CrossRef]
5. Khan, S.S.; Ning, H.; Wilkins, J.T.; Allen, N.; Carnethon, M.; Berry, J.D.; Sweis, R.N.; Lloyd-Jones, D.M. Association of body mass index with lifetime risk of cardiovascular disease and compression of morbidity. *JAMA Cardiol* **2018**, *3*, 280–287. [CrossRef] [PubMed]
6. Hall, M.; Carmo, J.; Silva, A.; Juncos, L.; Wang, Z.; Hall, J. Obesity, hypertension, and chronic kidney disease. *Int. J. Nephrol. Renovasc. Dis.* **2014**, *7*, 75–88. [CrossRef]
7. Strazzullo, P.; Barbato, A.; Galletti, F.; Barba, G.; Siani, A.; Iacone, R.; D'Elia, L.; Russo, O.; Versiero, M.; Farinaro, E.; et al. Abnormalities of renal sodium handling in the metabolic syndrome. Results of the Olivetti Heart study. *J. Hypertens.* **2006**, *24*, 1633–1639. [CrossRef]
8. Aurigemma, G.P.; Simone, G.D.; Fitzgibbons, T.P. Cardiac remodeling in obesity. *Circ. Cardiovasc. Imaging* **2013**, *6*, 142–152. [CrossRef]
9. Afshin, A.; Sur, P.J.; Fay, K.A.; Cornaby, L.; Ferrara, G.; Salama, J.S.; Mullany, E.C.; Abate, K.H.; Abbafati, C.; Abebe, Z.; et al. Health effects of dietary risks in 195 countries, 1990–2017: A systematic analysis for the Global Burden of Disease study 2017. *Lancet* **2019**, *393*, 1958–1972. [CrossRef]
10. He, F.J.; Tan, M.; Ma, Y.; MacGregor, G.A. Salt reduction to prevent hypertension and cardiovascular disease: JACC state-of-the-art review. *J. Am. Coll. Cardiol.* **2020**, *75*, 632–647. [CrossRef]
11. Strauss, M.; Smith, W.; Fedorova, O.V.; Schutte, A.E. The Na(+)K(+)-ATPase inhibitor marinobufagenin and early cardiovascular risk in humans: A review of recent evidence. *Curr. Hypertens. Rep.* **2019**, *21*, 38. [CrossRef] [PubMed]
12. Fedorova, O.V.; Zernetkina, V.I.; Shilova, V.Y.; Grigorova, Y.N.; Juhasz, O.; Wei, W.; Marshall, C.A.; Lakatta, E.G.; Bagrov, A.Y. Synthesis of an endogenous steroidal Na pump inhibitor marinobufagenin, implicated in human cardiovascular diseases, is initiated by CYP27A1 via bile acid pathway. *Circ. Cardiovasc. Genet.* **2015**, *8*, 736–745. [CrossRef]
13. Strauss, M.; Smith, W.; Wei, W.; Bagrov, A.Y.; Fedorova, O.V.; Schutte, A.E. Large artery stiffness is associated with marinobufagenin in young adults: The African-PREDICT study. *J. Hypertens.* **2018**, *36*, 2333. [CrossRef] [PubMed]
14. Fedorova, O.V.; Talan, M.I.; Agalakova, N.I.; Lakatta, E.G.; Bagrov, A.Y. Endogenous ligand of α1 sodium pump, marinobufagenin, is a novel mediator of sodium chloride–dependent hypertension. *Circulation* **2002**, *105*, 1122–1127. [CrossRef]
15. Elkareh, J.; Kennedy, D.J.; Yashaswi, B.; Vetteth, S.; Shidyak, A.; Kim, E.G.R.; Smaili, S.; Periyasamy, S.M.; Hariri, I.M.; Fedorova, L.; et al. Marinobufagenin stimulates fibroblast collagen production and causes fibrosis in experimental uremic cardiomyopathy. *Hypertension* **2007**, *49*, 215–224. [CrossRef] [PubMed]
16. Elkareh, J.; Periyasamy, S.M.; Shidyak, A.; Vetteth, S.; Schroeder, J.; Raju, V.; Hariri, I.M.; El-Okdi, N.; Gupta, S.; Fedorova, L. Marinobufagenin induces increases in procollagen expression in a process involving protein kinase c and fli-1: Implications for uremic cardiomyopathy. *Am. J. Physiol. Renal Physiol.* **2009**, *296*, F1219–F1226. [CrossRef]
17. Zhang, Y.; Wei, W.; Shilova, V.; Petrashevskaya, N.N.; Zernetkina, V.I.; Grigorova, Y.N.; Marshall, C.A.; Fenner, R.C.; Lehrmann, E.; Wood, W.H.; et al. Monoclonal antibody to marinobufagenin downregulates TGFβ; profibrotic signaling in left ventricle and kidney and reduces tissue remodeling in salt-sensitive hypertension. *JAHA* **2019**, *8*, e012138. [CrossRef] [PubMed]
18. Pratt, R.D.; Brickman, C.; Nawab, A.; Cottrill, C.; Snoad, B.; Lakhani, H.V.; Jelcick, A.; Henderson, B.; Bhardwaj, N.N.; Sanabria, J.R.; et al. The adipocyte Na/K-ATPase oxidant amplification loop is the central regulator of western diet-induced obesity and associated comorbidities. *Sci. Rep.* **2019**, *9*, 7927. [CrossRef]

19. Strauss, M.; Smith, W.; Kruger, R.; Wei, W.; Fedorova, O.V.; Schutte, A.E. Marinobufagenin and left ventricular mass in young adults: The african-PREDICT study. *Eur. J. Prev. Cardiol.* **2018**, *25*, 1587–1595. [CrossRef]

20. Obradovic, M.; Zafirovic, S.; Jovanovic, A.; Milovanovic, E.S.; Mousa, S.A.; Labudovic-Borovic, M.; Isenovic, E.R. Effects of 17β-estradiol on cardiac Na+/K+-ATPase in high fat diet fed rats. *Mol. Cell. Endocrinol.* **2015**, *416*, 46–56. [CrossRef]

21. Liu, C.; Bai, Y.; Chen, Y.; Wang, Y.; Sottejeau, Y.; Liu, L.; Li, X.; Lingrel, J.B.; Malhotra, D.; Cooper, C.J. Reduction of na/k-atpase potentiates marinobufagenin-induced cardiac dysfunction and myocyte apoptosis. *J. Biol. Chem.* **2012**, *287*, 16390–16398. [CrossRef] [PubMed]

22. Obradovic, M.; Bjelogrlic, P.; Rizzo, M.; Katsiki, N.; Haidara, M.; Stewart, A.J.; Jovanovic, A.; Isenovic, E.R. Effects of obesity and estradiol on Na+/K+-ATPase and their relevance to cardiovascular diseases. *J. Endocrinol.* **2013**, *218*, R13–R23. [CrossRef] [PubMed]

23. World Health Organization. *Obesity: Preventing and Managing the Global Epidemic*; World Health Organization: Geneva, Switzerland, 2000; p. 9. ISBN 9241208945.

24. Ekoru, K.; Murphy, G.; Young, E.; Delisle, H.; Jerome, C.; Assah, F.; Longo-Mbenza, B.; Nzambi, J.; On'Kin, J.; Buntix, F.; et al. Deriving an optimal threshold of waist circumference for detecting cardiometabolic risk in Sub-Saharan Africa. *Int. J. Obes.* **2017**, *42*. [CrossRef]

25. Iannello, S.; Milazzo, P.; Belfiore, F. Animal and human tissue Na, K-ATPase in obesity and diabetes: A new proposed enzyme regulation. *Am. J. Med. Sci.* **2007**, *333*, 1–9. [CrossRef]

26. Dzurba, A.; Ziegelhöffer, A.; Vrbjar, N.; Styk, J.; Slezák, J. Estradiol modulates the sodium pump in the heart sarcolemma. *Mol. Cell. Biochem.* **1997**, *176*, 113–118. [CrossRef] [PubMed]

27. Aryan, L.; Younessi, D.; Zargari, M.; Banerjee, S.; Agopian, J.; Rahman, S.; Borna, R.; Ruffenach, G.; Umar, S.; Eghbali, M. The role of estrogen receptors in cardiovascular disease. *Int. J. Mol. Sci.* **2020**, *21*, 4314. [CrossRef] [PubMed]

28. Belo, N.; Sairam, M.; Reis, A. Impairment of the natriuretic peptide system in follitropin receptor knockout mice and reversal by estradiol: Implications for obesity-associated hypertension in menopause. *Endocrinology* **2008**, *149*, 1399–1406. [CrossRef]

29. Jankowski, M.; Rachelska, G.; Donghao, W.; McCann, S.M.; Gutkowska, J. Estrogen receptors activate atrial natriuretic peptide in the rat heart. *Proc. Natl. Acad. Sci. USA* **2001**, *98*, 11765–11770. [CrossRef]

30. Fedorova, O.V.; Kashkin, V.A.; Zakharova, I.O.; Lakatta, E.G.; Bagrov, A.Y. Age-associated increase in salt sensitivity is accompanied by a shift in the atrial natriuretic peptide modulation of the effect of marinobufagenin on renal and vascular sodium pump. *J. Hypertens.* **2012**, *30*, 1817. [CrossRef]

31. Fedorova, O.V.; Talan, M.I.; Agalakova, N.I.; Lakatta, E.G.; Bagrov, A.Y. Coordinated shifts in Na/K-ATPase isoforms and their endogenous ligands during cardiac hypertrophy and failure in NaCl-sensitive hypertension. *J. Hypertens.* **2004**, *22*, 389–397. [CrossRef]

32. Bagrov, A.Y.; Agalakova, N.I.; Kashkin, V.A.; Fedorova, O.V. Endogenous cardiotonic steroids and differential patterns of sodium pump inhibition in NaCl-loaded salt-sensitive and normotensive rats. *Am. J. Hypertens.* **2009**, *22*, 559–563. [CrossRef] [PubMed]

33. Kennedy, D.J.; Shrestha, K.; Sheehey, B.; Li, X.S.; Guggilam, A.; Wu, Y.; Finucan, M.; Gabi, A.; Medert, C.M.; Westfall, K.; et al. Elevated plasma marinobufagenin, an endogenous cardiotonic steroid, is associated with right ventricular dysfunction and nitrative stress in heart failure. *Circ. Heart. Fail.* **2015**, *8*, 1068–1076. [CrossRef] [PubMed]

34. Kennedy, D.J.; Chen, Y.; Huang, W.; Viterna, J.; Liu, J.; Westfall, K.; Tian, J.; Bartlett, D.J.; Tang, W.H.; Xie, Z.; et al. CD36 and Na/K-ATPase-α1 form a proinflammatory signaling loop in kidney. *Hypertension* **2013**, *61*, 216–224. [CrossRef]

35. Vasan, R.S. Cardiac function and obesity. *Heart* **2003**, *89*, 1127–1129. [CrossRef]

36. Lang, R.M.; Badano, L.P.; Mor-Avi, V.; Afilalo, J.; Armstrong, A.; Ernande, L.; Flachskampf, F.A.; Foster, E.; Goldstein, S.A.; Kuznetsova, T.; et al. Recommendations for cardiac chamber quantification by echocardiography in adults: An update from the American Society of Echocardiography and the European Association of Cardiovascular Imaging. *Eur. Heart J. Cardiovasc. Imaging* **2015**, *16*, 233–271. [CrossRef] [PubMed]

37. World Health Organization. *Guideline: Sodium Intake for Adults and Children*; World Health Organization: Geneva, Switzerland, 2012; ISBN 9789241504836.

38. Fedorova, O.; Doris, P.; Bagrov, A. Endogenous marinobufagenin-like factor in acute plasma volume expansion. *Clin. Exp. Hypertens.* **1998**, *20*, 581–591. [CrossRef]

39. Grigorova, Y.N.; Wei, W.; Petrashevskaya, N.; Zernetkina, V.; Juhasz, O.; Fenner, R.; Gilbert, C.; Lakatta, E.G.; Shapiro, J.I.; Bagrov, A.Y. Dietary sodium restriction reduces arterial stiffness, vascular TGF-β-dependent fibrosis and marinobufagenin in young normotensive rats. *Int. J. Mol. Sci.* **2018**, *19*, 3168. [CrossRef]

40. Strauss, M.; Smith, W.; Wei, W.; Fedorova, O.V.; Schutte, A.E. Autonomic activity and its relationship with the endogenous cardiotonic steroid marinobufagenin: The african-PREDICT study. *Nutr. Neurosci.* **2019**, 1–11. [CrossRef]

41. Strauss-Kruger, M.; Smith, W.; Wei, W.; Bagrov, A.Y.; Fedorova, O.V.; Schutte, A.E. Microvascular function in non-dippers: Potential involvement of the salt sensitivity biomarker, marinobufagenin—The african-PREDICT study. *J. Clin. Hypertens.* **2020**, *22*, 86–94. [CrossRef]

42. Jablonski, K.L.; Fedorova, O.V.; Racine, M.L.; Geolfos, C.J.; Gates, P.E.; Chonchol, M.; Fleenor, B.S.; Lakatta, E.G.; Bagrov, A.Y.; Seals, D.R. Dietary sodium restriction and association with urinary marinobufagenin, blood pressure, and aortic stiffness. *Clin. J. Am. Soc. Nephrol.* **2013**, *8*, 1952–1959. [CrossRef]

43. Ogihara, T.; Asano, T.; Ando, K.; Sakoda, H.; Anai, M.; Shojima, N.; Ono, H.; Onishi, Y.; Fujishiro, M.; Abe, M.; et al. High-salt diet enhances insulin signaling and induces insulin resistance in dahl salt-sensitive rats. *Hypertension* **2002**, *40*, 83–89. [CrossRef]

44. Schutte, A.E.; Gona, P.N.; Delles, C.; Uys, A.S.; Burger, A.; Mels, C.M.; Kruger, R.; Smith, W.; Fourie, C.M.; Botha, S.; et al. The African Prospective study on the Early Detection and Identification of Cardiovascular Disease and Hypertension (African-PREDICT): Design, recruitment and initial examination. *Eur. J. Prev. Cardiol.* **2019**, *26*, 458–470. [CrossRef] [PubMed]

45. Ashwell, M.; Gunn, P.; Gibson, S. Waist-to-height ratio is a better screening tool than waist circumference and bmi for adult cardiometabolic risk factors: Systematic review and meta-analysis. *Obes. Rev.* **2012**, *13*, 275–286. [CrossRef] [PubMed]

46. Muntner, P.; Einhorn, P.T.; Cushman, W.C.; Whelton, P.K.; Bello, N.A.; Drawz, P.E.; Green, B.B.; Jones, D.W.; Juraschek, S.P.; Margolis, K.L.; et al. Blood pressure assessment in adults in clinical practice and clinic-based research: JACC scientific expert panel. *J. Am. Coll. Cardiol.* **2019**, *73*, 317–335. [CrossRef] [PubMed]

47. Unger, T.; Borghi, C.; Charchar, F.; Khan, N.A.; Poulter, N.R.; Prabhakaran, D.; Ramirez, A.; Schlaich, M.; Stergiou, G.S.; Tomaszewski, M.; et al. 2020 international society of hypertension global hypertension practice guidelines. *Hypertension* **2020**, *75*, 1334–1357. [CrossRef] [PubMed]

48. World Health Organization and the Pan American Health Organization Group for Cardiovascular Disease Prevention through Population-Wide Dietary Salt Reduction. Protocol for Population Level Sodium Determination in 24-h Urine Samples. 2010. Available online: https://www.paho.org/hq/dmdocuments/2013/24h-urine-Protocol-eng.pdf (accessed on 10 September 2020).

49. Fedorova, O.V.; Simbirtsev, A.S.; Kolodkin, N.I.; Kotov, A.Y.; Agalakova, N.I.; Kashkin, V.A.; Tapilskaya, N.I.; Bzhelyansky, A.; Reznik, V.A.; Frolova, E.V. Monoclonal antibody to an endogenous bufadienolide, marinobufagenin, reverses preeclampsia-induced Na/K-ATPase inhibition and lowers blood pressure in NaCl-sensitive hypertension. *J. Hypertens.* **2008**, *26*, 2414. [CrossRef]

50. Stevens, L.A.; Claybon, M.A.; Schmid, C.H.; Chen, J.; Horio, M.; Imai, E.; Nelson, R.G.; Van Deventer, M.; Wang, H.-Y.; Zuo, L.; et al. Evaluation of the chronic kidney disease epidemiology collaboration equation for estimating the glomerular filtration rate in multiple ethnicities. *Kidney Int.* **2011**, *79*, 555–562. [CrossRef] [PubMed]

Publisher's Note: MDPI stays neutral with regard to jurisdictional claims in published maps and institutional affiliations.

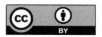

MDPI

St. Alban-Anlage 66

4052 Basel

Switzerland

Tel. +41 61 683 77 34

Fax +41 61 302 89 18

www.mdpi.com

Nutrients Editorial Office

E-mail: nutrients@mdpi.com

www.mdpi.com/journal/nutrients

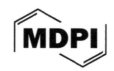